DIVIDED LEGACY

A HISTORY OF THE SCHISM IN MEDICAL THOUGHT

Volume I

DIVIDED LEGACY
A HISTORY OF THE SCHISM IN MEDICAL THOUGHT

Volume I

THE PATTERNS EMERGE
HIPPOCRATES TO PARACELSUS

Harris L. Coulter

Center
for
Empirical Medicine

Washington, D.C.
1994

Passage from Isaiah Berlin, *The Hedgehog and the Fox* (copyright 1957 by Mentor Books), used by permission of George Weidenfeld and Nicolson, World University Library.

Passages from George Boas, "Some Assumptions of Aristotle" (copyright 1959 by the American Philosophical Society), used by permission of the American Philosophical Society.

Passages from J. Chadwick and W.N. Mann, *The Medical Works of Hippocrates* (copyright 1950 by the Charles C. Thomas Co.), used by permission of Blackwell Scientific Publications, Ltd.

Passages from K. Deichgraeber, *Die Griechische Empirikerschule* (copyright 1965 by Weidmannsche Verlagsbuchhandlung), used by permission of Weidmannsche Verlagsbuchhandlung.

Passages from I.E. Drabkin, *Caelius Aurelianus On Acute Diseases and On Chronic Diseases* (copyright 1950 by the University of Chicago Press), used by permission of the University of Chicago Press.

Passages from Jolande Jacobi, ed., *Paracelsus: Selected Writings,* translated by Norbert Guterman (copyright 1951 and 1958 by Bollingen Foundation), used by permission of Princeton University Press.

Passages from G.S. Kirk and J.E. Raven, *The Presocratic Philosophers* (copyright 1962 by Cambridge University Press), used by permission of Cambridge University Press.

Passages from Kurt Leidecker, *Volumen Medicinae Paramirum* (copyright 1949 by The Johns Hopkins Press), used by permission of The Johns Hopkins Press.

Passages from Walter Pagel, *Paracelsus. An Introduction to Philosophical Medicine in the Era of the Renaissance* (copyright 1958 by S. Karger AG), used by permission of S. Karger AG.

Passages from Henry Sigerist, ed., *Four Treatises of Theophrastus von Hohenheim, Called Paracelsus,* translated by C. Lilian Temkin, George Rosen, Gregory Zilboorg, and Henry Sigerist (copyright 1941 by The Johns Hopkins Press), used by permission of The Johns Hopkins Press.

Passages from Fritz Steckerl, *The Fragments of Praxagoras of Cos and His School* (copyright 1958 by E.J. Brill), used by permission of E.J. Brill.

Passage from O. Temkin, *Soranus' Gynecology* (copyright 1956 by The Johns Hopkins Press), used by permission of The Johns Hopkins Press.

Second Printing, 1994

ISBN 0-916386-01-5 (Volume I)
1-55643-035-3 (Volume II)
0-913028-96-7 (Volume III paperback)
0-938190-57-1 (Volume III cloth)
1-55643-170-8 (Volume IV)

for Katya

INTRODUCTION: WHAT IS MEDICAL HISTORY?

> We suppose scientists to be wiser than men of experience . . . and this is because the former know the cause, but the latter do not. For men of experience know that the thing is so, but do not know why, while the others know the why and the cause.[1]

> You are dull of heart and blind of eye by reason of your anxiety to give good reasons for your opinions.[2]

To define the history of medicine we must first define "medicine." And this is clearly a difficult task. For medicine is the oldest scientific activity of man, and the most widely practiced. No civilization, ancient or modern, has done without it. And in recent years the dimensions of medical learning and medical services have increased exponentially from decade to decade.

Since no historical narrative, however multitomed, could encompass this huge volume of thought and activity, an attempt at definition must seek out the key elements, the ultimate determinants. When "medicine" has been thus defined, we will know better where to focus our history.

A clue to the problem is found in the realization that medicine was practiced before it became a pursuit of the intellect. When humans were living in caves, and before the discovery of writing, the sick were restored to health, broken bones were set, and women were aided in childbirth. Just as sick animals instinctively eat the grasses and herbs they require, so must early man have established vague and inchoate correspondences between his illnesses and the curative substances found in his surroundings—long before conscious thought was directed to these practices.

And the medical thought of all succeeding eras has also required constant correction by therapeutic experience.

Medical thought thus grows out of, and is governed by, therapeutic experience. Therapeutic theories in all their variety are attempts to make sense out of the healer's experience with the patient. Experience is chronologically prior to theory. Hence it is prior in importance. The meaning of "experience" has always been the key problem of medical thought—in the classical and medieval periods when the word, "experience," was widely employed in medical discourse and in more modern times when "experiment" has come to replace the older term.

The physician acquires experience initially from his observation of the patient. He may distinguish certain symptoms himself, and the patient may tell him about his feelings, sensations, and pains. The physician prescribes a medicine, a diet, or some other form of treatment, and the patient responds in a certain way which the physician can observe or elicit through questioning.

The physician may use more sophisticated techniques: X-rays, electrocardiograms, biopsies, and other tests and samplings of the patient's fluids and solids. All these procedures provide him with data.

Thus the physician's "experience" is nothing more or less than the information about the patient which he acquires through his five senses.

But none of this information is self-interpreting. Neither the symptoms, nor the patient's own account of his aches and miseries, nor the results of the most sophisticated measuring techniques, provide the physician with anything more than raw sensory data. He must still determine their *meaning.*

Do the observed changes mean that the patient is improving or getting worse? If the patient lives, is it because of the treatment or despite it? If he dies, is it because of the treatment or despite it? The physician has before him only the raw data of experience—whose meaning is a mystery.

The great medical thinkers have all sought a rule or rules permitting correct interpretation of the primary data of experience. History shows that the search for interpretative rules can be conducted along two alternative lines. One is to emphasize the paramount significance of the sensory data themselves and to base treatment in some way on these data. The other is to look for a higher order of reality assumed to be lurking behind the data of sense perception, treatment being guided by the physician's assumptions about this metaphysical reality.

Any therapeutic system emphasizes one or the other of these approaches, and the medical doctrines examined by us below may be classified in terms of how they incorporate these two elements of the physician's interpretation of his therapeutic experience.

* * * * * * * * *

These two attitudes toward reality are familiar to the student of philosophy, since they characterize two psychological types which become manifest whenever the human mind must organize a body of experience. Their existence, and the implications of this fact, have been pointed out by a number of thinkers. The German philosopher, William Windelband, voicing the Kantian tradition, described them as idiographic and nomothetic.[3] The first, he states, seeks particular facts, the second seeks general laws. In his view, idiographic knowledge is essentially historical, while nomothetic knowledge is scientific, and this polarity reflects the fundamental and insoluble problem of the relationship between the particular and the general. Thought is not in a position to resolve the problem: the law and the event remain side by side, "ultimate and incommensurable elements of our representation of reality."[4]

A more customary pair of terms for this dichotomy has been "empirical" and "rationalist." William James described as follows the difference between these two psychological types:

> In manners we find formalists and free-and-easy persons. In government, authoritarians and anarchists. In litera-

> ture, purists or academicals, and realists. In art, classics and romantics. You recognize these contrasts as familiar; well, in philosophy we have a very similar contrast expressed in the pair of terms, "rationalist" and "empiricist," "empiricist" meaning your lover of facts in all their crude variety, "rationalist" meaning your devotee to abstract and eternal principles. No one can live an hour without both facts and principles, so it is a difference rather of emphasis; yet it breeds antipathies of the most pungent character between those who lay the emphasis differently; and we shall find it extraordinarily convenient to express a certain contrast in men's ways of taking their universe, by talking of the "empiricist" and of the "rationalist" temper.[5]

More recently Sir Isaiah Berlin has analyzed the conflict in the character of Leo Tolstoy in these same terms. He expands on the saying of a Greek poet that "the fox knows many things, but the hedgehog knows one big thing," writing:

> . . . the words can be made to yield a sense in which they mark one of the deepest differences which divide writers and thinkers, and, it may be, human beings in general. For there exists a great chasm between those, on one side, who relate everything to a single central vision, one system less or more coherent or articulate, in terms of which they understand, think and feel—a single, universal organizing principle in terms of which alone all that they are and say has significance—and, on the other side, those who pursue many ends, often unrelated and even contradictory, connected, if at all, only in some *de facto* way, for some psychological or physiological cause, related by no moral or aesthetic principle; these last lead lives, perform acts, and entertain ideas that are centrifugal rather than centripetal, their thought is scattered or diffused, moving on many levels, seizing upon the essence of a vast variety of experiences and objects for what they are in themselves, without, consciously or unconsciously,

> seeking to fit them into, or exclude them from, any one unchanging, all-embracing, sometimes self-contradictory and incomplete, at times fanatical, unitary inner vision.[6]

These writers give modern expression to a division in thought which has always existed. It characterizes to some extent the opposition between Platonism and Aristotelianism, between nominalism and realism, between Lutheranism and Pietism. It crops up perennially in the history of philosophy, of religion, of education. But it has been almost entirely overlooked in the history of medicine. Of the very few efforts made to analyze medical history in terms of this duality the most interesting is Arturo Castiglioni's article, "Neo–Hippocratic Tendency of Contemporary Medical Thought."[7] He characterizes the two poles of the dichotomy as the "technico-morphological, chiefly analytical" and the "cosmical, vitalistic, and synthetical." "The first, which is doubtless the simplest and the most ancient, places foremost the local symptoms of diseases and considers the affection of each organ separately. This leads to localistic treatment based on the assumption of a cause" and to mechanistic thinking generally. The second tendency attributes the origins of life and of its functions to a superior vital energy: the *physis* of the Hippocratics being the most prominent example.[a] "This Hippocratic conception considers man as an indestructible part of the Cosmos, bound to it and subject to its laws: it may be called, therefore, a universal, cosmical, unitarian conception. Disease, according to it, is a general fact which strikes the whole organism and has its origins in a perturbation of natural harmony." Castiglioni goes on to note that "these two tendencies have a point of contact and at the same time are very different. They may alternate or modify each other and at times keep each other back. Thus, analytical doctrine returns in a period in which exaggerated

[a]On the *physis* see below, p. xiii.

metaphysical tendencies render absolutely necessary a very strict control of the method of reasoning, while a synthetic tendency with its vitalistic attitude appears . . . when a system has taken the inflexibility of a program so as to acquire the authority of a dogma."[8] Castiglioni classifies as representative of the analytical trend in medicine both Galen and the 19th-century German physiological school headed by Rudolph Virchow (1821-1902). As synthetic medical thinkers he mentions Hippocrates, Paracelsus (1493-1541), and Samuel Hahnemann (1755-1843).

No one has yet taken up Castiglioni's suggestion, and our task in this volume will be to apply his hypothesis to the Greek medical thinkers and to Paracelsus, with the aim of determining how correct and fruitful it is for the investigation and understanding of medical history. But, since this is a complicated undertaking, we should attempt at the outset to gain perspective by examining the fundamental operating assumptions of the two bodies of physicians in the ancient world who most dramatically represented this polarity: the Rationalist (Dogmatist) and Empirical schools in Greece and Rome. The former falls into what Castiglioni calls the "technico-morphological, chiefly analytical" tradition, while the latter is typically "cosmical, vitalistic, and synthetical."

The Rationalists assumed that the physician is capable of understanding and knowing the physiological and pathological processes occurring within the organism. They sought the reality underlying the patient's symptoms. Hence they were led to the further assumption that this underlying reality is subject to certain laws which are knowable *a priori* by the physician. They went so far as to maintain that the functioning of the living organism follows the rules of Aristotelian logic.

The Empirics maintained the contrary—that the physician can only know what he is taught by his own sense-perception and that of the patient. Hence they devoted paramount attention to the patient's symptoms – as the source and substance of the physician's experience. They denied the possibility of *a priori* knowledge of "hidden causes," meaning those physiological processes which do not lend themselves to sensory observation.

Their observation of symptom-patterns led them to the conclusion that the organism can manifest sickness and disease in an infinite number of different ways, each of which represents a different dynamic pattern taken by the body's innate healing power (the *physis,* the *natura*) in its effort to effect cure.

This conflict of assumptions, with its corollaries in Rationalist and Empirical doctrine, seems to us a fundamental psychological fact. Furthermore, our narrative will show that this dichotomy, which crystallized most strikingly in the Rationalist and Empirical schools, not only antedates the emergence of these schools—being found, most significantly, in the Hippocratic Corpus itself—but permeates all succeeding medical thought as well.

Medical thinkers in Western culture may be divided into these two traditions—those who attribute primary importance to the sensory data of experience being opposed to those who seek the reality assumed to lie behind the sensory data. The conflict and interaction between these two views forms the schism in medical thought which will be elaborated upon in this and the following volumes.

Not that every practitioner of medicine falls exclusively into one or the other tradition. The run-of-the-mill physician concerns himself essentially with the technical problem of applying given therapeutic rules to his patient's needs. He does not question the postulates and assumptions behind the rules he has learned because he is not aware of them. His practice is an eclectic and inconsistent mixture of the two bodies of doctrine. But the greatest thinkers fall on one or the other end of this spectrum of thought. They are great precisely because they have examined the underlying assumptions and on them have erected coherent bodies of doctrine. These are the thinkers with whom we will be primarily concerned.

* * * * * * * * *

Because these categories of thought and patterns of assumptions are generated by the encounter between the physician and his patient, a true history of medicine must be a history of clinical practice. A true history of medicine must be a history of therapeutics. The clashes over therapeutic practice strike the sparks which reveal the existence of these categories and assumptions.

The resulting doctrines take the following general form.

The Empirical tradition takes as the object of thought and speculation the whole organism in its environment. Here "environment" must be understood in its broadest sense and includes such factors as food, water, weather, and medicines —in a word, all the external influences which impinge upon the human organism. The Empirical physician aimed to analyze the interaction between the whole organism (as expressed by its reaction to stimuli) and the external environment:

environment (external, exciting causes)→whole organism *(physis, natura)*→visible signs of sickness and health

Characteristic of their holistic approach was the attempt to base treatment upon *all* of the patient's symptoms—in particular, the symptoms which were not common to all persons suffering from the given "disease" but were peculiar to the given patient.

The Rationalists considered the above model too imprecise in failing to spell out an analytical relationship between environmental influences and the patient's signs and symptoms. Hence they proposed the following model in which environmental causes produce the internal (proximate) causes which, in turn, yield the symptoms perceived by the physician:

environment (external, exciting causes)→internal (proximate) causes→visible signs of sickness and health

Characteristic of this analytical approach was the attempt to base treatment primarily upon the symptoms which the patient had in common with all others suffering from the same "disease." The Rationalist physicians slighted the peculiar symptoms of the individual patient.

The Rationalist viewpoint is represented by the quotation from Aristotle at the head of this Introduction. Medicine is primarily concerned with the proximate causes of disease (and health). These physicians in the ancient world accused the Empirical School of irrationality for rejecting this causal analysis and its corollary that physiological and pathological processes are subject to the laws of logic.

The Rationalist causal analysis of the organism left no metaphysical space for a spontaneous healing power.

The Empirics, on the contrary, rejected the proximate cause. The cornerstone of their doctrine was denial of the possibility of acquiring precise knowledge of these "obscure causes" and hidden processes. They held that, while such functions can be understood to some extent, therapeutics should not be based upon such crude knowledge. Being a life or death matter for the patient, it must be rooted in reliable data.

Their view is given in the second quotation at the head of this Introduction. The Rationalist concern for logical consistency makes them "blind of eye" to all that cannot be explained *a priori,* i.e., to the patient's unique and personal mode of illness which can be elicited only by close attention to his symptoms. The Rationalists are "dull of heart" because they lack the emotional involvement with the patient which such observation necessarily implies. A holistic medicine can be practiced only by a physician who feels sympathy and love for his patient and can thus appreciate him in his uniqueness.

The therapeutic philosophy of Paracelsus makes even more explicit the tie between a holistic medicine and the physician's charity or Christian love for his patient.

The conflict between the Rationalist and Empirical assumptions extends to every category of medical knowledge and therapeutic practice, e.g., the interpretation of the symptom, the relation between theory and practice, the meaning of disease "cause," the number of possible diseases, the role of the physician *vs.* that of the *physis,* etc.

The first two of these categories best illustrate the conflict between Rationalist and Empirical therapeutic method.

Rationalism views the symptoms as the direct effect of the operation of proximate causes. When these causes are morbid, the symptoms will also be morbid. Empiricism, however, takes the opposite view: symptoms are the signs of the *curative effort of the physis* and must be interpreted as positive or beneficial phenomena, not morbid.

This leads to different interpretations of the respective roles of theory and practice. In Empiricism the two are fused into a single doctrine. The object of medical thought is the spontaneous and reactive *physis*—the healing force of the body. "Theory" can be nothing more than observation of the different modes of the organism's reaction to external stimuli. But these (symptomatic) patterns are not only the "theory" of the *physis.* They are also its "practice." And the physician's practice must imitate that of the *physis.*

Since the symptoms represent the body's own curative effort, they are the physician's best guide. He need only ascertain how to aid this innate force for cure, and the Empirical physicians throughout history have concentrated their research on medicines which aid the *physis.*

The Rationalist tradition separates theory and practice. "Theory" means knowledge of the proximate causes, i.e., of physiology, and "practice" is the application of this theory. Since the proximate causes are assumed to be related analytically to both the (preceding) external causes and the (succeeding) symptoms, medical Rationalism identifies physiological theory with the analytical theories evolved in other areas of science.

The ancient Rationalist School identified physiological theory with Aristotelian logic. The proximate causes of disease were described in terms of the hot, the cold, the wet, and the dry, or a combination of these four qualities.

Medicines were analyzed in the same terms. For each disease, therefore, the appropriate medicine was the one with the "opposite" qualities. When diagnosis had been accomplished, the remedy could be found by logical deduction.

The 17th-century Iatrochemists substituted laboratory chemistry for Aristotelian logic. Medicines and physiological functions were analyzed in terms of "acids" and "alkalies." If an illness was seen as essentially "acid," the "alkaline" medicine, which neutralized acids in the laboratory, was the scientifically indicated remedy.

Their Iatromechanical colleagues viewed the human organism as a hydraulic system in which the heart, acting as a pump, was the source of all life and motion. Diseases were ascribed to obstructions in the veins and arteries, and medicines were selected for the ability to dissolve such obstructions.

In the late nineteenth century bacteriology emerged as the principal Rationalist therapeutic theory. Diseases were interpreted as the products of pathogenic microorganisms, and medicines which could kill the germ *in vitro* were thought to remove the associated disease *in vivo.*

It is seen that the gap between diagnosis and therapy in the Rationalist tradition has been filled by the doctrine of "contraries" (derived ultimately from Aristotle's "principle of contradiction"). The sciences of logic, chemistry, hydraulics, and bacteriology, although valuable for constructing theories of causation, do not in themselves yield therapeutic indications. But these physicians have always taken for granted that neutralizing or opposing the disease "cause" is equivalent to curing the patient.

The interpretation of symptoms as morbid phenomena is a necessary corollary of the principle of cure through contraries.

Medical research in the Rationalist tradition has always been concentrated in the "auxiliary sciences." The proximate causes of disease and health have been pursued farther and farther into the organism in the hope of discovering a better logical basis for the transition from diagnosis to therapy.

The Empirical thinkers have not been concerned with this problem, since therapeutics is the starting-point of their method, not its culmination. They have, in any case, rejected the doctrine of contraries as a logical formulation irrelevant to therapeutics.

Instead, the Empirical tradition has tended to espouse a theory of "similars"—meaning medicines which further and promote the inherent self-healing effort of the organism. When symptoms are viewed as signs of the curative process, medicines which intensify the symptoms must be understood as aiding this process.

Physicians of the Empirical tradition have generally rejected the causal knowledge elaborated in the auxiliary sciences and the therapeutics based upon this knowledge. The ancient Empirical School and Paracelsus rejected a therapeutics based upon Aristotelian logic. Thomas Sydenham (1624-1689), Georg Ernst Stahl (1660-1734), and Theophile Bordeu (1722-1776) all disputed the physical, chemical, and anatomical theories of their Rationalist contemporaries. And the homoeopathic school founded by Samuel Hahnemann consciously opposed much of the nineteenth-century physiological learning as the basis for medical practice.

In the Empirical tradition practice has preceded theory—meaning that the body's physiology and chemistry are understood through the practice of medicine. Empirical practice has been based largely upon the use of medicinal drugs. The Empirical School, Paracelsus, and Hahnemann were all famous for the depth and breadth of their pharmacological investigations.

* * * * * * * * *

We can now see that the question, "What is medicine?" has at least two answers. The Empirics have defined medicine as the minute observation of the sick person in order to understand the pattern of symptoms in sickness and health.

Medicine is first and foremost therapeutics, and therapeutic experience is the touchstone of truth.

The Rationalists have claimed the contrary: "medicine" means the correct comprehension of the body's various mechanisms (which they indeed regard as "mechanisms"). Therapeutics is secondary, being the derivative of the knowledge developed in the auxiliary sciences. Doctrinal coherence is the criterion of truth.

Clearly the medical historians of recent decades have sympathized with the Rationalist view, focussing on the development of knowledge in the auxiliary sciences. The systems of past medical thinkers are broken down into their components, and the value or relevance of these components are judged by their applicability to medicine in the twentieth century. To discuss the therapeutics of a medical thinker of the past has been regarded as almost indecent. Past practice is seen to embody faulty and defective procedures based upon faulty and defective knowledge, and its history is thus assumed to be the history of error. Far better, it is thought, to discover the germ of "scientific" truth in the older doctrines and draw a veil over the "unscientific" and often positively harmful practice.

A number of serious methodological objections may be made to this approach to medical history.

First, it slights the thinking of the Empirical physicians. Whole areas of thought and practice are skipped, or treated in the most cursory fashion, merely because the Empirics rejected the auxiliary sciences as sources of reliable therapeutic doctrine.

But these thinkers had excellent reasons for thus denying the relevance of the Rationalist learning of their times, and it is a mistake to ignore their contributions.

This raises the second objection. What criterion has been selected by medical historians for accepting or ignoring some element of an earlier therapeutic doctrine? While this question is not usually faced consciously, unconsciously the historian accepts the data which seem to him relevant to contemporary "medical science." But this is an unstable vantage-point, since the definition of "medical science" is continually shifting, and history written during one therapeutic vogue may be incomprehensible when another vogue has taken its place.

It is anachronistic to discuss the doctrine of a 14th-century physician in terms of its relevance to what the 20th century considers "scientific" in medicine. An evaluation of the constitutions of the 14th-century Italian cities in terms of their congruence with the 20th-century United States Constitution would hardly throw light on the organic development of Italian 14th-century politics, and such an approach is equally valueless for an understanding of 14th-century medicine. It does not yield a faithful picture of the doctrines themselves, which are organic unities and must be taken in their entirety.

The analytical knowledge contained in the "auxiliary sciences" is not as "hard" as some would believe. The practical function of such knowledge is determined by the therapeutic doctrine as a whole. Bits and pieces cannot be shifted from one era of history to another and still retain their meaning.

An example is William Harvey's (1578-1657) discovery of the greater circulation of the blood. Harvey himself thought that the expansion and contraction of the blood are prior to—hence the cause of—the movement of the heart. This discovery was taken up by Hermann Boerhaave (1668-1738), one of the founders of the hydraulic school of therapeutics mentioned above. His contemporary, Frederick Hoffman (1660-1742), also based therapeutics on Harvey's discovery, but he divided diseases into two classes: spasmodic (fevers, epilepsy) arising from excessive contraction (systole) of the heart, and atonic (cancer, chronic diseases) arising from too much dilatation (diastole).

Hence, to state (as in many histories of medicine) that Harvey discovered the circulation of the blood, and that this was incorporated into the systems of Boerhaave and Hoffmann, does justice to none of the three. Harvey himself was a vitalist, hence an Empiric, while the Rationalists, Boerhaave and Hoffmann, drew very different therapeutic consequences from Harvey's discovery.

Paracelsus hypothesized that diseases are rooted in the three principles: salt, sulphur, and mercury. His definition of these principles was obscure, as they possessed essentially cosmological significance. But with Sylvius de le Boe (1614-1672) these principles became materialized and identified with the acids and alkalies of laboratory chemistry. Thus the Iatrochemical School arose out of an interpretation of chemical elements differing from that of Paracelsus, and the same chemical terms have different meanings in the two doctrines.

In the ancient world, the Rationalist Galen's interpretation of the *physis* differed from that of the Empirics.

Since the Rationalist school of medical history is unjust even to past Rationalist thinkers, not to mention the Empirics, we propose an approach which will present the Rationalist and Empirical doctrines as whole entities interacting with one another. Nothing in medical thought is more certain than change. And, as we will show, such change often takes the form of an oscillation back and forth between the Rationalist and Empirical poles of the spectrum. Why not, then, seek solid historical ground in the laws and patterns of this change?

Furthermore, in the third volume of this series, we aim to bring out some of the social and economic—even political—determinants of medical thought, showing how the exigencies of medical practice in a given socio-economic context affect the physician's attitude toward medical and therapeutic doctrines. By introducing this socio-economic dimension we hope to cast light on the dynamics of change in therapeutic doctrines, permitting an analysis of the non-medical determinants of medical thought and thus making possible the elaboration of social policies to correct therapeutic doctrines when they have become distorted, exaggerated, and unscientific.

* * * * * * * * *

An investigation of medical history along these lines possesses both historiographic and practical value.

It provides a series of "common denominators" which make explicit the intellectual connections among these thinkers, relating them to one another in previously unrealized ways. For example, the intimate tie between ancient Rationalism and Methodism has not previously been noticed, nor that between one group of Hippocratic works, the ideas of the Empirical School, and the teachings of Paracelsus and Hahnemann. This method throws light on the organic development of medical thought.

It makes clear what were the issues agitating these thinkers and thus gives a contemporaneous account of their concerns and preoccupations.[b] It reflects accurately the true weight and importance of each thinker and each idea. It avoids the trap of anachronistic medical history.

It humanizes medical history by situating it in the general context of Western thought, thus showing it to be amenable to the sort of analysis which has been applied successfully to other areas of intellectual history. In particular, it brings to light the profound impact of formal philosophical doctrines on medical thought and speculation, as is shown below in our discussion of Aristotelianism and Scepticism.

To these considerations of a historiographic order may be added certain practical ones. The writer believes that an acquaintance with the attitudes of past physicians to perennial therapeutic problems will aid the physician of today in his own practice. How could it be otherwise? How could the

[b]The need for such a refocussing of medical history has been mentioned. See, for example, Erwin H. Ackerknecht, "A Plea for a 'Behaviorist' Approach in Writing the History of Medicine," *Journal of the History of Medicine and Allied Sciences* XXII (1967), 211-214.

thought and practice of so many millions of men and women have no value except for their minute contribution to the development of the "auxiliary sciences"? Only the man who knows no era but his own could exhibit such parochial arrogance.

The extraordinary development of medical specialization and of the "auxiliary sciences" in the last hundred years has turned medical thought increasingly to the technical disciplines subsidiary to therapeutics and has distracted the physician's attention from the fundamental identity between what he is seeking to do and what his colleagues of former times were also striving for. Overly concerned with investigating narrowly defined problems, he has lost sight of the fact that these problems, which loom large in any specialized approach to healing, are themselves ancillary to the main issues which have perplexed thinkers over the centuries and which have not yet found generally accepted solutions.

* * * * * * * * *

A major problem addressed in the following volumes is the relationship between the scientific and historical components of medical thought. If medicine is a science, therapeutic knowledge can be derived analytically from the existing body of doctrine. A science incorporates in itself what is useful in the thought and practice of the past and is consequently anti-historical in orientation.

But what is the value of a history which takes the past for granted and uses it only to prove the inevitability of the present?

A belief in the utility and value of medical history necessarily implies less than absolute confidence in the analytical knowledge of the "auxiliary sciences." Julius Petersen has made the valuable point that, as long as there remains a gap between medical theory and medical practice, between diagnosis and therapy, the physician will benefit from a knowledge of how his predecessors have confronted these same problems. He observes that since the knowledge contained in the "auxiliary sciences" is not self-interpreting, does not contain an unambiguous guide to its application, the physician will want to know how others have interpreted this knowledge and applied it.[9]

While tension between the historical and scientific components has always existed in medicine, in the age of Pasteur and Koch the analytical element completely overwhelmed the historical. The physician lost any feeling that a knowledge of medical history could be of practical use in the treatment of patients. The tremendous watershed in medical thought represented by the bacterial theory of disease seemed at one blow to nullify all past therapeutic speculation, and for many decades physicians strove to reconstruct medicine on the foundation offered by bacteriology.

The study of medical history virtually disappeared from the schools, and the scholars who remained saw it as a field of purely antiquarian endeavor. They were affected by the prevailing scorn and made the concession of treating medical history as little more than an account of the tiny contribution made by past thinkers to the currently accepted "scientific" truth. Rationalist thought acquired a profound ascendency over Empirical.

Many of the abuses observed in Rationalist therapeutics today owe their origin to this extreme development of analytical medicine.

It is clear that the conflict between the scientific and historical dimensions of medical thought parallels the conflict between the "auxiliary sciences" and therapeutics, or between the foci of the Rationalist and Empirical doctrines. The former stress logical analysis, while the latter stress history. The Empirical School's interest in ancient learning had its necessary corollary in a deeper concern for the (medical) history of the patient.

We do not agree with Windelband that in medicine the idiographic (historical) and nomothetic (scientific) components must remain incommensurable. The problem is precisely one of reconciling them, of finding the scientific laws enabling the physician to manipulate the idiographic descriptions of reality. This theme recurs frequently on the following pages as well as in volumes II and III of this work.

The problem is to determine the relationship between therapeutic method and scientific method, and since this is the fundamental issue discussed below, we may here indicate our interpretation of scientific method.

The purpose of scientific investigation is to increase man's understanding of natural processes and his control over them. Scientific method is the procedure employed to achieve this end. It is a set of rules for investigating physical reality and thus for controlling the physical world.

"Understanding" nature means perceiving certain laws and regularities in the succession of natural phenomena. It means only the ability to recognize these regularities and patterns and to predict or modify their occurrence.

Such patterns or laws are apprehended by elaborating hypotheses and testing them, or their logical corollaries, against the data of experience. When, after a suitable number of experiments or tests, the predictions implicit in the hypothesis are seen to be correct, the hypothesis is assumed to be true and, until disproved, is regarded as a correct characterization of a process in nature.

The concept of "cause" plays no role in scientific method. Knowledge of nature is not knowledge of causes but is an appreciation of the laws governing the occurrence of events. This should be emphasized, since "cause" as an element in "scientific medicine" will figure prominently in the ensuing narrative.

The all-important step in the scientific investigation of nature is formulation of the hypothesis. There are no rules governing this, and it must be considered an original act of creation.

The "facts" or "data" regarded as pertinent will, of

course, depend upon the hypothesis selected as the basis for investigation, and it will be seen that the Empirical and Rationalist traditions have presented different views of what data are pertinent to a scientific therapeutics. The former have emphasized symptomatic knowledge, and the latter have focussed on the underlying physiological or pathological mechanisms.

Consequently, the two traditions have attached different meanings to "medical science." Paracelsus discusses this in defining the words, *scientia, experimentum*, and *experientia.*

We feel that a scientific medicine must be holistic and that a holistic medicine (as mentioned above) must be founded on a relationship of love or empathy between the physician and the patient, since this is required for proper observation of the patient.

We conclude that the Empirical tradition contains the elements of a scientific approach to therapeutics, and, since we regard a scientific therapeutics as preferable to an unscientific one, any value judgments appearing below represent our preference for the former.

* * * * * * * * *

Returning, now, to our initial question: What is medical history? It is a description of the two opposed attitudes toward therapeutic method, Rationalist and Empirical. It is an account of how these attitudes interact with one another. It is an investigation of how closely each comes to the ideal represented by scientific method. Finally, it is an analysis of how economic, social, political, philosophical, and other non-medical factors influence the interaction between the Rationalist and Empirical formulations of therapeutic doctrine.

By illuminating the past, such a history helps prevent its recurrence. The search for a scientific therapeutics is inhibited by the social and economic forces affecting medical practice and the medical profession. Hence it must be renewed in each generation. We hope that our identification of the issues will contribute to the unending struggle for a solution.

NOTES

[1] Aristotle, *Metaphysics* 981a 25-30.

[2] An Empirical physician of the second century A.D., quoted by Galen (Richard Walzer, *Galen on Medical Experience,* Oxford, 1947, p. 110).

[3] William Windelband, *Geschichte und Naturwissenschaft: Rede zum Antritt des Rektorats der Kaiser-Wilhelms-Universitaet Strassburg* (Strasburg, 1904).

[4] *Ibid.,* p. 27.

[5] William James, *Pragmatism* (Cleveland and New York: World Publishing Company, 1965), pp. 20-21.

[6] Isaiah Berlin, *The Hedgehog and the Fox* (New York: Mentor Books, 1957), pp. 7-8.

[7] *Medical Life* XLI (1934), 115-146. A somewhat similar approach to medical history is seen also in Knud Faber's "Nosography in Internal Medicine" (*Annals of Medical History* IV [1922], 1-63) and Julius Petersen's *Hauptmomente in der geschichtlichen Entwicklung der medizinischen Therapie* (Copenhagen: Host, 1877).

[8] Castiglioni, "Neo-Hippocratic Tendency of Contemporary Medical Thought," pp. 127-128.

[9] Julius Petersen, *Hauptmomente,* Introduction.

THE PATTERNS EMERGE:
HIPPOCRATES TO PARACELSUS

TABLE OF CONTENTS

But it is particularly necessary, in my opinion, for one who discusses this art to discuss things familiar to ordinary folk. For the subject of inquiry and discussion is simply and solely the sufferings of these same ordinary folk when they are sick or in pain.

Ancient Medicine

PART ONE

GREEK MEDICINE IN GREECE

PART ONE

GREEK MEDICINE IN GREECE

The Western medical tradition originated in Greece and for many centuries was the monopoly of Greek thinkers and physicians. Even when medical works started appearing in Latin, early in the Christian era, they drew on the Greek heritage.

Although medicine had risen to the level of a self-conscious discipline in the Tigris and Euphrates valleys before the dawn of civilization in Greece, and was practiced in Egypt as well (the formerly mythical figure, Aesculapius, is now known to have been one of the pharaohs), the thought and practice of these cultures entered the mainstream of Western medicine only by way of Greece.

Thus a history of the Western medical tradition must commence with Greece in the fifth and fourth centuries B.C., that is, with the earlier writings of the Hippocratic Corpus which so profoundly marked all succeeding medical speculation.

Two other thinkers who greatly contributed to Western medicine were Plato and Aristotle who, as will be shown, influenced the Hippocratic writers and were influenced by them.

A major product of Greek medical speculation between 450 and 350 B.C. was the Rationalist School which had roots in the Hippocratic Corpus, was modified by the philosophies of Plato and Aristotle, and was perfected by the latter's medical followers.

CHAPTER I

THE HIPPOCRATIC CORPUS: STRUCTURE

The Hippocratic Corpus is the greatest puzzle of medical history. It is a heterogeneous collection of about seventy writings of varying length, covering all areas of medical thought and practice: surgery, gynecology, internal medicine, diet, hygiene, and therapeutic method. Philological and other evidence indicates that the works in the Corpus were written over a period of several centuries, and even the older part of the collection, dating from about 450-400 B.C., is seen from stylistic evidence to be the work of several authors.

For many centuries the whole Corpus was ascribed to Hippocrates—a historical figure mentioned by both Plato and Aristotle as the foremost physician of their time. As scholars came to realize, however, that the Corpus is full of doctrinal inconsistencies, they were forced to conclude that it was not the work of a single man. This, in turn, gave rise to the "Hippocratic problem"—which of the works are "genuine" and which are not, or, in other words, how one is to view the doctrinal structure of the Hippocratic Corpus as a whole and its ties to earlier and later medical thought. Several scholars have attempted a coherent doctrinal analysis of all or most of the works of the Hippocratic Corpus and have reached conclusions as to the "genuineness" of the various writings.[1]

Without belittling these efforts, which in many cases have clarified our understanding of the Hippocratic Corpus and embodied new insights into its various works, we are nonetheless proposing a different approach.

Our analysis accepts the results of the philological investigations of the Hippocratic Corpus and seeks to build upon them by invoking a new criterion—the criterion of the therapeutic systems contained in these works. We maintain that the guide to the affinities and distinctions among the Hippocratic works is to be found in the authors' views of the nature of the therapeutic process and, furthermore, that two distinctly contrasted views of the therapeutic process can be traced in the early works of the Hippocratic Corpus.

In a word, we hypothesize the existence of the Empirical-Rationalist polarity in the Greek medical thought of the fifth and fourth centuries B.C. Our investigation of the Hippocratic Corpus is designed to demonstrate the existence of this polarity—which is seen to be identical with the later ideologies of the Empirical and Rationalist schools.

Our analysis does not cover the whole of the Hippocratic Corpus. We have selected about twenty of the earliest writings—those dating from the late fifth and early fourth centuries B.C.[2] If examined from the standpoint of their assumptions about the nature of therapeutic method, these works are seen to fall into the following groups:

Group I: Prorrhetic I,[a] *Coan Prognosis, Epidemics I* and *III, Prognosis, Aphorisms,* and *Regimen in Acute Diseases (RAD I).* The doctrine of this group is that the organism is composed of an undefined number of humors, that disease consists in the isolation of one of these humors within the organism, and that cure is through coction of this humor by the organism and its evacuation as urine, sweat, sputum, or stool. The physician can follow and comprehend this process through observation of the patient's symptoms and inspection of his *secreta* and *excreta.* This information, and his prognosis of the future course of the disease, indicate the appropriate form of therapy. There is no discussion of internal (proximate) causes or of physiological mechanisms. The therapeutic techniques employed consist almost entirely of diet, exercise, hot baths and applications (to promote coction), and laxatives (to promote evacuation).

[a]Since *Prorrhetic I* is almost entirely incorporated in *Coan Prognosis,* no specific reference is made to it below.

Group II: The *Appendix to Regimen in Acute Diseases (RAD II), Affections, Diseases I-III,* and *Internal Diseases.* Within this group may be discerned, in addition to the above conception of therapy through coction and evacuation, an entirely different one: that of cure by countering the humor and nullifying its effects within the organism. Thus, cure through coction of the humor is paralleled by cure through contraries. While this group of works includes much dietary treatment, medicinal substances are also used very extensively. Employment of these substances is sometimes without any apparent rationalization or justification (i.e., purely "empirical"), but it is often justified in terms of an assumed opposition between the inherent property or power (*dynamis*) of the substance and the nature of the humor underlying the disease. Thus, medicinal substances are analyzed in terms of their *dynameis,* and this technique of analysis is also applied to diseases and to the organism. This group of works contains considerable speculation about the internal causes of disease. While some of these authors use prognosis, others diagnose the disease cause and analyze the organism's physiological mechanisms.

Group III: Airs Waters Places, The Sacred Disease, Nature of Man, Regimen in Health, Breaths, and *Regimen I-IV.* All of therapeutics is based on the concept of the proximate cause. The organism and its environment are analyzed in terms of hypothesized causal processes, and therapy consists in opposing the humor, element, quality, or *dynamis* causing the disease by administering a remedy of opposite quality or *dynamis.* Prognosis is not mentioned in these works, and the authors employ only diagnosis of the proximate cause of the disease.

Group IV consists of two works: *Ancient Medicine* and *The Art.* These two works provide a reasoned analysis and critique of the therapeutic doctrine of Group III. The idea of cure through opposition between qualities is rejected, and a philosophical justification is given for the ideas underlying the works of Group I. Thus, while in Group I these ideas are implicit, they are made explicit in Group IV. The authors of *Ancient Medicine* and *The Art* employ the philosophical language and the concepts which have emerged in Group III to refute the therapeutic ideas advocated in the works of this Group. Of particular interest is the redefinition of the words, *dynamis* and *aition.*

* * * * * * * * *

Two comments may be made at the outset. In the first place, this quadripartite division reflects the traditional classification of the Hippocratic writings. The works which we characterize as Group I have commonly been viewed as the "genuine" kernel of the Corpus,[3] those of Group II have been traditionally ascribed to the Cnidian School, those of Group III are usually viewed as differing in important respects from Groups I and II, while *Ancient Medicine* and *The Art* are ordinarily regarded as inspired by a philosophical outlook differing substantially from that of Groups I-III. The congruence between the traditional view of these works and our own analysis based on a new and specifically different criterion may be regarded as an additional argument in favor of the plausibility of our interpretation.

In the second place, this theoretical exposition of the Hippocratic writings to some extent reflects their historical development—or, at any rate, the organic development of the ideas which they set forth.

The Group I ideas seem to be historically prior to those of Groups II and III, while the ideas contained in the Group IV works emerged later than those of Groups II and III.

Groups I and IV represent the pure Empirical ideology. Group III sets forth the Rationalist ideology in its pristine form. Group II is an eclectic mixture of the two ideologies.

Some possible theories of the historical development of the Hippocratic writings are examined in the next chapter.

Group I

The therapeutic system embodied in this group of writings is based on certain assumptions about the functioning of the organism. To understand the therapeutic system one must first understand the operating assumptions.

The view of these authors is that the organism is composed of an indefinite number of humors. While the four humors: blood, phlegm, black bile, and yellow bile, which later became the theoretical basis for the medicine of Galen and the Rationalist School, are all to be found in these works,[4] they are not presented in a structured or schematic fashion.[5] Humors are not mentioned very frequently, in any case, and other varieties and types of humors are mentioned in addition to the four classic ones: "saltinesses," "bitter humors," "bitter bile," "bitternesses," "blacknesses," etc.[6]

Health consists in the even mixture or blending of these humors within the body. Disease arises when one of them becomes "raw" or "crude" and thus stands out from the rest—sometimes manifesting localized symptomatology but always afflicting the body as a whole.

This degeneration of the humor is usually due either to incorrect diet or to some change in the atmospheric conditions, but the causal relationship between the environmental factor and the change in the humor is not elucidated. The following is typical: "The man lying sick in the garden of Delearces had for a long time heaviness in the head and pain in the right temple. From some exciting cause he was seized with fever, and took to his bed."[7] Nor is the process of isolation of the humor (from the mixture characterizing the healthy organism) subjected to analysis. The physician knows because the patient starts to void discharges in their crude or unconcocted state. These works contain many references to "unconcocted discharges," "unmixed sputum," "unripe matters," "unconcocted evacuations," "unmixed stools," "unmixed blood," "unmixed vomit," "unconcocted stools," "unconcocted urine," "unripe urine," "crudenesses," etc.[8]

During the course of the disease the natural heat of the organism overcomes the crude humor by cooking it (i.e., coction) and making it palatable to the organism.[b] This is also described as "ripening" or "maturation" of the humor,[c] and such cooking or maturation terminates in the crisis which is characteristic of every disease process.[9]

The crisis may be successful or unsuccessful, that is to say, the crude matter may or may not be successfully concocted. The physician can tell by his observation of the discharges at the crisis and just after it. These works contain many references to: thick, thin, black, scanty urine, and to: watery, uncompounded, unconcocted, bilious, greasy, green, frothy, crude, scanty, or copious stools.[10] The sputum is also examined for signs of compounding.[11] The urine is a very important source of knowledge about the interior of the organism. Not only can it be thick, thin, scanty, unconcocted or concocted, but the physician can derive further information from observation of the sediment deposited. In general, the deposit of sediment is a good sign, especially if it is of the right color, while the absence of sediment or the suspension of matter in the urine is a bad sign.[12] The quality of the vomit, when the latter is spontaneous, is significant:

> That vomit is most useful which is most thoroughly compounded of phlegm and bile, and it must not be too thick nor brought up in too great quantity. Less compounded vomits are worse. And if that which is brought up be of the color of leeks, or livid, or black, in all cases vomit of these colors must be considered bad. If the

[b] This idea is apparently derived from ordinary observation of the cooking of food, whereby raw food is made acceptable to, and digestible by, the organism. This lends greater point to the observation, by the author of *Ancient Medicine,* that the prescription of diet for the healthy, and of medicine for the sick, are based on identical reasoning (*Ancient Medicine,* cap. VIIff; Jones, I, 25ff.).

[c] A simile taken from observation of the ripening of fruits and vegetables whereby nature makes them palatable to humans.

> same patient brings up vomit of all these colors, he is quite at death's door. Of the vomits, the livid indicates the earliest death, should the odor be foul; but all odors which are rather putrid and foul are bad in the case of all vomits.
>
> (*Prognosis,* cap. XIII: Jones, II, 29)

And the perspiration and menstrual blood are also examined for signs of coction.[13]

The patient may recover after the crisis, he may die, or he may recover partially. In the latter case the crude or partially concocted humor passes into an abscession or empyema—a localized swelling or inflammation—and the disease will drag on in this form for a further time.[14] Abscessions may terminate favorably or unfavorably. In the latter case they cause relapse:

> . . . in all dangerous cases you should be on the watch for all favorable coctions of the evacuations from all parts, or for fair and critical abscessions. Coctions signify nearness of crisis and sure recovery of health, but crude and unconcocted evacuations, which change into bad abscessions, denote absence of crisis, pain, prolonged illness, death, or a return of the same symptoms.
>
> (*Epidemics I,* Second Constitution, cap. XI: Jones, I, 163-165; see also *Aphorisms,* II: 12: Jones, IV, 111)

The most striking feature of this set of assumptions about the nature of the disease process is that "disease" is not radically different from "health." Rather, the two are on a continuum representing the degree of "crudeness" or "coction" of any one of the body's humoral constituents. The process of maintaining health is identical with the process of overcoming disease. And just as health is a condition of the whole organism, so is disease equally a condition affecting the whole organism. There is only one disease—the diseased organism.

The disease process is, in general outline, the same in all cases. It is a struggle between the strength of the disease and the strength of the body.[15] But this does not preclude the possibility that individual diseased states may be infinite in number. The organism has an endless number of ways of being sick. The physician must be able to understand this process from his observation of the symptoms:

> Do not regret the omission from my account of the name of any disease. For it is by the same symptoms in all cases that you will know the diseases that come to a crisis at the times I have stated.
>
> (*Prognosis,* cap. XXV: Jones, II, 55)

In these writings there is no identification of diseases with specific humors. Nor are diseases usually assigned specific names. I. M. Lonie has observed, *a propos* the above passage, that "the physician observes symptoms, not in order to identify a disease when a particular combination occurs, but in order to infer from them how the disease is progressing. Individual variations are numerous . . . but since all diseases are instances of the same fundamental process, these are in a sense insignificant . . . [what is said here] about sub-varieties of the same disease . . . the author of the *Prognosis* does in fact say about diseases in general: they are all 'the same disease,' because they are all instances of the same process . . ."[16]

This interpretation of disease as an infinitely varied process—thus, as "one" and "many" at the same time—distinguishes the doctrine of Group I from that of Groups II and III. As will be demonstrated below,[d] the latter doctrine defines a limited number of possible disease entities. In the Hippocratic works of Groups II and III diseases are neither "one" nor "infinite" but "finite" and "limited" in number.

The distinction is made clear by the comments which the author of *RAD I* makes on the *Cnidian Sentences.* He states: "the remedies [the Cnidians] used were few in number."[17] From this author's point of view, the assumption of an

[d] See below, pp. 41 and 51-52.

infinite variety of possible diseased states necessarily leads to the use of a very large number of different medicines and therapeutic procedures. The Cnidians, in his view, have cut down unduly on the number of possible diseases, and hence on the number of possible remedies.

He continues:

> Now were these remedies good, and suited to the diseases for which the Cnidians recommended their use, they would be much more worthy of recommendation, in that though few they were sufficient. But as it is this is not the case . . . Yet the many phases and subdivisions of each disease were not unknown to some; but though they wished clearly to set forth the number of each kind of illness their account was incorrect. There would be considerable difficulty in counting [diseases], if one infers the nature of the patients' diseases from the fact that one differs from another in some respect, and it is not thought to be the same disease if it does not have the same name.
>
> (*RAD I,* cap. III: Jones, II, 63-65. The translation of the last sentence is from I. M. Lonie, *op. cit.,* p. 63)

This passage, especially the last sentence, has been the subject of much dispute. The customary interpretation—as given, for instance, by Werner Jaeger[18] —is that the Cnidians carried the subdivision of diseases too far, and that the author of *RAD I* advised them to reduce this number. But this is untenable in view of the preceding criticism of the Cnidians for using too few remedies. The author of *RAD I* would have criticized the Cnidians for using too *many* remedies, rather than too few, if he had thought they carried the subdivision of diseases too far. Nor would he have noted that the "many phases and subdivisions of each disease were not unknown to some." Jaeger attempts to graft onto the works of Group I a doctrine which does not suit them, even though entirely applicable to the works of Groups II and III.

The contrast is not between the Cnidians who hypothesized the existence of too many diseases, and the author of *RAD I* who wanted to "establish the exact number of types of each disease . . . to reduce the several forms of a disease to one *eidos.*"[19] The actual opposition is between the concept of the disease as an *eidos* (entity) separate and apart from the body, and that of disease as the diseased organism which can yield an infinite number of different morbid manifestations and hence requires an infinitely varied curative technique.

Thus the Group I works take a holistic view of the living organism in sickness and in health—symbolized by the references in these works to the *physis* (unitary vital force) of the organism as the criterion or standard by which the physician must be guided.[20]

This holistic approach to medicine, which was later to distinguish the Empirical School, is the key to understanding the therapeutic system of the Group I writings. A holistic therapeutics is the necessary complement of a vitalistic view of the organism—of the conviction that the organism's own reactive powers are the first line of defense against illness.

Such a holistic approach has two corollaries: (1) the symptoms have no absolute significance in themselves but must be interpreted in function of what they reveal about the struggle between the organism's vitality and the disease; (2) at the same time, the symptoms are the physician's *only* source of knowledge of the disease process, since it is not possible to obtain analytical *a priori* knowledge of the holistic vital reactive organism.

The first of these corollaries has been illustrated by the preceding discussion. The disease process is understood through an evaluation of the patient's discharges. While coction is always to be understood as intrinsically beneficial, and "crudeness" as intrinsically harmful, many other symptoms have no absolute significance in themselves. Specifically, fevers, inflammations, swellings, hemorrhages, diarrhoeas, and other painful and, at first glance, pathological manifestations often have positive significance in that they indicate progress in the coction and evacuation of the morbific cause:

> When the stools are bilious, they cease if deafness supervenes; when there is deafness, it ceases when bilious stools supervene.
>
> (*Aphorisms,* IV: 28: Jones, IV, 143)
>
> A sufferer from ardent fever is cured by the supervening of a rigor.
>
> (*Aphorisms,* IV: 58: Jones, IV, 151)
>
> In cases of chronic lientery, acid eructations supervening which did not occur before are a good sign.
>
> (*Aphorisms,* VI: 1: Jones, IV, 181)
>
> When the head aches, and the pain is very severe, a flow of pus, water, or blood, by the nostrils, ears, or mouth, cures the trouble.
>
> (*Aphorisms,* VI: 10: Jones, IV, 183)
>
> Whenever tremors occur in ardent fevers, delirium removes these tremors.
>
> (*Aphorisms,* VI: 26: Jones, IV, 185)
>
> In a case of angina, it is a good thing when a swelling appears on the outside of the trachea.
>
> (*Aphorisms,* VI: 37: Jones, IV, 187)
>
> In cases of enlarged spleen, dysentery supervening is a good thing.
>
> (*Aphorisms,* VI: 48: Jones, IV, 191)
>
> When in the case of a white phlegm violent diarrhoea supervenes, it removes the disease.
>
> (*Aphorisms,* VII: 29: Jones, IV, 199)
>
> In protracted fevers, swelling or pain in the joints may occur; they are not without profit.
>
> (*Coan Prognosis* II: 115: Chadwick and Mann, 227)

> . . . in this constitution there were four symptoms especially which denoted recovery—a proper hemorrhage through the nostrils, copious discharges by the bladder of urine with much sediment of a proper character; disordered bowels with bilious evacuations at the right time; the appearance of dysenteric characteristics. The crisis in many cases did not come with one only of the symptoms described above, but in most cases all symptoms were experienced, and the patients appeared to be more distressed; but all with these symptoms got well.
>
> (*Epidemics I,* Third Constitution, cap. XIX: Jones, I, 175)

Hemorrhages, especially nosebleed (epistaxis), are usually favorable, as are hemorrhoids.[21] Fever, whether occurring alone or supervening on another disease, is a favorable indication.[22] Cessation of diarrhoea, epistaxis, or expectoration is a particularly bad sign when not accompanied by improvement in the patient's condition.[23]

Moreover, the new symptoms associated with abscession and empyema—however painful they may be—are positive signs which must be welcomed by the physician:

> . . . in all cases where the fevers cease neither with signs of recovery nor on critical days, a relapse may be expected. If a fever be protracted, although the patient is in a state indicating recovery and pain do not persist through inflammation or any other obvious cause, you may expect an abscession, with swelling and pain, to one of the joints, especially to the lower ones.
>
> (*Prognosis,* cap. XXIV: Jones, II, 49)

> . . . whenever from pneumonia an abscession takes place to the ears, while gatherings occur in the lower parts and fistula forms, the patient recovers . . . abscessions to the legs in severe and critical pneumonia are all beneficial.
>
> (*Prognosis,* cap. XVIII: Jones, II, 39)

> The only good sign, the most striking that occurred, which saved very many of those who were in the greatest danger, was when there was a change to strangury, into which abscession took place. . . . Rapid and great was the complete change that occurred in their case. For the bowels, even if they were perniciously loose, quickly recovered; their appetite for everything returned, and hereafter the fever abated . . . they all survived, and I know of none that died.
>
> (*Epidemics I,* Second Constitution, cap. X: Jones, I, 163)

A skin disease indicates that an internal disorder is leaving the body through the skin. Hence the appearance of a rash is favorable, and the disappearance of a skin disorder without concomitant improvement in the patient's well-being is one of the most unfavorable signs—indicating that the disease has turned inward:

> When erysipelas that spreads externally turns inwards it is not a good thing; but it is good when internal erysipelas turns outwards.
>
> (*Aphorisms,* VI: 25: Jones, IV, 185)
>
> In cases of angina, if swelling or redness appear on the breast, it is a good sign, for the disease is being diverted outwards.
>
> (*Aphorisms,* VII: 49: Jones, IV, 205)
>
> [In angina] when throat and neck are both red, the illness is more protracted, and recovery is most likely should neck and chest be red and the erysipelas does not turn back inwards. Should, however, the erysipelas disappear neither on the critical days nor with the formation of an abscess on the exterior, and if the patient should not cough up pus easily and without pain, it is a sign of death or of a relapse of the redness. The most hopeful sign is for the redness to be determined as much as possible outwards; but if it be determined to the lungs, it

> produces delirium, and such cases usually result in empyema.
>
> (*Prognosis,* cap. XXIII: Jones, II, 47)

While all symptoms indicate a struggle between the illness and the forces of the organism, some indicate a weakening of the latter and ascendency of the disease:

> When a convalescent has a good appetite without improving his bodily condition, it is a bad sign.
>
> (*Aphorisms,* II: 31: Jones, IV, 117)
>
> In every disease it is a good sign when the patient's intellect is sound and he enjoys his food; the opposite is a bad sign.
>
> (*Aphorisms,* II: 33: Jones, IV, 117)
>
> Should black bile be evacuated at the beginning of any disease, whether upwards or downwards, it is a mortal symptom.
>
> (*Aphorisms,* IV: 22: Jones, IV, 141)
>
> Blood evacuated upwards, whatever be its nature, is a bad sign; but evacuated downwards it is a good sign, and so also black stools.
>
> (*Aphorisms,* IV: 25: Jones, IV, 141)
>
> There is no hope for a dropsical patient should he suffer from cough.
>
> (*Aphorisms,* VII: 47: Jones, IV, 205)

Max Neuburger has written that "the symptomatic picture is composed of signs of damage and defense . . . the organism does not behave passively toward injuries received, but strives to equalize these through self-regulation."[24] In the Group I Hippocratic works the symptom has no absolute value but takes on significance only as a clue to the process of struggle between the force of the disease and the forces of the organism.

It is even permissible to disregard some symptoms when they do not fit the overall pattern of the struggle:

> One must not trust improvements that are irregular, nor yet fear overmuch bad symptoms that occur irregularly; for such are generally uncertain and are not at all wont to last or grow chronic.
>
> (*Aphorisms,* II: 27: Jones, IV, 115)

The second important corollary of a holistic approach to the organism is the doctrine that the physician has no source of knowledge of the patient other than sense-perception. As has already been noted above, all indications for prognosis and treatment have been based upon sensory observation. And while this thesis, which was also fundamental to the Empirical ideology, is not given abstract expression in these Hippocratic writings, it is clear that the authors of the Group I works took it for granted. For these writings contain no physiological speculation about the origins and course of diseases. The occasional statements about the interior of the organism found in these writings are either statements of a very general nature:

> [In consumption] the things about the lungs spread downwards.
>
> (*Epidemics III,* Constitution, cap. XIII: Jones, I, 167)

or they are immediate inferences from what is observable to the physician's senses:

> In those who, having pain in the right hypochondrium, spit out a foamy blood, the expectoration is from the liver; and most of them succumb.
>
> (*Coan Prognosis,* XX: 402: Chadwick and Mann, 254)

> Water . . . increases the bile of the naturally bilious and is injurious to the hypochondrium . . . It enlarges the spleen, and the liver, when inflamed; it causes a gurgling

inside without penetrating downwards. For it travels slowly owing to its being cool and difficult of digestion.
(*RAD I,* cap. LXII: Jones, II, 117-118)[e]

Blood or pus in the urine indicates ulceration of the kidneys or bladder.
(*Aphorisms,* IV: 75: Jones, IV, 155)

When the urine is thick, and small pieces of flesh-like hairs pass with it, it means a secretion from the kidneys.
(*Aphorisms,* IV: 76: Jones, IV, 155)

When the patient has a spontaneous discharge of blood and urine, it indicates the breaking of a small vein in the kidneys.
(*Aphorisms,* IV: 78: Jones, IV, 157)

When the urine contains a sandy sediment, there is a stone in the bladder.
(*Aphorisms,* IV: 79: Jones, IV, 157)

When the scum on the urine is greasy and massed together, it indicates acute disease of the kidneys.
(*Aphorisms,* VII: 35: Jones, IV, 201)

When a patient passes in the urine blood and clots, suffers strangury and is seized with pain in the perineum and pubes, it indicates disease in the region of the bladder.
(*Aphorisms,* VII: 39: Jones, IV, 201)

Even such statements as these, however, are rare in Group I. These physicians do not speculate about physiological processes but obtain their therapeutic indications from sensory evidence:

Exacerbations and constitutions will be made plain by the diseases, by the seasons of the year, and by the correspondences of periods to one another, whether they come every day, every other day, or at a longer interval.

[e]See below, pp. 120-121 for further discussion of *RAD I.*

> Moreover, there are supervening symptoms; for example, in pleurisy, if expectoration supervene immediately on the commencement of the disease, it means a shorter illness, if afterwards, a longer one. Urine, stools, sweat, by the manner in which they supervene, show whether the disease will have a difficult crisis or an easy one, whether it will be short or long.
>
> (*Aphorisms,* I: 12: Jones, IV, 105)

> The following were the circumstances attending the diseases, from which I framed my judgments, learning from the common *physis* of all and the particular *physis* of the individual, from the disease, the patient, the regimen prescribed, and the prescriber—for these make a diagnosis more favorable or less; from the constitution, both as a whole and with respect to the parts, of the weather and of each region; from the custom, mode of life, practices and ages of each patient; from talk, manner, silence, thoughts, sleep, or absence of sleep, the nature and time of dreams, pluckings, scratching, tears; from the exacerbations, stools, urine, sputa, vomit, the antecedents and consequents of each member in the succession of diseases, and the abscessions to a fatal issue or a crisis, sweat, rigor, chill, cough, sneezes, hiccoughs, breathings, belchings, flatulence, silent or noisy, hemorrhages, and hemorrhoids. From these things must we consider what their consequents also will be.
>
> (*Epidemics I,* Third Constitution, cap. XXIII: Jones, I, 181)

This is necessary when disease is viewed as an affliction of the *whole* body. In these works the disease is described as "moving around the body" and ultimately "settling" in some part:

> If convalescents from diseases have pain in any part, the abscessions form in that part.
>
> (*Aphorisms,* IV: 32: Jones, IV, 143)

> But if previous to an illness a part be in a state of pain, the disease settles in that part.
> (*Aphorisms,* IV: 33: Jones, IV, 143)
>
> And on whatever part of the body there is sweat, it means that the disease has settled there.
> (*Aphorisms,* IV: 38: Jones, IV, 145)
>
> And in whatever part of the body there is heat or cold, in that part is the disease.
> (*Aphorisms,* IV: 39: Jones, IV, 145)
>
> Those who survive angina, should the disease turn to the lungs, die within seven days, or, should they survive these, develop empyema.
> (*Aphorisms,* V: 10: Jones, IV, 161)

No distinction is made between physical and mental disease, as they pass into and out of one another and are read by the same signs:

> Varicose veins or hemorrhoids supervening on madness remove it.
> (*Aphorisms,* VI: 21: Jones, IV, 185)
>
> For madness to be followed by dysentery, dropsy, or [increase of the maniacal symptoms, bringing it to a crisis] is a good sign.
> (*Aphorisms,* VII: 5: Jones, IV, 195)

Because knowledge of the inner workings of the body is inaccessible to the physician, these works call for prognosis instead of diagnosis: "Declare the past, [know *(ginoskein)*] the present, foretell [*prolegein*] the future."[f] Prognosis is a natural technique for understanding disease when disease is

[f]*Epidemics I,* Second Constitution, cap. XI (Jones, I, 165). Another function of prognosis was to elicit the patient's confidence (*Prognosis,* cap. I: Jones, II, 7). By his correct prognosis the physician proves to his patient that he knows what he is doing: "for in this way you will justly win respect . . . while you will be blameless if you learn and declare beforehand those who will die and those who will get better." This point was developed, and perhaps over-emphasized, by Edelstein in his work, *Peri Aeron und Die Sammlung der Hippokratischen Schriften* (Berlin, 1931). While the physician, of course, wanted to gain the patient's confidence, for

seen as a process with a beginning, a middle, and an end. By forecasting not only whether the patient will live or die, but also the *whole course of the disease*, the physician obtains the information he needs about the efforts which the organism is making to combat the disease, and this enables the physician himself to combat it in the correct way: "he will carry out the treatment best if he know beforehand from the present symptoms what will take place later."[25]

Typical of the prognostic efforts of these physicians are the following passages from the *Coan Prognosis:*

> When fear and unexplained despondency follow chilling, a convulsion results.
> (*Coan Prognosis* I: 4, Chadwick and Mann, p. 219)
>
> At the beginning of a fever, the presence of black bile in the vomit or in the stools is a bad sign.
> (*Coan Prognosis* II: 68, Chadwick and Mann, p. 223)
>
> A headache accompanied by drowsiness and heaviness brings on a liability to spasms.
> (*Coan Prognosis* IV: 170, Chadwick and Mann, p. 231)
>
> Coma-like sleep and acute chilling are fatal signs.
> (*Coan Prognosis* IV: 177, Chadwick and Mann, p. 232)

economic reasons if for no other, Edelstein's surmise that prognosis was a particular characteristic of the therapeutic method of the itinerant physicians of this period, who stayed only a short while in any given location and thus needed a short-cut technique for eliciting confidence, is an exaggeration. The function of prognosis grows out of the whole system of medicine presented in these writings. It corresponds to diagnosis in the Rationalist medical tradition. Abjuring any claim to comprehend the inner processes of the organism, these physicians obtained the information they needed for cure by observing all external signs of the disease process. They not only predicted whether the disease would, or would not, be fatal, they predicted *all the stages* of the disease in order to know what sort of treatment to administer—to promote the disease's passage through these stages.

After all, curing a patient is a better way of eliciting his confidence than forecasting correctly the date of his death.

See pp. 66-67, 88 below for further discussion of prognosis and diagnosis.

The work, *Prognosis,* is devoted entirely to this subject. Furthermore, the author observes that, in the same geographical regions, the symptoms always have the same meaning and that the physician should therefore be able to foretell the outcome of any disease without difficulty.[26] This is viewed by many commentators as one of the first statements of the regularity and predictability of natural phenomena, thus the beginning of the scientific outlook.

The physician's therapeutic activity is based upon the preceding interpretation of the organism's functioning in sickness and health. His own task is therefore, to second the efforts of the organism.[g] This means, in general, helping the body in its efforts to concoct the *materies morbi* and to evacuate it.[h] Thus the physician should be careful not to purge the body when the humors are still crude:

> Purge or otherwise disturb concocted, not crude humors, and avoid the onset of a disease . . .
> (*Aphorisms,* I: 22: Jones, IV, 109)

And, above all, he should avoid procedures which violate the course followed by the body itself:

> In disorders of the bowels, and in vomitings that are spontaneous, if the matters purged be such as should be purged, the patient profits and bears up well. If not, the contrary. So too artificial evacuations, if what takes place is what should take place, profit and are well borne. If not, the contrary . . .
> (*Aphorisms,* I: 2: Jones, IV, 99)

[g]A nineteenth-century French physician attacked these works on the ground that "attendre qu'il plaise a la nature de nous delivrer de nos maux, c'est laisser l'economie en proie a la douleur, c'est donner le temps aux alterations de devorer nos visceres, c'est, en un mot, nous conduire surement a la mort" (quoted in Jones, I, xvii-xviii). This view is identical with that of one of the leading Methodist physicians. See below, p. 299.

[h]See Max Neuburger, *History of Medicine,* Vol. I (London, 1910), pp. 142ff. and "The Doctrine of the Healing Power of Nature Throughout the Course of Time," pp. 868ff.

> ... But reduction of flesh must not be carried to extremes, as such action is treacherous; it should be carried to a point compatible with the *physis* of the patient ...
>
> (*Aphorisms,* I: 3: Jones, IV, 101)
>
> What matters ought to be evacuated, evacuate in the direction to which they tend, through the appropriate passages.
>
> (*Aphorisms,* I: 21: Jones, IV, 107)
>
> Judge evacuations, not by bulk, but by their conformity to what is proper, and by the ease with which the patient bears them ...
>
> (*Aphorisms,* I: 23: Jones, IV, 109)
>
> If the matters purged be such as should be purged, the patient benefits and bears up well; otherwise the patient is distressed.
>
> (*Aphorisms,* I: 25: Jones, IV, 109)
>
> In purging, bring away from the body such matters as would leave spontaneously with advantage; matters of an opposite character should be stopped.
>
> (*Aphorisms,* IV: 2: Jones, IV, 135)
>
> If matters purged be such as should be purged, the patient benefits and bears up well; otherwise, the patient is distressed.
>
> (*Aphorisms,* IV: 3: Jones, IV, 135)

The physician must be careful not to interfere during the crisis:

> Do not disturb a patient either during or just after a crisis, and try no experiments, neither with purges nor with other irritants, but leave him alone.
>
> (*Aphorisms,* I: 20: Jones, IV, 107)

Particularly to be avoided is any sort of excess. The gradual and gentle mode of treatment is usually the best:

> A restricted and rigid regimen is treacherous, in chronic diseases always, in acute, where it is not called for. Again, a regimen carried to the extreme of restriction is perilous; and in fact repletion, carried to extremes, is perilous.
> (*Aphorisms,* I: 4: Jones, IV, 101)

> Excess and suddenness in evacuating the body, or in replenishing, warming, cooling, or in any other way disturbing it, is dangerous; in fact all excess is hostile to the *physis.* But "little by little" is a safe rule, especially in cases of change from one thing to another.
> (*Aphorisms,* II: 51: Jones, IV, 121)

But:

> For extreme diseases extreme strictness of treatment is most efficacious.
> (*Aphorisms,* I: 6: Jones, IV, 103)

> It is when the disease is at its height that it is necessary to use the most restricted regimen.
> (*Aphorisms,* I: 8: Jones, IV, 103)

Generally, the physician should take care not to do more harm than good: "As to diseases, make a habit of two things—to help, or at least to do no harm" (*Epidemics I,* Second Constitution, cap. XI: Jones, I, 165). And this means, in particular, not to suppress the spontaneous efforts of the body:

> When menstruation is too copious, diseases ensue; when it is suppressed, diseases of the womb occur.
> (*Aphorisms,* V: 57: Jones, IV, 173)

> When a patient has been cured of chronic hemorrhoids, unless one be kept, there is a danger lest dropsy or consumption supervene.
> (*Aphorisms,* VI: 12: Jones, IV, 183)

> A woman does not get gout unless menstruation is suppressed.
> (*Aphorisms,* VI: 29: Jones, IV, 187)

> After spitting of pus, consumption and flux; and when the sputum is checked, the patients die.
>
> (*Aphorisms,* VII: 16: Jones, IV, 197)

The therapeutic techniques at his disposal are relatively few: "purging of sputum or evacuation of the bowels or venesection, purges, and regimen."[27] These works make little mention of drugs. Hellebore is mentioned in *Coan Prognosis* and elsewhere as an emetic and laxative,[28] and two passages in *RAD I* allude to some herbal remedies and "the rest of the compound medicines."[29i] The most important therapeutic procedure used by these physicians is regimen. The doctrine of regimen is discussed in detail in *Regimen in Acute Diseases,* and there it is seen that the function of regimen, as of the other therapeutic techniques of Group I, is to assist the organism in the coction and evacuation of crude humors:

> . . . it has not been ascertained why, in acute diseases some physicians think that the correct treatment is to give unstrained barley gruel throughout the illness; while others consider it to be of first-rate importance for the patient to swallow no particle of barley, holding that to do so is very harmful, but strain the juice through a cloth before they give it. Others again will give neither thick gruel nor yet juice, some not before the seventh day, others at no time until the disease reaches a crisis. Now certainly physicians are not at all in the habit of even raising such questions; even when they are raised, perhaps nothing is learned.
>
> (*Regimen in Acute Diseases,* caps. VII-VIII: Jones, II, 69)

Since, as the author notes, this difference of views gives the profession a bad name—like that of the priests and diviners—he proposes to fill in the gap with a doctrine of regimen, and this work is a discussion of when and how to administer barley juice and barley gruel in acute diseases (pleurisy,

[i]See discussion of *RAD I* below, pp. 120-121.

pneumonia, phrenitis, *causus*[j], and the like).[30] The doctrine itself is relatively simple, consisting of a description, based on certain commonsense parallels with observable processes occurring outside the body, of the ways in which these substances promote evacuation of the bowels: "the gluten of [barley gruel] is smooth, consistent, soothing, lubricant, moderately soft, thirst-quenching, easy of evacuation . . . and it neither has astringency nor causes disturbance in the bowels nor swells up in them. During the boiling, in fact, it has expanded to the utmost of its capacity."[31] [k] If the signs indicate an early crisis, the barley gruel should be given in greater quantities to promote the crisis.[32] And the more completely the bowels are to be purged, the more of it is to be given.[33] The rules for administering the pure juice are "practically" the same as for the gruel.[34] "In their essence the facts are on the whole as stated."

Since the aim of therapy is to promote coction and crisis, and since this is the normal procedure of the body, it is not surprising that cure through similars appears in these writings.[l] Fever is evidence of coction, hence a beneficial phenomenon, and is not to be suppressed; instead, it is intensified through the application of hot water.[35] Heating the body is a major therapeutic technique generally.[36] In tetanus, where the body is cold and stiff, heat is produced by applying cold water to the affected part.[37] Most of the other therapeutic techniques discussed—emetics, purges, and the like—are also to be considered treatment through similars in that they are designed to further a natural impulse of the

[j] *Causus:* A fever prevalent in ancient Greece.

[k] This sort of physiological analogy, which is as far as any work of Group I goes in the direction of analyzing the mechanisms of the organism, should be compared with similar analogies in *Ancient Medicine,* cap XXII (Jones, I, 57) and *The Art,* cap. X (Jones, II, 207) and contrasted with the sort of physiological explanation found in Groups II and III (see further discussion below, pp. 37-40, 52-56, and 80-82).

[l] See Castiglioni, *History of Medicine,* p. 173.

organism. The purpose of hellebore is to cause evacuation. Enemas, clysters, and cold water also cause bowel movements.[38] Wine is also an evacuant and is used as an expectorant besides.[39] Hydromel is an expectorant, laxative, or diuretic.[40] Oxymel is a diuretic and expectorant.[41]

This prejudice in favor of similars is given general application in that diseases are considered less serious when similar to the constitution (*physis*) of the patient, his age, and the season:

> In diseases there is less danger when the disease is more nearly related to the patient in respect of *physis,* habit, age, and season, than when there is no such relationship.
> (*Aphorisms,* II: 34: Jones, IV, 117)

> If phrenitis attacks those beyond forty years of age, they rarely recover; for the risk is less when the disease is related to the *physis* and the age.
> (*Aphorisms,* VII: 82: Jones, IV, 215)

However, not all the treatment in these writings is by similars. Presumably because some symptoms indicate that the strength of the body is being overcome by the force of the disease, these works occasionally call for measures which counteract the symptoms. An astringent wine checks diarrhoea.[42] Vomiting of blood is treated with styptics or refrigerants.[43] The flesh of moist persons should be dried out through starving.[44] Parts of the body that are chilled should be heated.[45] Inflammations and hemorrhages are treated by cold applications.[46] The pain of a sprained joint is relieved by cold water.[47]

Some of the measures advocated seem to be purely "empirical," i.e., not justified by similars or contraries. Thus, bloodletting is called for in strangury and dysuria, as well as for certain kinds of pain.[48]

What is striking is that none of these remedies are analyzed in abstract terms. Similarity or contrariety are judged from sense-perceptible evidence. Success or failure of treatment is determined in terms of the effect of the whole remedy upon the whole organism. In all of the Group I writings there is only one reference to a medicine acting directly upon some humoral component of the organism (as opposed to action upon the organism as a whole):

> acidities from vinegar benefit those who suffer from bitter bile more than those who suffer from black. For the bitternesses are dissolved and turned to phlegm by it, not being brought up; but the blacknesses are fermented, brought up and multiplied, vinegar being apt to raise blacknesses.
>
> (*RAD I,* cap. LXI: Jones, II, 117)[m]

While this is a departure from the therapeutic doctrine of the other Group I works, it still differs from the structured humoralism of the Group III writings with their advocacy of cure through "contrary qualities." In these latter works bile (considered "hot" and "dry") would be treated with a "cold" "wet" medicine, not with vinegar.

By the same token *Aphorisms* II: 22 – "Diseases caused by repletion are cured by depletion; those caused by depletion are cured by repletion, and in general contraries are cured by contraries"–is not to be interpreted in the sense attributed to it by the later Rationalist tradition, but means only that food is the cure for hunger and vice-versa.

The Group I therapeutic doctrine thus regards disease as "one" and "many" at the same time–"one" because all diseases are subject to the same process of cure through coction and "many" because coction can occur in a great variety of different ways. Hence the kinds of treatment are also extremely varied:

> . . . one ought to have an eye to season, district, age, and disease, to see if the treatment is, or is not, proper in the circumstances.
>
> (*Aphorisms,* I: 2: Jones, IV, 99)

[m]See discussion of *RAD I* below, pp. 120-121.

> To some food should be given once, to others twice; in greater quantity or in less quantity; a little at a time. Something too must be conceded to season, district, habit, and age.
>
> (*Aphorisms,* I: 17: Jones, IV, 107)

The good physician is the one who can adjust the variety of specific treatments to the infinity of different ways taken by the organism in its combat against disease. This demands a knowledge of "the *physis* common to all" and of "the *physis* of the individual."[49] The Group I therapeutic doctrine aims at individualization and specificity of treatment founded upon a profound understanding of the different patterns of response of the body to morbific stimuli.

But this doctrine is in no way an intellectual abstraction. It is a precisely defined set of rules:

> The course I recommend is to pay attention to the whole of the medical art. Indeed, all *acts* that are good or correct should be in all cases well or correctly performed; if they ought to be done quickly, then they should be done quickly, if neatly, neatly; if painlessly, they should be managed with the minimum of pain; and all such *acts* ought to be performed excellently, in a manner better than that of one's fellows.
>
> (*RAD I,* cap. IV: Jones, II, 65)

The test of the skillful physician is his ability to perform these acts correctly. This doctrine is a *method,* a set of rules for the physician's guidance. The rules and the method are copied from the method taken by the body in *its* struggle with disease.

Since the body can act for cure in many different ways, this therapeutic method must be no less infinitely subtle and diversified: "Life is short, the art long, opportunity fleeting, experiment treacherous, judgment difficult . . ."[50] The physician's own freedom of choice and action is severely restricted for he is "the servant of the art."[51] He must act "according to rule."[52] He is bound by the art which is itself patterned on the art of the organism.

Such a method can be learned only by long observation, practice, and experience. Once mastered, it imposes a rigorous discipline on the practitioner who must, therefore, be a moral and conscientious individual. The subtle gradations of therapy cannot be written down in detail in the books, and the physician who fails to do his job correctly answers only to his conscience.

"Hippocratic medicine is essentially individualistic,"[n] and in two senses: for not only is treatment individualized, but the doctrine finds its focus, its *fons et origo,* in the individual practitioner.

Group II

In this Group a holistic approach to the organism and its treatment coexists with another doctrine—that of cure through opposition between qualities. All six treatises of Group II contain a mixture of these two doctrines, although, as we will see, not in the same proportion.

Of all the works of this group the *Appendix to Regimen in Acute Diseases* [*RAD II*] contains the most discussion of coction. For example, the word, "coction" *(pepsis),* which appears in no other work of Group II, is mentioned here in four places.[53] And the analysis of disease and cure is in general reminiscent of Group I. The discussion, in Chapters 1, 3, 5, 8, 10, 11, 12, 13, and 14, for instance, covers all aspects of the coction theory, with crisis, resolution through some bodily discharge, and the possibility of empyema.

The word, "coction," does not appear in the other Cnidian treatises, but "maturation" of the humors, which is

[n]Castiglioni, *History of Medicine,* p. 177.

virtually the same as coction, figures quite prominently in *Diseases I.* Empyema forms in the chest after a pleurisy when the disease has been severe and there is neither maturation nor expectoration on the critical days.[54] Tumors develop in the lung when phlegm or bile collect there and pus forms; in a crude state they produce a light pain and a dry cough, but when there is ripening, the pain becomes acute if the maturation and rupture are very prompt and the pus is evacuated through expectoration; if the cavity dries out, the patient is cured completely.[55] Peripneumonia occurs when the lung attracts to itself bile and phlegm; there they rot and form pus, and if this corrupt matter is expectorated on the critical days, the patient recovers; but if the lung, in addition to the matters collected there initially, receives more, and if the abundance of this influx prevents maturation and expectoration, the patients usually die; if they last twenty-two days and the fever falls, but without expectoration, then an empyema forms; it forms particularly in those cases where the pleurisy or peripneumonia has been most intense.[56]

The same concept occurs in *Diseases III* and *Affections,* but with a different emphasis:

> . . . [in pleurisy] give drinks and soups; the drinks will be acidulated so as to clean the matters to be expectorated from the ribs; when the expectoration becomes purulent, the side should be heated up from the outside, so as to mature what is sticking to the ribs; prior to this time this technique would not have been successful, as it would have dried up [the patient].
>
> (*Affections,* cap. 7: VI, 215, L.)

> . . . [in pleurisy] if the expectoration leaves a residue on the tongue which turns to pus, this will give rise to dry coughs, fever, shivering, orthopnoea. . . . If you get such a patient in the first ten days, you will heat him up by regimen and hot baths, and you will infuse into the lung that which will bring forth the pus; you will use all the

remedies which have that property. . . . You will dry out the head, so that nothing will flow from it. If the infusion in the lung does not mature and bring forth the pus, an abscess will form in the lung.

(*Diseases III,* cap. 16: VII, 151-153, L.)

Now the *physician* is the agent who brings about the maturing, and no longer the organism itself.[57] This is a sign of the shift in emphasis, in the transition from Group I to Group II, to the *physician* as the agent of cure. The idea of maturation does not appear in *Diseases II* and *Internal Diseases.*

Other bits and pieces of the doctrine of Group I are to be found scattered through Group II: diseases cure themselves from the inside to the outside,[58] the process of cure involves the appearance of new symptoms,[59] prognostic signs,[60] cure through spontaneous evacuation of the *materies morbi,*[61] fever and sweating as favorable prognostic signs,[62] and the general idea that disease is resolved through an eruption or evacuation, with consequent suppuration or empyema if the evacuation is not complete.[63]

These, however, are mere traces of the doctrine of Group I. While these traces are fairly prominent in *Diseases I* and *Affections,* they are less frequent in the other works of this group. The theory of coction gradually yields to a different therapeutic doctrine—one based on the logical analysis of diseases and remedies in terms of a hypothesized opposition among qualities.

Whereas in Group I the theory of coction was the integrating concept, in Group II (and, *a fortiori,* in Group III) therapeutics is based upon the doctrine of contraries. The component parts of the theory of coction are split apart and then restructured into a quite different doctrinal edifice based upon the assumption that contrariety is the governing force in physiology and medicine.

* * * * * * * * *

In examining this new doctrine the best place to begin is with the humor. In Group I the humor is defined by its sense-perceptible qualities. This is characteristic also of the *Appendix to Regimen in Acute Diseases.* Here "bile" is mentioned only once or twice,[64] "black bile" also,[65] while phlegm is not mentioned at all. Instead we find a series of the same characterizations of the humoral components of the body noted in the works of Group I: acrid and bilious humors, sharp and hot fluxes, humors, fluxes, cold fluxes, abundant and viscous flux, hot and acrid flux, sharp and hot fluxes, atrabilious humors, phlegmatic diseases, etc.[66]

Such sensory descriptions of the humoral causes of disease do not figure prominently in the remaining works of Group II.[67] Instead there is a new formulation—the vague etiological agent, "bile-and-phlegm" or "bile-phlegm."

Thus in *Diseases I* "bile-phlegm," as the internal (proximate) cause of disease, is contrasted with the kinds of external causes which figure in Group I:

> All diseases come, as regards what is in the body, from bile and phlegm, and as regards what is outside, from fatigue and wounds, excessive heat, cold, dryness, or wetness. Bile and phlegm are always in the body to a greater or lesser degree and determine diseases by the intermediary of the food and drink, or of excess heat or excess cold.
>
> (*Diseases I,* cap. 2: VI, 143, L.)

If we now take the works of Group II in their traditional order,[68] we will find that the vague entity, "bile-phlegm," gradually disappears, and an increasing number of diseases are attributed to a single abstractly defined humor or two or three abstractly defined humors. In *Diseases I* some sixteen out of twenty-six cases have "bile-phlegm" as their etiological agent. In *Affections* about thirteen out of thirty cases are ascribed to this cause, about nine out of seventy-five in *Diseases II,* and three out of fifty-four in *Internal Diseases.* The "bile-phlegm" concept does not appear in *Diseases III.*

By the same token, in proceeding from *Diseases I* to *Internal Diseases* we find increasingly frequent ascription of diseases to an individual humor. The first diseases to be so attributed seem to have been the ones with the most striking or precisely defined characteristics, in the sense of symptoms or localization. For example, in *Diseases I* attributed to individual humors are paralysis (black bile),[69] loss of hearing (phlegm),[70] phrenitis (bile or phlegm),[71] and empyema of the lung (phlegm),[72] while to "bile-phlegm" are attributed abscess of the spleen,[73] lung tumors,[74] "fever and shivering,"[75] melancholy,[76] etc. In *Affections* they are earache (phlegm),[77] phrenitis (bile),[78] various skin diseases (phlegm),[79] nasal polyps (phlegm),[80] jaundice (bile),[81] etc., while to "bile-phlegm" are ascribed such less easily defined entities as: sudden pains without fever,[82] diseases of the spleen,[83] tertians,[84] quartans,[85] sciatica,[86] arthritis,[87] gout,[88] etc. The very few cases ascribed to "bile-phlegm" in *Internal Diseases* are a kidney disease,[89] two obscure rheumatic diseases,[90] and a series of diseases described as "thick"—which Littre calls "general nervous diseases."[91] In this work nearly all the diseases are rather precisely ascribed to one, two, or three humors.[92]

In the transition from *Diseases I* to *Internal Diseases* the simple abstraction, "bile-phlegm," becomes differentiated. Thereby the humoral descriptions seem to become more concrete and explicit, but, since they are even further removed from sensory observation, they are actually even more abstract than "bile-phlegm" itself.

Similarly, the physiological explanations given of diseases become increasingly complex as we go through the Cnidian works in their traditional order. All of these works are characterized by a partiality for physiological explanation, and in this respect they all differ from the works of Group I, but various degrees of complexity of the explanations may be distinguished, the proportion of complicated explanations to simple increasing during the passage from *Diseases I* and *Affections* to the other works of this group.

Most of the explanations in *Diseases I* are in terms of "bile-phlegm" or some simple humor and its heating, cooling, wetting, drying or other effect on the *whole* body. Pulmonary empyema is caused by phlegm descending from the head to the lungs and corrupting there, ulcerating the lung.[93] Empyema in the chest occurs when the phlegm from the head rots there and becomes pus.[94] Fever arises when the body is heated by bile and/or phlegm.[95] Pleurisy and peripneumonia without expectoration are caused by dryness.[96] Peripneumonia is caused when the bile and phlegm are put into motion and heated,[97] etc.

Similar explanations are found in the other works of this group, but in progressively smaller proportion to more complex explanations.

Erysipelas forms in the lung when it is dried out and attracts blood, especially from the large veins.[98] Empyema in the lung comes from a burst vein; then the blood rots and forms pus.[99] The veins of the head disgorge their contents and draw in phlegm, causing headache or apoplexy.[100] *Causus* arises when the small veins which have been dried out during the summer draw into themselves sharp and bilious humors.[101] Angina in the back of the throat is caused by a copious viscous flux from the head to the jugular vein; this is cold and blocks up the air and the blood, causing suffocation.[102] Hepatitis is caused when the bile of the liver becomes, "according to our way of reasoning," filled with phlegm and blood.[103] A pulmonary aneurysm causes dry cough, shivering, and fever.[104] Phthisis arises when the spinal marrow becomes full of blood and bile.[105]

Finally, there are several cases, concentrated particularly in *Internal Diseases,* in which the physiological explanations are very involved. Dropsy occurs when the patient has an impure body after some lengthy disease; the stomach fills with water, and the flesh melts.[106] Ileus is the effect of calcination of fecal matters in the intestine: phlegm accumulates around them, and the intestine swells around this mass.[107] Ileus is caused by heating of the upper stomach, while the lower one is cold: the intestine is dried up and condensed by phlegm, so that neither food nor air can go through it, and the stomach is hard.[108] Phthisis arises when the head becomes filled with phlegm which descends to the chest and the lungs: the head filled with phlegm heats up, and the phlegm corrupts there since it cannot be discharged; then when it is thickened and corrupted, and the veins are unduly filled, there is fluxion onto the lung, and the lung, having received it, is irritated by the phlegm which is salty and putrid.[109] Phlegm is transformed into a dropsy when the fat melts and, through the heat in the phlegm, becomes water; as long as fat remains in the lower abdomen the patient is curable; the curable cases may be distinguished from the incurable as follows: if there is no fever, the patient can get up and move around, and the navel does not stick out, then there is fat in the stomach, and the patient can be saved.[110] Dropsy also occurs when phlegm gets into the liver and suffuses it with humidity; this causes heat and gas, and, after some time, fills the liver with water.[111] Dropsy arises when in summer one is thirsty and drinks a lot of water all at once: the lung is filled up and, in turn, passes the water into the chest; this causes great heat which melts the fat in the bronchia; when the fat has started to melt abundantly, dropsy is not long in coming.[112]

Through these increasingly complex physiological explanations external and environmental (exciting) causes, in particular, those of climatic origin, are converted into internal (proximate) causes.

The works of Group I limit themselves to observing that such-and-such weather conditions predispose to such-and-such diseases,[113] and no analytical relationship is hypothesized between such external conditions and the internal pathological process. But in Group II this connection is made, as is seen from the passage quoted above (see p. 36) from *Diseases I.*[114] And there are many other passages which seek to establish a precise causal relationship between the environment and some hypothesized process occurring within the body. In *Affections* it is stated that bile and phlegm cause disease when they become excessively dry, wet, hot, or cold from food, drink, fatigue, wounds, smell, hearing, sight, or from heat and cold.[115] Heat, fever, fatigue, or intemperance dry out the lungs, which causes erysipelas.[116] Fatigue causes phlegm to descend from the head into the lungs and provoke empyema.[117] Intoxication causes the black bile in the head to flow down to the neck and chest, cooling the blood and causing the patient to become paralyzed and to lose his voice.[118] When the head is heated by the sun, by fire, by fatigue or by foods, it attracts to itself the phlegm from the body and then, in turn, disgorges it onto the lungs.[119] Excess eating of such fish as *cephale* and eels, whose fat is contrary to the human constitution, causes a phlegmasy to form in the lungs.[120]

This is the sign, and the concomitant, of a shift in the physician's orientation—from the concern with the whole organism which characterizes the works of Group I to an emphasis on the disease. This necessarily involves hypostatization of disease as an entity and intellectual effort directed at distinguishing one disease entity from another.

Thus these authors lose sight of other factors which must be borne in mind at all times by the physician:

> Much of what the physician should know besides, without the patient's telling him, they have omitted; this knowledge varies in varying circumstances, and in some cases is important for the interpretation of symptoms.
>
> (*RAD I,* cap. I: Jones, II, 63)

These were the age of the patient, his habits, seasonal and climatic factors, and the geographical region—in a word, all the elements which were slighted by the Cnidians in their effort to pinpoint the (humoral) causes of diseases.[o]

The works of the Cnidian group are characterized by emphasis on disease names, and this school was known in

[o]This was the opinion of the Empirical School (K XV 728).

antiquity for its habit of classifying diseases into categories. Galen writes that they described seven diseases caused by bile, twelve diseases of the bladder, four diseases of the kidneys, four stranguries, three forms of tetanus, four forms of jaundice, and three forms of phthisis.[121] The author of *Regimen in Acute Diseases,* as has been noted (above, p. 14), criticizes them for being misled by the names of diseases.[p] From the point of view of the author of this work the Cnidians erred in attempting to single out individual entities from the infinite variety of symptoms characterizing the disease process. Thus they lost sight of the process itself. And by doing so they prescribed too few remedies, neglecting the infinitely subtle adjustments of regimen which are needed if the physician is really to cope with the infinite variety of possible disease processes.[q]

Galen, who had available a copy of the basic text of the Cnidian School, the *Cnidian Sentences,* accuses them of incorrect subdivision of disease categories, of neglecting the signs of coction and also of failing to take an indication from the patient's habits.[122]

Finally, the Cnidian involvement with the internal causes of diseases led them to neglect prognosis. The author of *Regimen in Acute Diseases* is alluding to this when he states:

[p]*RAD I,* caps. 2-3 (Jones, II, 63-65). This is to be contrasted with the passage from *Prognosis* given above (p. 13): "Do not regret the omission from my account of the name of any disease. For it is by the same symptoms in all cases that you will know the diseases that come to a crisis at the times I have stated" (cap. XXV: Jones, II, 55). This has traditionally been considered a remark directed at the Cnidian School.

[q]*RAD I,* cap. II (Jones, II, 63). In Lonie's words, "the early Cnidians appear to have regarded a disease as a static collection of symptoms, over against which the physician stood with a rigid system of treatment . . . The primary importance of symptoms was to identify: as the symptoms varied, so did the disease and its name; and as the name varied, so did the treatment. The attitude implied by both *RAD* and the *Prognostikon* is altogether different. The physician, as it were, stands side by side with the disease; he looks toward the end which it should naturally reach, assisting it at each stage in its progress toward this end, and checking it and diverting it when it takes an unfavorable turn. This difference of attitude is fundamental." Lonie, "The Hippocratic Treatise Peri diaites okseon," p. 64.

> And whenever they interpret symptoms with a view to determining the right method of treatment in each case, my judgment in these matters is in many things different from their exposition.
>
> (*RAD I,* cap. II: Jones, II, 63)

The Cnidians could elicit the symptoms from which the patient was suffering at the time, but, not employing prognosis, they were not able to take into consideration the all-important fact of the future course of the disease.[r]

* * * * * * * * *

The conflict, in Group II, between two concepts of the disease process leads to advocacy of two rival approaches to therapy and two different rationalizations of the curative powers of remedies: one centering on the need to promote coction and the other aiming to counteract the quality of the peccant matter by opposing to it a remedy with the contrary quality.

In Group I the organism cured itself through (1) heating and concocting the crude humor and (2) evacuating it. The physician could assist the organism in this but was guarded in

[r]This is discussed by Lonie, "The Hippocratic Treatise Peri diaites okseon," pp. 52, 59, 63ff. It is true that the author of *Diseases I* (cap. 6: VI, 151, L.) characterizes skill in medicine as the ability to prognose correctly the course of disease. He then, however, complains of the difficulty of making a correct prognosis because of the differences in the patients' constitutions and in environmental conditions (VI, 171, L.). There is no further discussion of prognosis in Group II, although the idea of the sign indicating approaching crisis is occasionally mentioned (see *Diseases III,* caps. 6, 15, 16: VII, 125ff., 137ff., 143ff., L.). The frequent mention in Group II of the number of days a given disease is supposed to last is a lifeless formalization of the prognostic doctrine of Group I (which was perpetuated in the Rationalist tradition [*infra,* pp. 316-317]). Physiological explanations are given of the typical prognostic sign of the works of Group I—sediment in the urine: the kidney attracts phlegm and, instead of casting it out again, retains it; the humor solidifies there and turns into little stones like sand (*Internal Diseases,* cap 14: VII, 203, L.). In a kidney disease caused by bile and phlegm, if the sediment in the urine is thick, reddish, and floury, the disease is caused by bile. If the sediment is thick and white, the disease is caused by phlegm (*Internal Diseases,* cap. 17: VII, 207 L.).

his intervention, bearing in mind that cure was essentially by the organism itself.

We have noted that this concept appears to break down in Group II. And with disappearance of the coction theory, which relied on the curative powers of the organism, there is increased emphasis on the curative effort of the physician. *RAD II,* which in many respects seems to be a bridge between Group I and Group II, contains several references to the conflict between the view that the organism cures and the opposed view that the physician cures. The author defends the former view, almost as though he were arguing in opposition to physicians who have departed from it. In Chapter 3 he states: "physicians who try to resolve phlegmatic diseases by purging at the outset of the disease do not deliver the body of what is tense and inflamed, since the disease in its crudeness does not permit this; instead, they only melt down the healthy parts of the body which were resisting the disease; the body being weakened, the disease gets the upper hand, and when this has happened, cure is impossible."[126] [s] In Chapter 7 he again tells the physician to refrain from moving too hastily and advises him to follow the natural processes of the organism.[124] And in Chapter 23 he repeats this—the physician "must not purge in any of these cases, since purging will be dangerous, will not be advantageous, and will prevent the crisis and the evacuation which would otherwise occur of themselves."[125]

The works of Group II contain the following references to therapeutic procedures associated with coction.

When strangury is caused by excess heat in the head, which melts the phlegm and causes it to pass into the urinary tract, the cure is to heat the head further with a hot-water bottle.[126] In peripneumonia when the patient is not expectorating properly, he should be given a steam bath.[127] In pleurisy the treatment is to heat up the side of the body so as

[s]The Group I writings generally oppose purging at the outset of the disease before the morbific cause has been concocted *(Aphorisms,* I: 22: Jones, IV, 109)

to mature the bile and phlegm inside.[128] In a *causus*-like fever, in which the patient is burning hot and has bilious urine and a burnt and dry sputum, the treatment is to wash him in hot water several times a day.[129] In phrenitis, where the patient is feverish and delirious, the cure is to heat him with wet applications and warming drinks.[130] In erysipelas of the lung caused by excess blood in the lung, the patient being feverish and having a swollen chest, part of the treatment consists in washing him with hot water and giving him hot drinks.[131]

In addition to this system there appears another one—which gives greater scope to the activist orientation of the physician. This is the doctrine of cure through contraries. This doctrine is logically incompatible with coction, and the duality of their therapeutic procedure is consciously recognized by these writers: Do not "wet that which should be dried, dry that which should be moistened . . . do not fail to cool that which should be cooled, heat that which should be heated, ripen that which should be ripened."[132]

In Group II as much emphasis is laid on cure through contraries as on cure through promotion of coction. Thus, if there is pus in the lower stomach, apply potter's clay to the outside to dry up the disease.[133] In empyema of the lung, characterized by rotten blood and pus, prescribe a diet which makes the patient as dry and bloodless as possible.[134] In a case of dry fever with vomiting of bile, give cold and emollient foods but nothing sharp or salty.[135] In a leucophlegmasy dry out the patient through diet.[136] In a phlegmatic disease the patient should eat sharp, oily, sweet, and acid things, as these draw out the phlegm and dry up the body.[137] In a dropsy, dry out the stomach with the appropriate regimen.[138] When the body is torpid due to the blood being cooled off by the phlegm, the cure is to heat up the patient.[139] In a case of ileus, which is caused by heating of the upper stomach while the lower stomach is cold, the cure is to evacuate blood from the head and the arm in order to cool off the upper stomach, and to heat up the lower stomach with sitzbaths.[140] In a headache with fever due to phlegmasy, give cold foods, refresh the head with cooling remedies, and apply potter's clay to cool off the head.[141] Inflamed wounds need cold applications, while putrid and filthy wounds need sharp and biting applications.[142] In dropsy the regimen should make the patient thin and dry.[143] When a bilious person has an enlarged spleen, he should be given a moistening diet.[144] In a *causus* due to bile, when the patient is cold outside and hot inside, the treatment is with cold drinks.[145] Toothache caused by phlegm at the roots of the teeth is cured by cauterizing the teeth and thus drying up the phlegm.[146]

In cure through contraries the physician substitutes his own knowledge and activity for that of the organism. The ultimate stage in this substitution is reached with advocacy of an *operation* to extract the pus (empyema) from the lungs, kidneys, and other organs. In Group I, as will be recalled, empyema was one final stage of the process of natural cure by the organism. In Group II, however, the physician can abort this natural process through his own intervention.[147] Another technique of active intervention which makes its appearance in Group II is infusion of a liquid into the lung to provoke coughing and thus extract the pus.[148]

The existence of these two theories of cure is reflected in the various proposed explanations of the healing powers of remedies. Sometimes remedies are explained in terms of a capacity to provoke urine, stool, sweat, expectoration, etc.[149] [t] At other times the remedy is justified in terms of its heating, cooling, moistening, or drying qualities.[150]

Sometimes the writer tries to explain the action of a remedy in terms of both theories at once:

[t]Barley water, wine, and hydromel are prescribed very frequently in this connection, thus justifying the reproach of the author of *Regimen in Acute Diseases* that the Cnidians prescribe these same remedies for everything (cap. VI: Jones, II, 67).

> Purifying remedies are used as follows: bilious patients get chylogogues, phlegmatic patients get phlegmagogues, melancholic patients get medicines which purge black bile, dropsical patients ones which purge water. The medicinal substances which evacuate neither bile nor phlegm should, when introduced into the body, manifest their *dynamis* either by cooling, heating, drying, moistening, contracting, or loosening.
>
> (*Affections*, cap. 36: VI, 247, L.)

> Give these refrigerants in cases of *causus* when you judge them to be indicated; they have many properties; some are diuretic, others are purgative, some are both one and the other, others are neither one nor the other, but cool in the same way as when you pour cold water into a jar of boiling water or set this jar out in the fresh air.
>
> (*Diseases* III, cap. 17: VII, 157, L.)

> Of the medicines given for the spleen, some purge through the bladder and thus empty the spleen. Others do not promote any perceptible evacuation of the spleen, but even so it is emptied.
>
> (*Affections*, cap. 20: VI, 231, L.)

The emergence of this theory of cure through opposition between abstract qualities can be understood as reflecting the parallel rise of a new class of physicians—who disliked the slow and perhaps cumbersome technique of cure through promotion of coction and preferred the more rapid diagnostic and curative technique afforded by the doctrine of contraries. This theme will be elaborated upon at greater length below, but evidence in its favor is found even in these Cnidian writings.

This development has been well depicted by Lonie, who writes: "we tend to regard it as a characteristic of the Cnidian School, as opposed to the school of Cos, to give detailed rules of treatment which could be applied *au pied de la lettre* irrespective of the individual constitution of the patient, to which other works in the collection pay so much regard. Certainly the physician who had mastered the detailed therapies of *On Internal Diseases* and carried them in his head would be armed against all contingencies. Prepared to apply his remedies swiftly and mechanically, he need never appear at a loss in the sickroom; and he must have aroused awe and admiration by the complexity of his prescriptions."[151]

A distinguishing characteristic of the Group I doctrine was absolute reliance upon sense-perception and renunciation of any claim to comprehend the essence of morbid processes. But such an attitude denies any qualitative distinction between physicians and laymen. Both work with the same materials, and the physician differs from the layman only in his possession of greater skill and experience. Such an attitude is consistent with the view of medicine as a craft and the physician as craftsman.

In the Cnidian works, however, we see emerging the idea that the physician is more than a craftsman. The doctrine of contraries, with its implication of knowledge beyond that which is sense-perceptible, suggests the existence of a class of physicians claiming knowledge which was qualitatively different from that of the layman. This is brought out strikingly in *Affections* which notes that there are two roads to the knowledge of medicines--accidental discovery and use of the intellect. The properties which can be discovered accidentally are the emetic, diuretic, and evacuant properties.[152] These accidental discoveries can be made as well by the non-professional as by the professional.[153] But (the author continues) the obscure properties must be learned by reasoning from the evident ones: that is, the heating and cooling powers are determined by observing the laxative and diuretic ones and reasoning from them.[154] Here the professional is superior to the non-professional.[155]

Examples of this reasoning process are as follows: laxative foods heat up rapidly in the stomach and, when heated, are consumed, melt, and provoke a prompt evacuation. Constipating foods, on the other hand, heat up slowly; when heated, they dry out, condense, and thus, having become hard, do not provoke stools. Laxative foods have a lot of juice and are naturally hot. Diuretic foods are drying and cold (since, when the urine leaves the body, the latter becomes colder and drier).[156] Hot dry foods tighten up the stomach by absorbing the humors there; wet foods relax it. Astringent foods dry and contract the body, causing constipation.[157]

On the basis of this doctrine certain foods, formerly viewed as only diuretic or evacuant, could now be associated directly with some humoral component of the organism. Raw leeks and grenadines are productive of phlegm.[158] Greasy and sweet foods cause moistness and phlegm, as do cheese, sesame, and raisins.[159]

The physician's latitude in coping with disease is extended by a final doctrine of the Cnidian works, namely, that the inherent qualities of foods can be altered through preparation. Hot foods can be made cold, cold ones hot, wet ones dry, and dry ones wet. This is, in fact, a necessity, as the author points out, since the diet in disease should in any case not deviate very far from what the patient customarily eats when in health.[160][u]

This is an exquisite example of how the Group I precept that diet in illness should not differ greatly from diet in health is adjusted to the doctrine of cure through contraries.[161] Thus, confronted with a patient presenting a phlegmatic disease whose customary diet consists of cold wet foods, the physician processes these customary foods to make them hot and dry.

Needless to say, this conflict between two systems of therapeutics was productive of some logical confusion. If an

[u]The author goes on: "do not be at a loss and because you cannot avail yourself of means within your grasp . . . fail to be of use to the patient. Extend your investigations judiciously beyond what is (usually) given to the patient, and you will hit upon some remedy " *Affections,* cap. 39 (VI, 249, L.).

inflammation is caused by phlegm, is the physician supposed to give a refrigerant against the inflammation, a heating remedy to warm up the phlegm, or a heating remedy to promote coction of the phlegm? In the case of a bilious disease, does he give a refrigerant to cool the bile or a heating remedy to promote coction of the bile? This confusion is quite apparent in some of the cases. For example, if there is a pleurisy or peripneumonia without expectoration, caused by dryness which prevents the bile and phlegm from maturing, the cure is to give drinks which moisten the lung and thereby promote expectoration.[162] If the lungs swell due to heat, the cure is to give diuretics *which are not heating* (but the physician then goes on to prescribe heating the patient after all).[163] When there is bile on the brain causing a heavy fever and shivers, the correct treatment is by refrigerant remedies *and* the steam bath.[164] In an angina with fever and pain in the head, the cure is through a hot sponge bath; then, if the phlegmasy descends to the chest, apply cold wet beet leaves and give cold drinks to promote expectoration.[165] In leucophlegmasy, when the body is swollen by a white edema, first give purgatives which evacuate the water or phlegm, and then prescribe a drying regimen.[166] In swelling of the gall bladder, purge if that is necessary; if it is not, use a drying diet.[167] There are two types of cataplasms for tumors: those which mature and those which resolve the tumor.[168]

Thus the emergence in the Cnidian works of a therapeutic theory based upon contraries reflects the existence of a self-conscious professional group of physicians which aimed to distinguish its procedures, based upon abstract analysis of the human organism and of curative substances, from the Group I approach based upon coction.

Acceptance of the doctrine of contraries thus signified: (1) superiority of the physician to the organism as the agent of cure and (2) superiority of the professional to the layman as the agent of cure. The physician now possessed abstract knowledge beyond the comprehension of the layman lacking the necessary education (as opposed to therapeutic experience). And he no longer had to obey the laws of the organism; reinterpretation of the coction theory in terms of contraries permitted the physician to dominate the therapeutic process, instead of being subordinate to it, by the judicious administration of remedies with the necessary contrary qualities.

Group III

While the Group II writings are a battleground between the holistic theory of coction and the analytical doctrine of contraries, Group III presents the latter doctrine in a perfected form. All elements of the theory of coction are transvalued and reorganized under the guiding principle of contrariety.

These works make almost no reference to the theory of coction, and they specifically deny the unity and holism of the organism which that theory presupposes:

> Some physicians say that a man is blood, others that he is bile, a few that he is phlegm. Physicians . . . all add the same appendix. For they say that a man is a unity, giving it the name that severally they wish to give it; this changes its form and its *dynamis,* being constrained by the hot and the cold, and becomes sweet, bitter, white, black, and so on. But in my opinion, these views . . . are incorrect.
>
> (*Nature of Man,* cap. II: Jones, IV, 7)

Coction is mentioned as a physiological process only once and there accorded a limited role:

> Feverishness of the bowels must be accompanied by feverishness of the bladder. For when it is abnormally heated, its mouth is inflamed. In this condition it does not expel the urine, but concocts it and heats it within

> itself. The finest part is separated off, and the clearest part passes out as urine, while the thickest and muddiest part forms solid matter.
>
> (*Airs Waters Places,* cap. IX: Jones, I, 97)

In another passage from the same work coction is removed not only from the focus of the physician's attention, but even outside the body entirely: "the heat of the sun produces coction, just as all other things always become sweeter through coction " (cap. VIII: Jones, I, 93).[V]

These physicians are striving for an analytical theory of the organism which will permit medical practice to be based upon knowledge of proximate causes. Two classes of such causes are developed: the humors and the *pneuma* (air, wind, breath).

Most of the Group III writings are still influenced by the "bile-phlegm" physiology and pathology discussed above, which is too vague to serve as a useful instrument of analysis. In *Nature of Man* (*The* Physis *of Man*), however, this is converted into the quadripartite humoral doctrine which was to be the foundation of Rationalist therapeutics for the next two millenia:

> The body of man has in itself blood, phlegm, yellow bile, and black bile; these make up the nature [*physis*] of his body, and through these he feels pain or enjoys health. Now he enjoys the most perfect health when these elements are duly proportioned to one another in respect of compounding, *dynamis,* and bulk, and when they are perfectly mingled. Pain is felt when one of these elements is in defect or excess, or is isolated in the body without being compounded with all the others. For when an element is isolated and stands by itself, not only must the place which it left become diseased, but the place where it stands in a flood must, because of the excess, cause pain and distress. In fact, when more of an element flows

[V]See below p. 114, note.

> out of the body than is necessary to get rid of superfluity, the emptying causes pain. If, on the other hand, it be to an inward part that there takes place the emptying, the shifting and the separation from other elements, the man certainly must, according to what has been said, suffer from a double pain, one in the place left, and another in the place flooded.
>
> (*Nature of Man,* cap. IV: Jones, IV, 11-13)

This passage is of profound importance because it is the first attempt by a Hippocratic writer to define the *physis.* In Group I the existence of a vital power in the body is taken for granted. While it is sometimes called the *physis,*[169] mention is also made of the "strength" of the body or its *dynamis.*[170] *Nature of Man,* however, makes *physis* a term of art and then dissolves it into its humoral components.

Henceforth the vital power of the body is nothing more than the mixture of the four humors. Group III presents a humoral doctrine without coction!! Disease is only the excess or deficiency of one of the humors.

The idea of a humor being deficient has no parallel in Group I. The concept of humoral "excess," however, may be related to the suggestion in Group I that blood can at times be in excess, the patient being relieved by spontaneous hemorrhage.[171] The "isolation" of a humor most resembles the Group I idea that a humor stands out because of its "crudeness." But in Group III this "isolation" of the humor is not associated with "crudeness," nor has restoration of the proper *krasis* anything to do with coction.

Instead, the dyscrasia or separation of the humors is enlisted to support a doctrine of localized diseases. While in Group I disease was always an affliction of the whole organism, now various pains, tumors, inflammations, etc., are attributed to isolation of the peccant humor.

The traditional fever classes—quotidian, tertian, quartan, and continued—are also adjusted to the quadripartite humoral doctrine, *Nature of Man* explaining them in terms of the total amount of black or yellow bile in the organism. Continued fever is from "the most abundant and purest bile, and its crises occur after the shortest interval. For since the body has no time to cool, it wastes away rapidly, being warmed by the great heat." "The quotidian next to the continued comes from the most abundant bile, and ceases quicker than any other, though it is longer than the continued, proportionately to the lesser quantity of bile from which it comes. . . ." "The tertian is longer than the quotidian and is the result of less bile." "The quartans are in general similar, but they are more protracted than the tertians in so far as their portion is less of the bile that causes heat, while the intervals are greater in which the body cools. It is from black bile that this excessive obstinacy arises. For black bile is the most viscous of the humors in the body, and that which sticks fast the longest. Hereby you will know that quartan fevers participate in the atrabilious element; because it is mostly in autumn that men are attacked by quartans. . . ." (cap. XV: Jones, IV, 39-41).

Regimen in Health gives a more stringently analytical interpretation of these fevers. The diseases of winter are ascribed to phlegm, localized in the upper half of the body (above the diaphragm), and treated with emetics, while the fevers of summer are localized below the diaphragm, ascribed to bile, and treated with clysters (cap. V: Jones, IV, 51).

These authors had another technique for isolating and defining the proximate causes of disease: assimilating them to the atmospheric air (*pneuma*) which was already recognized as a major *external* (exciting) cause of disease. By identifying the external air (wind) with the air in the body (breath) they transformed *pneuma* from an external cause into an internal (proximate) cause.[w]

[w]The pneumatic doctrine, which plays a very important role in Rationalist therapeutics generally, was first devised by Philistion of Locri and the Sicilian School (see below, p. 106). Pneumatism is discussed very thoroughly in C.R.S. Harris, *The Heart and the Vascular System in Ancient Greek Medicine* (Oxford, At the Clarendon Press, 1973).

This is done in *Breaths* and *Sacred Disease* where the conflict between the two types of causes is seen in the use of two different words for cause: *prophasis* and *aition.*

Aition does not appear in the Group I works, which only use *prophasis* (meaning external, exciting, cause).[172] Introduction of the new word–which has a more abstract sense than *prophasis* and becomes the technical term for "cause" in Aristotle's metaphysics[x] –signifies an extension of the concept of causality from the perceptible exciting causes (wind, weather, accidents, wounds, etc.) of Group I to proximate causes operating within the body beyond the reach of the senses.

In *Sacred Disease* the conflict between the two types of causes takes the form of a contrast between divine causes (*aitia*) and all natural causes both external and internal (*prophasies*).[173] The author writes that all diseases have natural causes and none are caused divinely: epilepsy has "the same *physis* and *prophasis* as other diseases."[174] It is caused by the *pneuma* entering the body and moving around inside: "this disease is born and grows from the things that come to the body and leave it."[175] "This disease styled sacred comes from the same *prophasies* as others, from the things that come to and go from the body, from cold, sun, and from the changing restlessness of the *pneumata.*"[176]

But, carried away by his own argument, he even characterizes humoral causes as *prophasies;* "those who are mad through phlegm are quiet and neither shout nor make a disturbance; those maddened through bile are noisy, evil-doers, and restless, always doing something inopportune. These are the *prophasies* of continued madness."[177]

The author's theory that the *pneuma* is the *prophasis* of the disease, both *qua* wind and when it has entered the body, leads him to call the humors themselves *prophasies,* since the *aitia* have been preempted by the Gods.

[x] *Physics* 194b 23-195a 3. See below, pp. 127-128.

Invoking the *pneuma* and the now hypostatized humors, the author can propose a precise physiological explanation of epilepsy. Through the veins running to the liver and spleen the body takes in *pneuma* from the outside.[178] Epilepsy occurs when the phlegm in the brain, with which man is born and which remains with him unless purged away in childhood, descends from the brain and enters these veins, interrupting the flow of air through them: "The patient becomes speechless and chokes; froth flows from the mouth; he gnashes his teeth and twists his hands; the eyes roll and intelligence fails, and in some cases excrement is discharged."[179] The symptoms of epilepsy are described in detail, and each is related in some way to the blockage, by phlegm, of the *pneuma* in the veins.

Breaths also projects *pneuma* to the inside of the body but leaves aside problems of divine causation and can use *aition* to characterize all the forms—external and internal—taken by the *pneuma* as a causal agent.[180] "*Pneuma* in the body is called breath, outside the body it is called air."[181] Outside it causes epidemic diseases, and when it enters the body with the food it causes the diseases usually ascribed to regimen.[182] The author concludes:

> so breaths are seen to be the most active agents during all diseases; all other things are but secondary and subordinate causes. This, then, as the *aition* of diseases I have now expounded. I promised to declare the *aition* of diseases, and I have set forth how *pneuma* is lord not only in things as wholes, but also in the bodies of animals.
>
> (*Breaths,* cap. XV: Jones, II, 253)

This work gives a similar explanation of epilepsy: air is taken into the organism with the food and, making its way into the veins, blocks the flow of blood. "The progress of the blood through the body proving irregular, all kinds of irregularities occur. The whole body is torn in all directions; the parts of the body are shaken in obedience to the trembling and disturbance of the blood; distortions of every kind occur in every manner."[183]

Both *Sacred Disease* and *Breaths* account for a number of ailments and diseases through combinations of humors and *pneuma.*[184]

Thus environmental air is the device which unifies external (exciting) and internal (proximate) causes. In *Sacred Disease* the air is called *prophasis* while in *Breaths* it is called *aition,* but the outcome is the same: emergence of the idea that a definable and palpable cause can be discerned within the body.[y]

* * * * * * * * *

An important consequence of these efforts to pinpoint the proximate causes of diseases is the development of a structured relationship between the organism and its environment—also based upon the idea of contrariety.

We have already noted that the Group I writers considered the disease less severe when related to the constitution of the patient, his age, and the season. Little else of a structured nature can be discerned in these works in respect of the relationship between diseases and seasons: certain constitutional types are more likely to fall ill in winter, others in summer[185]; some diseases are worse in some seasons, others in others[186]; in normal seasons the associated diseases are also normal, while in abnormal seasons the diseases are also abnormal[187]; continuation of the same weather is healthy, while a change of weather is liable to bring on disease[188]; and those who are sick in one season will recover when the season changes.[189]

While *Aphorisms* states that acute fevers occur during droughts[190] and that a rainless autumn benefits those with moist constitutions[191] (suggesting a relationship of con-

[y]On the use of *aition* and *prophasis* in Group III see also *Nature of Man,* caps, IX and XIII, and *Airs Waters Places,* caps. IV, IX, XII, XVI, XXII (Jones, I, 77, 97, 107, 115, 127 and IV, 25, 27, 29, 37).

trariety), this is a minor theme and could as well be based upon empirical observation as upon logical analysis.

The beginning of a structured relationship between seasons and diseases is definitely to be noted, however, in Group II—particularly in *RAD II* and *Internal Diseases.* Erysipelas of the lung is due to an influx of blood and is frequent in summer.[192] Hepatatis is from black bile and occurs in the autumn.[193] Disease of the spleen is due to the sun's setting in motion the bile.[194] Another splenetic disease is caused by influx of blood in the springtime.[195] Still another splenetic disease is caused by black bile in the autumn.[196] A jaundice is due to yellow bile in the summer.[197] Another one is caused by phlegm in the winter.[198] Typhus occurs in summer when the bile is set in motion.[199] One type of angina occurs in winter or spring when a cold and viscous flux descends from the head to the back of the throat, and another arises in summer or autumn when a hot and acrid flux plays the same role; it is the season which makes it dangerous.[200]

This doctrine cannot be discerned in the other Cnidian works. Although the author of *Diseases I* writes that phlegm is the coldest humor, blood is the hottest, and bile is a little colder than blood,[201] and for that reason diseases should be treated only in their proper seasons,[202] his suggestion is not followed in *Diseases I* or in the other Cnidian works. This probably reflects the "bile-phlegm" pathology which inhibits identification of either one of the pair with a quality or a season. Bile and phlegm are equally subject to being heated up (an impossibility in later Rationalist humoralism).[z] Thus, in apoplexy the veins of the head are heated and draw in phlegm,[203] in headache the bile and phlegm are heated and in turn heat up the blood,[204] pleurisy is caused by strong drink which heats and moistens the bile and phlegm.[205]

[z]Philolaus of Croton, who was a contemporary of Socrates, also claimed that phlegm is by nature hot (W.H.S. Jones, *Medical Writings of Anonymous Londinensis* [Cambridge University Press, 1947], XVIII: 20).

The development of an analytical relationship between diseases and seasons culminates in *Nature of Man* which aligns the four humors with the elements (heat, cold, wetness, and dryness) and with the four seasons:

> Phlegm increases in a man in winter; for phlegm, being the coldest constituent of the body, is closest akin to winter . . . . That winter fills the body with phlegm you can learn from the following evidence. It is in winter that the sputum and nasal discharge of man is fullest of phlegm . . . . And in spring too phlegm still remains strong in the body, while the blood increases. For the cold relaxes and the rains come on, while the blood accordingly increases through the showers and the hot days. For these conditions of the year are most akin to the nature of the blood, spring being moist and warm . . . . And in summer blood is still strong, and bile rises in the body and extends until autumn. In autumn blood becomes small in quantity, as autumn is opposed to its nature, while bile prevails in the body during the summer season and during autumn . . . . But in summer phlegm is at its weakest. For the season is opposed to its nature, being dry and warm. But in autumn blood becomes least in man, for autumn is dry and begins from this point to chill him. It is black bile which in autumn is greatest and strongest. When winter comes on, bile, being chilled, becomes small in quantity, and phlegm increases again because of the abundance of rain and the length of the nights.
>
> (*Nature of Man,* cap. VIII: Jones, IV, 19)

From this analysis the author draws two conclusions: (1) that the diseases of winter cease in summer while those of summer cease in winter; and (2) that diseases are most powerful in their own seasons.[206]

Thus the logical therapeutic doctrine of Group III runs counter to the Group I doctrine on the very important point:

are diseases intensified or moderated by the similar seasonal influence? Whereas Group I concludes that the similar seasonal influence is beneficial (*Aphorisms,* II: 34), Group III, with its stress on contrariety, is forced to conclude that the similar influence is harmful.

The analytical relationship between organism and environment developed in the Group III writings makes it possible to "explain" why particular environmental influences have a particular effect upon the body. The contrast between Groups I and III in this respect is strikingly illustrated by parallel passages in *Aphorisms* and *Airs Waters Places.* Where the former states:

> As for the seasons, if the winter be dry and northerly and the spring wet and southerly, of necessity occur in the summer acute fevers, eye diseases, and dysentery, especially among women and those with moist constitutions.
> (*Aphorisms,* III: 11: Jones, IV, 125)

the latter adds:

> For whenever the great heat comes on suddenly while the earth is soaked by reason of the spring rains and the south wind, the heat cannot fail to be doubled, coming from the hot, sodden earth and the burning sun; men's bowels not being braced nor their brain dried—for when spring is such the body and its flesh must necessarily be flabby—the fevers that attack are of the acutest type in all cases, especially among the phlegmatic.
> (*Airs Waters Places,* cap. X: Jones, I, 99)

Whereas in the *Aphorisms* we find:

> But if the winter prove southerly, rainy, and calm, and the spring dry and northerly, women whose confinement is due in the spring suffer abortion on the slightest provocation, or, if they do bear children, have weak and unhealthy offspring, so that they either die at once or live with puny and unhealthy bodies. Among the rest prevail

> dysentery and dry diseases of the eyes, and, in the case of the old, catarrhs that quickly prove fatal.
>
> (*Aphorisms,* III: 12: Jones, IV, 125)

Airs Waters Places adds this interpretation:

> Phlegmatics are liable to dysenteries, and women also, phlegm running down from the brain because of the humidity of their *physis.* The bilious have dry ophthalmia because of the warm dryness of their flesh. Old men have catarrhs because of their flabbiness and the wasting of their veins, so that some die suddenly, while others become paralyzed on the right side or the left. For whenever, owing to the winter being southerly and the body warm, neither brain nor veins are hardened, a northerly, dry, cold spring supervening, the brain, just at the time when it ought to have been relaxed along with the spring and purged by the cold in the head and hoarseness, congeals and hardens, so that the heat of summer having suddenly supervened and the change supervening, these diseases befell.
>
> (*Airs Waters Places,* cap. X: Jones, I, 101)

* * * * * * * * *

While Group I assumed that the internal operations of the organism and the relations between organism and environment form an organic whole which the physician comes to understand through his therapeutic experience, the physicians of Group III have analyzed this whole into its component parts.

The *physis* of the body is analyzed into four humors, each possessing its own *physis.* The humors are viewed as liquids possessing powers (*dynameis*): "these elements are not all one . . . each of them has its own *dynamis* and its own *physis*" (*Nature of Man,* cap. V: Jones, IV, 15).

Since these physicians aimed to base medical practice on an analysis of the organism, of medicines, and of foods, all of these had to be reduced to the same common denominator. Hence *dynamis* is also used to denote the capacity of the drug or food to affect the organism, and the words, *arete* (virtue) and *poiotes* (quality), are discarded.[207] This hypostatization of the "power" of a drug or food resembles the hypostatization of the proximate cause symbolized by the substitution of *aition* for *prophasis.*

The outcome is stress on the "knowing" part of medicine:

> Knowledge of the cause [*aition*] of a disease will enable one to administer to the body what things are advantageous.
>
> (*Breaths,* cap. I: Jones, II, 229).

> He who aspires to treat correctly of human regimen must first acquire knowledge and discernment of the *physis* of man in general—knowledge of its primary constituents and discernment of the components by which it is controlled. For if [the physician] be ignorant of the primary constitution, he will be unable to gain knowledge of their effects; if he be ignorant of the controlling thing in the body, he will not be capable of administering to a patient suitable treatment.
>
> (*Regimen I,* cap. II: Jones, IV, 227).

Having broken medicine up into pieces, like Humpty-Dumpty, these physicians now wanted to put it back together—guided by the intellect and assuming contrariety as the overall integrating concept:

> The physician must set himself against the established character of diseases, of constitutions, of seasons, and of ages; he must relax what is tense and make tense what is relaxed. For in this way the diseased part would rest most, and this, in my opinion, constitutes treatment.
>
> (*Nature of Man,* cap. IX: Jones, IV, 25)

> Those with physiques that are fleshy, soft, and red, find it beneficial to adopt a rather dry regimen for the greater

> part of the year. For the *physis* of these physiques is moist. Those that are lean and sinewy, whether ruddy or dark, should adopt a moister regimen for the greater part of the time, for the bodies of such are constitutionally dry. Young people also do well to adopt a softer and moister regimen, for this age is dry, and young bodies are firm. Older people should have a drier kind of diet for the greater part of the time, for bodies at this age are moist and soft and cold. So in fixing regimen pay attention to age, season, habit, land, and physique, and counteract the prevailing heat or cold. For in this way will the best health be enjoyed.
>
> (*Regimen in Health,* cap. II: Jones, IV, 47, 49)

> For in this disease [epilepsy] as in all others it is necessary, not to increase the illness, but to wear it down by applying to each what is most hostile to it, not that to which it is conformable. For what is conformity gives vigor and increase; what is hostile causes weakness and decay. Whoever knows how to cause in man by regimen moist or dry, hot or cold, he can cure this disease also . . .
>
> (*Sacred Disease,* cap. XXI: Jones, II, 183)

The passage from *Regimen in Health* is a parallel with *Aphorisms* I: 2, and *Breaths,* cap. I, states that: "opposites are the cure for opposites . . . Medicine is subtraction and addition, subtraction of what is in excess, addition of what is wanting" (Jones, II, 299)—a precise parallel with *Aphorisms* II: 22.[a] The spirit of these pronouncements, however, is very different in the Group III writings where the physician's attention is centered on abstractly conceived proximate causes. For it is assumed that the physician can reason his way to a knowledge of these causes and of hidden physiological and pathological processes generally. The author of *Breaths* asserts that "[wind] is invisible to sight though visible to reason [*logismos*]" (cap. III: Jones, II, 231), thus

[a]See above p, 31.

laying a foundation for the claim that *pneuma* in the body is also visible to reason. He notes further: "to judge of the most obscure and difficult diseases is more a matter of opinion than of art, and therein there is the greatest possible difference between experience and inexperience. Now of these obscure matters one is the *aition* of diseases, what the beginning and source is whence come affections of the body" (cap. I: Jones, II, 229). The author of *Regimen I,* discussing the elements of the body, notes that men "trust eyes rather than mind, though these are not competent to judge even things that are seen. But I use mind to expound thus" (cap. IV: Jones, IV, 235). "Men do not understand how to observe the invisible through the visible" (cap. XI: Jones, IV, 249).

Thus observation and experience are subordinated to the physician's knowledge of theory. He reasons his way to an understanding of the balance of hot, cold, wet, and dry within the organism and applies the contrary remedy. It is assumed that the mere application of a drug or food of opposed *dynamis* neutralizes the *dynamis* of the humor which is in excess. There is no consideration here of coction or of "crude" or "matured" humors. Even when allusion is made to evacuant medicines, as

> If you were to give a man a medicine which withdraws phlegm, he will vomit you phlegm; if you give him one which withdraws bile, he will vomit you bile. Similarly, too, black bile is purged away if you give a medicine which withdraws black bile.
>
> (*Nature of Man,* cap. V: Jones, IV, 15)

> When the drug enters the body, it first withdraws that constituent of the body which is most akin to itself, and then it draws and purges the other constituents . . . just as things that are sown and grow in the earth, when they enter it, draw each that constituent of the earth which is nearest akin to it.
>
> (*Nature of Man,* cap. VI: Jones, IV, 17)

there is no suggestion that the humors have to undergo any preparation before they are ready for evacuation.

These works discuss how the desired *dynameis* of foods are developed:

> These things therefore the author must know, and further the *dynamis* possessed severally by all the foods and drinks of our regimen, both the *dynamis* each of them possessed by nature and the *dynamis* given them by the constraint of human art. For it is necessary to know both how one ought to lessen the *dynamis* of these when they are strong by nature, and when they are weak to add by art strength to them . . .
>
> (*Regimen I,* cap. II: Jones, IV, 227)

> Freshly cooked meal and flour are drier than those which are stale, because they are nearer the fire with which they were prepared; for as they grow stale the heat exhales and the cold succeeds. Hot bread dries, cold dries less, yesterday's bread somewhat less, and causes a certain amount of leanness.
>
> (*Regimen I,* cap. XLIV: Jones, IV, 315)

> the articles of diet to be used are such as are of a drying nature, of a warming character, assorted and undiluted; wheaten bread is to be preferred to barley cake, and roasted to boiled meats . . . vegetables should be reduced to a minimum, except such as are warming and dry.
>
> (*Regimen III,* cap. LXVIII: Jones, IV, 369-371)

There is some confusion between the evacuant properties of remedies and these assumed *dynameis:* heat, cold, wetness, and dryness:

> barley in its own nature is cold, moist, and drying [sic], but it has *something purgative from the juice of the husks* . . . When it is parched the moist and purgative quality is removed by the fire, and that which is left is cool and dry. When, therefore, it is necessary to cool and

dry, barley meal thus used will do it, no matter how the cake is prepared . . .

(*Regimen I,* cap. XL: Jones, IV, 307)

Water is cooling and moist. Wine is hot and dry, and it has *something purgative from its original substance.* Dark and harsh wines are more dry, and they pass well neither by stool nor by urine, nor by spittle. They dry by reason of their heat, consuming the moisture out of the body . . . the sweet dark wines are moister and weaker; they cause flatulence because they produce moisture.

(*Regimen I,* cap. LII: Jones, IV, 325)

The concept of "something purgative from its original substance" is a survival of the Group I attitude toward medicines—in which they were all viewed as unanalyzable whole entities. The author of *Regimen I* has not succeeded in reducing the purgative effect of barley or wine to an interplay of the hot, the cold, the wet, and the dry and must perforce fall back upon the view that something remains over and above these four *dynameis.*[b]

Other elements of the Group I doctrine are given a different interpretation—reflecting the different assumptions underlying the works of Group III. Crisis, for instance, is analyzed in *Nature of Man* in terms of the amount of bile in the body causing the fever.[208] The use of hot baths and applications is justified in *Breaths* not to promote coction but because "by the heat of the fomentation the wind is rarefied and passes through the body, thus affording some relief of the pains."[209] We have already seen the Group I idea that disease is caused by improper regimen presented in *Breaths* in terms of air entering the organism with the food. In this group, also, physiological explanations are given of the Group I concepts of abscession, empyema, and sediment in the urine:

[b]Galen, in the same way, proposes a category of medicines which cure by their "whole substance." This holistic concept remains in the background, ready to fill in the gaps of Rationalist analysis. See *infra,* p. 314.

> ... [patients who have empyema in the lung] must have been in their youth hard-working, diligent, and industrious; afterwards when delivered from their labors they must have put on soft flesh very different from their former flesh, and there must be a wide difference between the previous condition and the hypertrophied condition of their body, so that there is no longer harmony. Accordingly when a disease seizes men in such a condition, at first they escape, but after the disease the body in time wastes and serous matter flows through the veins wherever it finds the broadest passage ... When the flux is to the chest the patients suffer suppuration, because since the purging is along an upward passage and abides a long time in the chest it rots and turns to pus.
>
> (*Nature of Man,* cap. XII: Jones, IV, 35)

> Patients whose urine contains a deposit of sand or chalk suffer at first from tumours near the thick vein, with suppuration; then, since the tumours do not break quickly, from the pus there grow out pieces of chalk, which are pressed outside through the vein into the bladder with the urine.
>
> (*Nature of Man,* cap. XIV: Jones, IV, 39)

> ... their digestive organs are hard, and the slightest cause inevitably produces in many patients abscesses, the result of a stiff body and hard digestive organs. For their dryness, combined with the coldness of the water, makes them liable to internal lacerations.
>
> (*Airs Waters Places,* cap. IV: Jones, I, 77)

Finally, where Group I employs prognosis, Group III uses diagnosis, as is to be expected from the opposed structures of their medical doctrines (see above, p. 23 and note). If they allude to the idea of forecasting the disease course, these works relegate it to a subordinate role. Thus, *Nature of Man* seems to link such forecasts to knowledge of the external exciting cause:

> Diseases which arise soon after their origin, and whose *prophasis* is clearly known, are those the history of which can be foretold with the greatest certainty. The patient himself must bring about a cure by combating the *prophasis* of the disease, for in this way will be removed that which caused the disease in the body.
>
> (*Nature of Man,* cap. XIII: Jones, IV, 37)

From the author's point of view, both prognosis and exciting causes fall outside the analytical structure of medicine. And in *Regimen I* prognosis is entirely separated from the therapeutic process: "I have discovered [the secret of regimen] as well as the forecasting [*prodiagnosis*] of an illness before the patient falls sick, based upon the direction in which is the excess."[210] Similarly in *Regimen III:* "prognosis before illness and diagnosis of what is the matter with the body, whether food overpowers exercise, whether exercise overpowers food, or whether the two are duly proportioned."[211] *Regimen IV* discusses prognosis from dreams—removing it still further from the therapeutic process.[212]

These physicians thus present an analytical theory of medicine identical to that of the later Rationalist School. Their denial, noted above, that the organism is a unity shows that the Group III doctrine is regarded as an explicit contrast to the therapeutic method of the Group I writers and physicians. "Since then [blood, phlegm, yellow bile, and black bile] are so different from one another in essential form and in *dynamis,* they cannot be one, if fire and water are not one" (*Nature of Man,* cap. V: Jones, IV, 15).[c]

Nature of Man notes, furthermore, that the unitarian view of the organism is held by the majority of the profession: "Most physicians maintain views like these, if not identical with them" (cap. II: Jones, IV, 7). The physicians of Group

[c]This argument seems directed specifically against the position defended by *Ancient Medicine.* See below. p. 70 and note.

III must therefore represent a professional minority bent on reform.

Group IV

The two works, *Ancient Medicine* and *The Art,*[d] the most interesting writings of the whole Hippocratic Corpus, are a reaction to the ideas developed in Group III and a reformulation, in technical philosophical language, of the doctrines and assumptions of Group I.

There are several reasons for supposing that the Group IV authors were aware of, and opposed to, the ideas presented in Group III.

In the first place, they employ the technical and philosophical medical language of Group III—specifically, the words *physis, aition* and *dynamis,* to refute the Group III doctrines.[e]

Even more to the point, however, the author of *Ancient Medicine* forthrightly rejects the new doctrine of contraries:

[d]The word, *tekhne,* is more properly translated "applied science" than "art." But since "applied science" is cumbersome, we have preferred to leave *tekhne* (in most places) untranslated.

[e]Jones notes that the language of cap. XV of *Ancient Medicine* is "strikingly like the terminology of Plato, far too much so to be a mere coincidence." If the Hippocratic work was written before the appearance of Plato's system, this would mean that many of the Platonic terms, and even the doctrine of the Ideas, were "well-known to educated men a generation at least before Plato" (Jones, I, 6).

Jones himself, however, maintains that *Ancient Medicine* must be dated prior to Plato because the word, *sophistes,* is used there (cap. XX) in its "early sense of 'philosopher,' which implies that the writer lived before Plato attached to the word the dishonorable meaning it has in later Greek" (Jones, I, 5). He overlooks the possibility that the author of *Ancient Medicine* might have rejected Plato's redefinition of *sophistes.* We believe that this was, in fact, the case, and support for this view is found in the parallels between the ideas of *Ancient Medicine* and *The Art,* which is clearly written by a Sophist.

Bourgey (*Observation et Experience,* p. 67), calls for a post-Platonic dating on the ground that the word, *philosophia (Ancient Medicine,* cap. XX), was introduced by Plato and used only after Plato.

> But I want to return to the theory of those who prosecute their researches in the *tekhne* after the *novel* fashion, building on a postulate. For if there be such a thing as heat, or cold, or dryness, or moistness, which injures a man, it necessarily follows that the scientific healer will counteract cold with hot, hot with cold, moist with dry, and dry with moist . . . for, according to the theory of the *new* school, if the injury was caused by one of the opposites, the other opposite ought to be a specific.
>
> (*Ancient Medicine,* cap. XIII: Jones, I, 35)

> I am at a loss to understand how those who maintain the other view, and *abandon the old method* to rest the *tekhne* upon a postulate, treat their patients on the lines of their postulate. For they have not discovered, I think, an absolute hot or cold, dry or moist, that participates in no other form. But I think that they have at their disposal the same foods and the same drinks as we all use, and to one they add the attribute of being hot, to another, cold, to another, dry, to another, moist, since it would be futile to order a patient to take something hot, as he would at once ask, "What hot thing?" So that they must either talk nonsense or have recourse to one of these known substances.
>
> (*Ancient Medicine,* cap. XV: Jones, I, 41)[f]

The Art, likewise, attacks certain persons "who have made an art of vilifying the *tekhne's*" and who think that they are thus "making a display of their own knowledge." "The present discussion will oppose those who thus invade the *tekhne* of medicine" (cap. I: Jones, II, 191).

These writers seem clearly to be attacking a medicine based upon philosophy—presumably the Platonic-Aristotelian idealist philosophy which was emerging at this time. They are defending the concept of medicine as a skill learned through

[f]His characterization of the "old" approach as a "method" is not accidental. See above, p. 32; below, pp. 72, 92-93.

practice, a skill which is "not commonly considered a *tekhne* . . . for it is inappropriate to call anyone an artist [i.e., technician] in a craft in which none are laymen, but all possess knowledge through being compelled to use it." (*Ancient Medicine,* cap. IV: Jones, I, 21).

In other words, they are defending the doctrine of the Group I writers—that medicine is founded on the *physis* which operates through coction—against the inroads being made by the philosophers of this new school who promised Rationalist short-cuts to cure and thought in this way to elevate medicine from a craft ("in which none are laymen") to a learned profession.

The writer of *Ancient Medicine* observes that the "ancients" (the Group I authors) first developed the method of making discoveries in medicine through experience, by testing one thing after another and retaining what proved useful (caps. III, XIV: Jones, I, 19, 37). This experience was based on the hypothesis that the body functions as a whole entity which cures itself of disease through coction and evacuation.[g] This is precisely parallel to the Group I view set forth above—that medicine is a skill practiced by craftsmen whose justification lies in its results. *The Art* describes physicians as "craftsmen" or "experienced craftsmen" and states that medicine is shown to be a *tekhne* by experience: it cures and people entrust themselves to it (caps. IV, VIII: Jones, II, 195, 203). This cannot be proved logically but is demonstrated from "the expositions of those versed in the *tekhne,* expositions set forth in acts, not by attention to words" (cap. XIV: Jones, II, 217).

[g]The author of *Ancient Medicine* nowhere states in so many words that the organism must be viewed holistically. This is seen, however, from the whole course of his argument. Furthermore, his question: "If a humor that is sweet assumes another form, not by admixture, but by a self-caused change, what will it first become, bitter or salt, or astringent or acid?" (cap. XXIV: Jones, I, 63) seems to be the view attacked in *Nature of Man* (see above, p. 50), and which, this author asserts, typifies those who assert that "a man is a unity."

The contrast which this author draws between deeds and words is not accidental. For in the Group II and III works one notes an increasing emphasis on the verbal side of medicine, on logical demonstration of the correctness of therapeutic procedures. This is seen, for example, in *Diseases I,* where the writer talks in a surprising way about talking:

> He who would, as regards treatment, interrogate accurately, reply to questions, and contradict appropriately, should note the following: first, whence come all the diseases of men; then, what are the pathological necessities which cause them to be long or short, mortal or not mortal . . . [then] what is done or said conjecturally by the physician to the patient, or by the patient to the physician; what in medicine is done or said precisely, what is right and what is not right; what is end, beginning, middle or any other determination of this sort which is rightly demonstrated to exist there or not to exist . . . that one should think of things which can be done, talk about them, and, if necessary, perform them but about nonfeasible things one should not think, not talk, and one should not perform them . . . These are the points which you should remember and retain faithfully in your discourse; any time the interlocutor makes a mistake in his discourse, his questioning, or his replies—stating that a complicated disease is simple or a serious disease is mild, or if he states the impossible to be possible, or makes any other mistake of this sort—by these notions you will catch him in his reply.
>
> (*Diseases I,* cap. I: VI, 141-143, L.)

The author of *Nature of Man,* in discussing the controversies among philosophers over the nature of the organism, notes that none of them are convincing:

> The fact that, while adopting the same idea, they do not give the same account, shows that their knowledge too is at fault. The best way to realize this is to be present at

> their debates. Given the same debaters and the same audience the same man never wins in the discussion three times in succession, but now one is victor, now another, now he who happens to have the most glib tongue in the face of the crowd. Yet it is right that a man who claims correct knowledge about the facts should maintain his own argument always, if his knowledge be knowledge of reality and if he set it forth correctly.
>
> *(Nature of Man,* cap. I: Jones, IV, 3, 5)[h]

These passages reflect the idea that the criterion of truth is correct discourse rather than correct action. The opposition between Group I and Group III is, *inter alia,* between the view that experience is the criterion of truth and the view that logical consistency is the touchstone.

The Art defends the Group I doctrine, asserting that experience demonstrates medicine to be a *tekhne* and not a matter of mere luck. The proof is in the act: "It is conceded that of those treated by medicine some are healed . . . Again, how is it possible for patients to attribute their recovers to anything else except the *tekhne,* seeing that it was by using it and serving it that they recovered" (cap. IV: Jones, II, 195). Moreover, the *tekhne* is not a body of theory but a series of rules for practice, a method of curing: "I will define what I conceive medicine to be. In general terms it is to do away with the sufferings of the sick, to lessen the violence of their diseases, and to refuse to treat those who are overmastered by their diseases" (cap. III: Jones, II, 193). That the medical *tekhne* exists is proven by the fact that people can observe these procedures: "I do not know how a man could regard as non-existent what he can both see with his eyes and with his mind think that it exists . . . the existent is always seen and known, and the non-existent is neither seen nor known." He is arguing against those who insisted that medicine had to have definitions and a logical structure before it could be

[h]Note the contrast with *RAD I,* cap. IV (Jones, II, 65) quoted above at p. 32.

granted the right to existence as a *tekhne:* "I for my part think that the names also of the *tekhne's* have been given them because of their real essences: for it is absurd—nay impossible—to hold that real essences spring from names. For names are conventions, but real essences are not conventions but the offspring of nature [the *physis*]" (cap. II: Jones, II, 193).[i]

The style of *The Art* indicates that it was by a Sophist.[j] These were practical men, teachers of rhetoric for use in politics and the courts. They were castigated by Plato who wanted to deflect philosophy from this practical goal and make it the province of a leisured class who would use it to explore the nature of thought and of ideas. It is not unlikely that a Sophist wrote this defence of the old method in medicine out of sympathy with the physicians whose practical justification of the validity of their *tekhne* was being contested by a new group; influenced by the same philosophical currents which were opposing the Sophists, these newcomers were maintaining that medicine needed some other justification than mere practical success, specifically,

[i]This sentence could be construed to mean that the *tekhne* of medicine is generated by, and reflects, the working of the *physis.*

[j]The possibility that Akron of Agrigentum wrote *The Art,* while unprovable, is worthy of consideration. This shadowy figure, born about 470 B.C., is mentioned by several ancient authors as a founder of the Empirical School, and he was so regarded by the Empirics themselves.

According to Suidas he exercised the profession of Sophist in Athens (i.e., in the late fifth century when *The Art* was written), examined the question of breaths or air *(pneumata),* and wrote on medicine *(peri iatrikes)* and regimen in health *(peri trophes hygieinon).*

The Art was written by a Sophist, sets forth views identical with those of the Empirical School, and states that the cavities of the body are filled with air *(pneumata)* (cap. X: Jones, II, 207).

The evidence is only circumstantial but is at least an answer to the question why the Empirics regarded Akron as a founder of their school.

His fragments have been collected in Max Wellmann, *Die Fragmente der Sykelischen Aerzte* (Berlin, 1901), pp. 108-109. See, also, Adriana Amerio, "Considerazioni su Acrone Agrigentino," *Medicina nei Secoli* III (1966), Supp. al #4, 33-37.

that it needed to be suffused with metaphysics in order to claim legitimacy as a *tekhne*.

The author of *Ancient Medicine* is combating this same view: that the object of medicine must be analyzed and defined before medicine can be practiced:

> Certain physicians and philosophers assert that nobody can know medicine who is ignorant what man is; he who would treat patients properly must, they say, learn this. But the question they raise is one for philosophy; it is the province of those who, like Empedocles, have written on natural science, what man is from the beginning, how he came into being at the first, and from what elements he was originally constructed. But my view is, first, that all that philosophers or physicians have said or written on natural science no more pertains to medicine than to painting.
>
> (*Ancient Medicine,* cap. XX: Jones, I, 53)

The course which these two writers follow is to give (1) a reasoned justification, and a restatement, of the assumptions and principles of the works of Group I, and (2) a refutation of the new ideas of the philosophically oriented physicians.

The primary assumption of Group I was that the organism cures itself through coction of the *materies morbi.* This is set forth explicitly in *Ancient Medicine* as the theory of cure: "there is in man salt and bitter, sweet and acid, astringent and insipid, and a vast number of other things, possessing *dynameis* of all sorts, both in number and in strength. These, when mixed and compounded with one another, are neither apparent nor do they hurt a man; but when one of them is separated off, and stands alone, then it is apparent and hurts a man" (cap. XIV: Jones, I, 39). This generally happens through a change in the diet (caps. X, XI: Jones, I, 29-33). The sickness disappears when the crude humor is overcome by the body's heat: "pains, burning, and intense inflammation prevail until the discharges are concocted and become thicker, so that rheum is forced from them. This coction is the result of mixture, compounding, and digestion . . . but so long as these bitter particles are undissolved, undigested, and uncompounded, by no possible means can the pains and fevers be stayed . . . No relief from these symptoms is secured until the acidity is purged away, or calmed down and mixed with the other humors" (cap. XIX: Jones, I, 49-51).

Note that the author asserts the humoral components of the organism to be infinite, or, at any rate, "vast," in number.

We have already seen that he specifically attacks the doctrine of contraries. For this is not medicine, and medicine cannot be practiced in this way: "they are most open to censure because they blunder in what is a *tekhne,* and one which all men use on the most important occasions, and give the greatest honors to the good craftsmen and practitioners in it" (cap. I: Jones, I, 13).

The author aims to refute the postulate that the *dynameis* are entities which the physician can manipulate logically, and his argument leads to a fundamental critique of the whole view of the *dynamis* developed in Group III. He contradicts outright the trend of thought exemplified by the statement in *Nature of Man* that "each element has its own *dynamis* and its own nature."[k] The author of *Ancient Medicine* takes the holistic attitude that the humors and their *dynameis* may not be separated. "What I mean is roughly that a *dynamis* is an intensity and strength of the humors."[l]

[k]*Nature of Man,* cap. V (Jones, IV, 15). In this discussion we follow the original and perceptive observations of H. W. Miller, "*Dynamis* and *Physis* in: *On Ancient Medicine,*" *Transactions of the American Philological Association,* 83 (1952), 184-197. See Plamboeck, pp. 74-89.

[l]*Ancient Medicine,* cap. XXII (Jones, I, 57). Miller states that the *dynamis* "is conceived simply as the 'humor' or substance in activity. A 'humor' and a *dynamis* are two aspects of the same simple entity, the one as substantial, the other as active. But it is the *dynamis* which actualizes the 'humor' or substance, and thereby makes known its essential nature" (*ibid.,* p. 194). "In [the author's] empirical conception of *physis,* the concept of *dynamis* is far more basic than that

Thus, the organism does not consist of four elements, each with its own *dynamis,* but of an infinite number of elements, i.e., an infinite number of *dynameis.* "The strongest part of the sweet is the sweetest, of the bitter the most bitter, of the acid the most acid, and each of all the component parts of man has its extreme. For these [the ancients] saw are component parts of man, and that they are injurious to him; for there is in man salt and bitter, sweet and acid, astringent and insipid, and a vast number of other things, possessing *dynameis* of all sorts both in number and in strength" (cap. XIV: Jones, I, 39).

The purpose of this line of thought is to get the physician away from the "fallacy of misplaced concreteness,"[m] of thinking he knows something about the organism when he has given names to its imaginary components, and to direct his attention to the dynamic process of health and disease. Thus the author shows that *"dynamis"* has no meaning aside from its operational significance for the process of healing. He takes up the concepts of cold and heat, the foundation stones of the opposing trend in medicine: "I believe that of all the *dynameis* none hold less sway in the body than cold and heat." The reason is that these in themselves are ephemeral phenomena. "For instance, if a man in health will cool his body in winter, either by a cold bath or in any other way, the more he cools it (provided that his body is not entirely frozen) the more he becomes hotter

of substance, for the simple substances are identified, characterized, and known in essence only through their specific *dynameis.* The author's conception of the interrelationship of *dynamis* and substance is less sophisticated than that implied by the terms 'quality' or 'property.' The primary entities of *physis* are substances which *are dynameis,* substances in their natural 'power' of activity. But the substances are revealed only in their activity, i.e., as *dynameis* . . . It is the *dynamis* alone which makes possible knowledge of the essential nature of the substance" (*ibid.,* p. 192). We would only dispute Miller's view that this approach is "less sophisticated" than the other.

[m]R. Joly calls it *"surdetermination."* (*Le Niveau de la Science Hippocratique* [Paris: Societe d'Edition "Les Belles Lettres," 1966], pp. 36-40).

than before when he puts his clothes on and enters his shelter. Again, if he will make himself thoroughly hot by means of either a hot bath or a large fire, and afterwards wear the same clothes and stay in the same place as he did when chilled, he feels far colder and besides more shivery than before." "So ready is cold to pass into heat and heat into cold . . . What important or serious consequence, therefore, could come from that thing on which quickly supervenes its exact opposite, spontaneously annulling its effect. Or what need has it of elaborate treatment?" (cap. XVI: Jones, I, 43, 45).

Heat and cold have meaning only as clues to the vital processes of which they are the signs. It is the process which is significant, and not the heat or cold which characterizes it. "Men are not feverish merely through heat . . . it could not be the sole cause of the harm; the truth being that one and the same thing is both bitter and hot, or acid and hot, or salt and hot, with numerous other combinations, and cold again combines with other *dynameis.* It is these things which cause the harm. Heat, too, is present, but merely as a concomitant, having the strength of the directing factor which is aggravated and increases with the other factor, but having no *dynamis* greater than that which properly belongs to it" (cap. XVII: Jones, I, 45-47).

He proves his point by discussing the case of a man with a cold. His nose is indeed hot and inflamed. "But in some way the heat of the nostril ceases, not when the discharge takes place and the inflammation is present, but when the running becomes thicker and less acrid, being matured and more mixed than it was before, then it is that the heat finally ceases. But in cases where the evil obviously comes from cold alone, unaccompanied by anything else, there is always the same change, heat following chill and chill heat, and these supervene at once, and need no coction. In all other instances, where acrid and unmixed humors come into play, I am confident that the cause is the same, and that restoration results from coction and mixture" (cap. XVIII: Jones, I, 47).

The author of *Ancient Medicine* has thus reaffirmed the theory of coction and at the same time given a refutation of the new humoralism, of the view set forth in *Nature of Man* that cure can take place in the absence of coction.

He also objects to the new doctrine that medicine consists in the physiological investigation of disease causes. Clearly the cause of disease is going to be very difficult either to determine or to define. The author indicates his bewilderment: "We must surely consider the causes [*aitia*] of each complaint to be those things the presence of which of necessity produces such and such a complaint, which ceases when they change into another combination . . . For what shall we call it? Combinations of [things] that exhibit a *dynamis* that varies with the various factors?"[n]

The author considers the whole concept of the internal (proximate) cause to be so problematical that medicine may not be based on it. "All who . . . narrow down the causal principle of diseases and of death among men and make it the same in all cases, postulating one thing or two, all these obviously blunder in many points even of their statements" (cap. I: Jones, I, 13). One reason is that such causal speculation can never be demonstrated one way or the other: "If a man were to learn and declare the state of these, neither to the speaker himself nor to his audience would it be clear

[n]*Ancient Medicine,* cap. XIX (Jones, I, 49, 51). The second part of this quotation is about half a page removed from the first part, and is situated in the middle of another discussion. The editor realizes that it is either in the wrong place or an interpolation (Jones, I, 50, 51). The problem is to determine the antecedent of "it" (*auto*). Jones leaves the question open after noting that it cannot mean either "health" or "disease." In his later translation of *Ancient Medicine* he again tackles this problem, deciding that *auto* refers to the whole preceding discussion of coction ("Philosophy and Medicine in Ancient Greece," *Bulletin of the History of Medicine* [Baltimore, 1946], p. 83). This is not acceptable, however, since coction cannot be defined as "combinations of [things] that exhibit a *dynamis* that varies with the various factors." "It" *(auto)* can only refer to *aition* (Jones I, 48, line 18). The sentence is a perfect definition of *aition* from the viewpoint of the author of *Ancient Medicine* and makes clear the opposition between his own philosophy and that of Group III.

whether his statements were true or not. For there is no test the application of which would give certainty" (cap. I: Jones, I, 15).

Another reason is that people's *physies*° differ greatly, and the assumption of a limited number of possible causes does violence to the facts: "There are many . . . structural forms, both internal and external, which differ widely from one another with regard to the experiences of a patient and of a healthy subject, such as whether the head be large or small, the neck thin or thick, long or short, the bowels long or round, the chest and ribs broad or narrow, and there are very many other things, the differences between which must all be known, so that knowledge of the causes [*aitia*] of each thing may ensure that the proper precautions are taken" (cap. XXIII: Jones, I, 61). "Cheese does not harm all men alike; some can eat their fill of it without the slightest hurt, nay, those it agrees with are wonderfully strengthened thereby. Others come off badly. So the *physies* of these men differ, and the difference lies in the constituent of the body which is hostile to cheese, and is roused and stirred to action under its influence. Those in whom a humor of such a kind is present in greater quantity, and with greater control over the body, naturally suffer more severely. But if cheese were bad for the human *physis* without exception, it would have hurt all" (cap. XX: Jones, I, 55).

Medicine is, therefore, not to be based upon *a priori* knowledge of causes. The practice is not based upon theory; the theory arises out of the practice. Knowledge in medicine is not the basis, but the outcome, of practice. "I also hold that clear knowledge of the *physies* can be acquired from medicine and from no other source, and that one can attain this knowledge when medicine itself has been properly comprehended, but till then it is quite impossible—I mean, to possess this information, what man is, by what causes [*aitias*]

°Plural of *physis*.

he is made, and similar points accurately" (cap. XX: Jones, I, 53).

This is a refutation of the view in *Nature of Man* that *a priori* knowledge of the *physis* is possible, since the latter consists of nothing more than four humors. *Ancient Medicine* asserts that the physician can acquire such knowledge not directly, but indirectly—in the practice of medicine.

Hence the physician cannot claim arcane knowledge of physiological processes. This raises a problem since he may want to have some conception of these internal matters, many diseases being concealed from observation. "Some, but only a few diseases, have a seat where they can be seen; others, and they are many, have a seat where they cannot be perceived . . . These are those which are determined to the bones or to the cavities. The body has of these not one but several. There are two that take in food and discharge it, with several others besides these, known to men who are interested in these things . . ." (*The Art,* caps. IX, X; Jones, II, 207). "While some diseases arise from *dynameis,* others arise from structures [*skhemata*]. 'Structures' are the conformations to be found in the human body, some of which are hollow, tapering from wide to narrow; some are expanded, some hard and round, some broad and suspended, some stretched, some long, some close in texture, some loose in texture and fleshy, some spongy and porous" *(Ancient Medicine,* cap, XXII: Jones, I, 57).

These authors endeavor to provide a solution to this problem. In Group I the issue of the organism's physiological mechanisms is not even raised, but Group IV must face up to it because Group III has given an incorrect analysis of the procedure for comprehending the organism's physiological processes. The authors of *Ancient Medicine* and *The Art* give precisely the answer one would expect—the only legitimate knowledge of these processes is that which may be inferred from external signs or from direct analogy with the exterior.

The Art contrasts "open" and "hidden" diseases. "Those

that can be perceived produce eruptions on the skin, or manifest themselves by color or swelling; for they allow us to perceive by sight or touch their hardness, moistness, heat, or cold [and thus] what are the conditions which, by their presence or absence in each case, cause the diseases to be of the nature they are. Of all such diseases in all cases the cures should be infallible, not because they are easy but because they have been discovered . . . Now such being its nature, the *tekhne* must be a match for the open diseases" (caps. IX, X: Jones, II, 207).

The same procedure is advocated for the hidden diseases, those "which are determined to the bones or to the cavities." "Without doubt no man who sees only with his eyes can know anything of what has here been described. It is for this reason that I have called them obscure, even as they have been judged to be by the *tekhne.* Their obscurity, however, does not mean that they are our masters, but as far as is possible they have been mastered, a possibility limited only by the capacity of the sick to be examined and of researchers to conduct research. More pains, in fact, and quite as much time, are required to know them *as if they were seen with the eyes:* for what escapes the *eyesight* is mastered by the *eye* of the mind, and the sufferings of patients due to their not being quickly *observed* are the fault, not of the medical attendants, but of the *physis* of the patient and of the disease. The attendant, in fact, as he could neither *see* the trouble with his eyes nor learn it with his ears, tried to track it by reasoning [*logismos*] . . . For the delay thus caused not the *tekhne* is to blame, but the *physis* of the human body. For it is only when the *tekhne sees* its way that it thinks it right to give treatment, considering how it may give it, not by daring but by judgment, not by violence but by gentleness. As to our human constitution, if it admits of being *seen* it will also admit of being healed" (cap. XI: Jones, II, 209-211). "Now medicine, being prevented, in cases of empyema and of diseased liver, kidneys, and the cavities generally, from *seeing* with the *sight,* with which all men *see* everything most perfectly, has nevertheless discovered other means to help it. There is clearness or roughness of the voice, rapidity or slowness of respiration, and for the customary discharges, the ways through which they severally pass, sometimes smell, sometimes color, sometimes thinness or thickness furnishing medicine with the means of inferring what condition these symptoms indicate, what symptoms mean that a part is already affected, and what that a part may hereafter be affected. When this information is not afforded, and the *physis* herself will yield nothing of her own accord, medicine has found means of compulsion, whereby the *physis* is constrained, without being harmed, to give up her secrets; when these are given up she *makes clear,* to those who know the *tekhne,* what course ought to be pursued. The *tekhne,* for example, forces the *physis* to disperse phlegm by acrid foods and drinks, so that it may form a conclusion *by vision* concerning those things which were invisible before. Again, when respiration is symptomatic, by uphill roads and by running, it compels the *physis* to *reveal* symptoms. It brings on sweats by the means already stated, and forms the conclusions that are formed through fire when it makes hot water give out steam. There are also certain excretions through the bladder which indicate the disease better than those which come through the flesh . . . Now as the relation between secretions and the information they give is variable, and depends on a variety of conditions, it is accordingly not surprising that disbelief in this information is prolonged [and] treatment is curtailed, for extraneous factors must be used in interpreting the information before it can be used by medical intelligence" (cap. XIII: Jones, II, 213-217).[p]

This remarkable passage is a restatement of the fundamental assumption of the works of Group I—that the physician ascertains the internal processes of the organism

[p]Note the emphasis on *visibility.*

from his observation of visible symptoms. Some of these symptoms are presented spontaneously, and some have to be elicited by the physician. This information is tedious and difficult to acquire; philosophical short-cuts and instantaneous diagnosis are not allowed. Furthermore, the symptoms are not self-interpreting but must be understood in the light of a preexisting body of doctrine concerning the nature of disease and health ("extraneous factors"). The newer school of physicians lack interest in this technique and patience to pursue it ("disbelief in this information is prolonged").

Of particular interest is the author's treatment of the relationship between sense-perception and reasoning (*logismos*). The problem of comprehending the inner workings of the organism is solved by making them visible to sight. *Logismos* must thus be based upon visibles. The contrast with the treatment of the same issue in *Breaths* and *Regimen I* could hardly be greater: in these works sense-perception is made dependent upon *logismos* ("[wind] is invisible to sight though visible to *logismos*," "[men] trust eyes rather than mind, though these are not competent to judge even things that are seen").[q]

Thus, where *Breaths* and *Regimen I* subordinate sense-perception to *logismos, The Art* subordinates *logismos* to sense-perception.

The problem of extrapolating from the visible is also discussed in *Ancient Medicine.* Having noted that some diseases arise from "structures," the author admits that knowledge of what occurs in the corporal structures may be obtained by reasoning from analogy with structures of the same shape outside the body. "Now which structure is best adapted to draw and attract to itself fluid from the rest of the body, the hollow and expanded, the hard and round, or the hollow and tapering? I take it that the best adapted is the broad hollow that tapers. One should learn this thoroughly

[q]See above, pp. 62-63.

from *unconcealed* objects that can be *seen.* For example, if you open the mouth wide, you will draw in no fluid; but if you protrude and contract it, compressing the lips, and then insert a tube, you can easily draw up any liquid you wish . . . Of the parts within the human frame, the bladder, the head, and the womb are of this structure. These obviously attract powerfully and are always full of a fluid from without" (cap. XXII: Jones, I, 57). "If a man can in this way conduct with success inquiries outside the human body, he will always be able to select the very best treatment" (cap. XXIV: Jones, I, 63). As in *The Art,* stress is placed upon perception of the visible.

These two authors then turn to the problem of how to ascertain the curative powers of foods and medicines, and how to match them to the patient's disease.

They accept the Group I view that the fundamental curative process is coction and evacuation: "coction is the result of mixture, compounding, and digestion" (*Ancient Medicine,* cap. XIX: Jones, I, 49); "restoration results from coction and mixture" (cap. XVIII: Jones, I, 49); "a man is in the best possible condition when there is complete coction and rest, with no particular *dynamis* displayed" (cap. XIX: Jones, I, 53).

The types of treatment employed resemble those in the Group I works: "purgation . . . spontaneous or by medicine" (cap. XIX: Jones, I, 51); adjustment of the diet (caps. III, V, *et passim:* Jones, I, 17, 19, 21, 23, etc.): "fasting . . . abundant diet . . . excess of drink . . . abstinence therefrom . . . bathing . . . refraining therefrom . . . violent exercise . . . rest . . . keeping awake . . . or a combination of all these things" *(The Art,* cap. V: Jones, II, 197); "medicines purgative or astringent . . . regimen and other substances . . . drugs" (cap. VI: Jones, II, 199).

Mention is made of treatment by similars: "medicine has also discovered foods and drinks of such a kind that, becoming warmer than the natural heat, melt the matters I spoke of and make them flow away" (cap. XIII: Jones, II, 217).

The physician confronted with a new patient decides what treatment to adopt on the basis of his prior experience:

> The physician sets about his task with healthy mind and healthy body, having considered the case and past cases of like characteristics to the present, so as to say how they were treated and cured.
>
> (*The Art,* cap. VII: Jones, II, 201)

The author of *Ancient Medicine,* furthermore, makes it clear that, in the absence of previous experience, the physician can only experiment. Attacking the view that the medicinal properties of substances can be deduced logically from their sensory ones, in chapters VI to XVI he discusses the discovery of the appropriate diet for the healthy person and for the sick and comes to the conclusion that the two processes are identical: "What difference then can be seen between the purpose of him we call physician, who is an acknowledged handicraftsman [*kheirotekhnes*], the discoverer of the mode of life and of the nourishment suitable for the sick, and his who discovered and prepared originally nourishment for all men, which we now use, instead of the old savage and brutish mode of living? My own view is that their reasoning was identical and the discovery one and the same. The one sought to do away with those things which, when taken, the *physis* of man in health could not assimilate because of their brutish and uncompounded character, the other those things which the temporary condition of an individual prevented him from assimilating" (cap. VII: Jones, I, 25).[r] And this method was trial and error: "those who sought for and discovered medicine . . . I think, lessened the bulk of the foods, and, without altering their character, greatly diminished their

[r]As we have stated above (p. 11, note) the idea that humors are concocted by the organism is taken from cooking—indicating the close parallel between cooking and the Group I therapeutic theory.

quantity. But they found that this treatment was sufficient only occasionally, and although clearly beneficial with some patients, it was not so in all cases, as some were in such a condition that they could not assimilate even small quantities of food. As such patients were thought to need weaker nutriment, slops were invented by mixing with much water small quantities of strong foods, and by taking away from their strength by compounding and boiling. Those that were not able to assimilate them were refused even these slops, and were reduced to taking liquids, these moreover being so regulated in composition and quantity as to be moderate, and nothing was administered that was either more or less compounded than it ought to be" (cap. V: Jones, I, 21-23). "For it is necessary to aim at some measure. But no measure, neither number nor weight, by reference to which knowledge can be made exact, can be found except bodily [perception]" (cap. IX: Jones, I, 27).[s]

The reason for this is that no two substances are identical. Every medicine and every article of regimen is a specific, and the physician who arranges them into categories on the basis of some fancied quality is over-simplifying:

> Of course I know also that it makes a difference to a man's body whether bread be of bolted or of unbolted flour, whether it be of winnowed or of unwinnowed wheat, whether it be kneaded with much water or with little, whether it be thoroughly kneaded or unkneaded, whether it be thoroughly baked or unbaked, and there are countless other differences. Barley-cake varies in just the same way. The *dynameis,* too, of each variety are powerful, and no one is like to any other.
>
> (*Ancient Medicine,* cap. XIV: Jones, I, 37)

"For the trouble caused by each of these things is also peculiar to each, and so with surfeit or such and such food" (cap. XXI: Jones, I, 57). But the newer physicians ignore this

[s]Jones translates *aisthesis* as "feeling."

fact. "How could he who has not considered these truths, or who considers them without learning, know anything about human ailments?" "For each of these differences produces in a human being an effect and a change of one sort or another, and upon these differences is based all the dieting of a man, whether he be in health, recovering from an illness, or suffering from one. Accordingly, there could surely be nothing more useful or more necessary to know than these things, and how the first discoverers, pursuing their inquiries excellently and with suitable application of reason to the *physis* of man, made their discoveries. . . . For they did not consider that the dry or the moist or the hot or the cold or anything else of the kind injures a man or that he has need of any such thing, but they considered that it is the strength of each thing, that which, being too powerful for the *physis* of man, it cannot assimilate, that causes harm, and this they sought to take away" (cap. XIV: Jones, I, 37).

The author resorts to an analogy with coction to explain why some foods are beneficial to the organism and others harmful. He states:

> . . . of the foods that are unsuitable for us and hurt a man when taken, each one of them is either bitter or salt, or acid, or something else uncompounded and strong, and for this reason we are disordered by them, *just as we are by the secretions separated off in the body*.But all things that a man eats or drinks are plainly altogether free from such an uncompounded and potent humor, e.g., bread, cake, and suchlike, which men are accustomed constantly to use in great quantity, except the highly seasoned delicacies which gratify his appetite and greed. And from such foods, when plentifully partaken of by a man, there arises no disorder at all or isolation of the *dynameis* resident in the body, but strength, growth, and nourishment in great measure arise from them, for no other reason except that they are well compounded and have

nothing undiluted and strong, but form a single, simple whole.

(*Ancient Medicine,* cap. XIV: Jones, I, 39)

In other words, foods which are strong and uncompounded have to be prepared (concocted) beforehand by the cook. If they were introduced into the body in their crude state, the body would have to concoct them, and this might be beyond its power.[t]

The use of "whole" in the above passage reveals the author's view that medicines must be taken as unanalyzable whole entities. It may also be seen as symbolizing his holistic orientation generally.

A final element of the Group I doctrine mentioned in Group IV is prognosis: "medicine, because its results may be forecasted, has reality, as is manifest now and will be manifest forever" (*The Art,* cap. VI: Jones, II, 201; see *ibid.,* caps. VII and XIII).

Thus these two works are an attack on hypostatized humors as proximate causes of disease, and they restate the Group I therapeutic doctrine of cure through coction and evacuation. Cure through "contraries" is rejected in favor of a therapeutic procedure designed to assist the body's natural curative power.

Scientific Method in the Hippocratic Corpus

The preceding analysis makes it clear that the contrast within the Hippocratic Corpus is not the one usually alleged—between the schools of Cos and Cnidos—but rather between Groups I and IV on the one hand, and Group III on the other. Group II (the Cnidian works) is an eclectic mixture of elements found in Groups I and III.

This is the first historically recorded conflict between the two medical ideologies which we have called Rationalist and

[t]The parallel may be drawn here with Paracelsus' definition of alchemy as an "external bowel," meaning that the alchemist concocts medicines for use by the organism. See *infra,* p. 430.

Empirical. It is identical with the later conflict between the Rationalist and Empirical Schools, and not surprisingly, since this conflict is rooted precisely in the division of the Hippocratic tradition.

The writings of Groups I and IV present the following doctrine: the organism is viewed as an unanalyzable whole which copes with morbific stimuli through a process of coction and evacuation; symptoms are significant for what they tell about this process; the physician must rely entirely upon sensory data in reaching conclusions about the processes of disease and health; while he takes into account the impact of environmental (exciting) causes, he is barred from knowledge of internal (proximate) causes; medical knowledge and therapeutic procedures arise out of experience in the sense that any therapeutic technique is proved correct only by its outcome; the reliability of medical knowledge may be tested only by the results of therapy; the aim of therapy is to assist the organism to combat the disease along the lines already selected by the organism; the medicines and techniques employed to this end may be described as operating on the basis of "similarity" in that they stimulate the organism to continue along the path which it has already chosen.

The doctrine presented in Group III has the following form: the internal processes of the body are knowable *a priori;* the functioning of the organism as well as its relations with the environment are analyzable in terms of chains of causes passing from the external exciting causes to the internal (proximate) causes and ultimately to the symptoms; medical doctrine is a body of logically coherent theory reflecting the essentially logical structure of the human organism; the aim of medical diagnosis is to discover the disease "cause," and the aim of therapeutics is to counteract or oppose this cause by the appropriate "contrary" medicine; the emphasis on "contrariety" leads to an interpretation of symptoms as harmful, morbific, phenomena.

This latter doctrine reduces the organism to its components and thereby reduces the importance of the organism's inherent reactive power. The former view is premised upon the existence of precisely such a spontaneous force within the organism.

In terms of the idiographic-nomothetic polarity posited in the Introduction, Groups I and IV emphasize the variety of the phenomena, while Group III stresses the supposed underlying structure of reality. The best example of the opposition between these two viewpoints is the contrast between the assertion in *Ancient Medicine* that the organism consists of an indefinite number of humoral elements and that in *Nature of Man* that it consists of four humors only.

In our opinion the true Hippocratic doctrine is presented in Groups I and IV, the reason being that the medical doctrine of these writings is a scientific approach to therapeutics. It is an embryonic formulation of scientific method, and that is why it is valid for all time. That is why it has been a perennial source of inspiration for physicians.

The doctrine of the Group III writings shows the impact of idealist philosophy on medical thought. It is not a scientific approach to medicine or to the investigation of the organism.

The conflict between the two approaches is related to the changing social status of the physician in Greece during this period.[213]

The theory of coction underlying the Group I writings is the therapeutic doctrine of physicians who are not differentiated from craftsmen (*kheirotekhnes*) and whose sense-based knowledge is not qualitatively different from that of laymen. The theory of contraries, on the other hand, is the doctrine of physicians who are aspiring for a better social status than that of craftsmen (i.e., laymen) and who thus claim to base medical practice on hidden (proximate) causes.

If we attempt to analyze the relevance of the two approaches to what is now regarded as scientific method we will find August Comte's hypothesis of the three stages of the history of the mind to be very useful. Comte states that man initially interpreted phenomena in terms of divine causation, then replaced divine by metaphysical causes, and finally—in the "positivist" stage—has abandoned the search for causes and concentrates on formulating rules governing the succession of the observed phenomena. In the theological stage the mind seeks the "intimate nature" of things, their first and final causes. The second, metaphysical, stage is only a modification of the first: supernatural agencies are replaced by abstract objectified forces viewed as capable of engineering the observed phenomena. In the "positivist" stage the mind recognizes the impossibility of obtaining absolute notions and hence "renounces the search for the origin and destination of the universe, also knowledge of the intimate causes of phenomena, attempting solely to discover, by a proper combination of reasoning and observation, their effective laws, that is, their invariable relations of succession and similarity. Explanation of the facts, if we reduce it to its actual terms, is henceforth nothing more than a link established between the various particular phenomena and certain general facts whose number is gradually reduced by the progress of science."[214]

If this perceptive generalization is applied to our analysis of the Hippocratic Corpus, it will immediately be seen that the doctrine of Group III is Comte's second, metaphysical, stage of the mind.[u] The approach outlined in Groups I and IV is identical with the "positivist" last stage of the mind—characterized by the effort to establish the "invariable relations of succession and similarity" among the phenomena.

[u]*Sacred Disease* is a perfect example of the replacement of divine causation by metaphysical causation—the hypothetical presence of air in the veins. The importance of this passage for the origin of scientific medicine has been greatly overemphasized (see, for example, M. Pohlenz, *Hippokrates und die Begruendung der wissenschaftlichen Medizin* [Berlin, 1938], p. 85.)

The doctrine set forth in Group III corresponds to the view that "science" is knowledge of causes. This view was widespread in the nineteenth century, and at that time these works of the Hippocratic Corpus were viewed as the truly scientific ones. More recently, however, "science" has been regarded as a search, not for causes, but for the general laws governing natural phenomena, and in the light of this conception of scientific method the works of Groups I and IV are seen to be the truly scientific works of the Hippocratic Corpus.

Contemporary discussions of scientific method have departed from the former emphasis on induction of general rules from the consideration of individual "facts" and stress the elaboration of hypotheses and their verification or rejection through experiment.[215] And in this respect the works of Groups I and IV are completely scientific, since they base investigation upon a hypothesis: that the organism is a vital entity interacting with its environment. In this system practicing medicine is equivalent to engaging in scientific research, since it is investigation of the organism under the guidance of a hypothesis. As the author of *Ancient Medicine* states: "clear knowledge of the *physies* can be acquired from medicine and from no other source."

This writer of genius claims to base "knowledge" on a defined method–in the strongest possible contrast to the doctrine of Group III that therapeutic method is based upon *a priori* knowledge of reality. The viewpoint expressed in *Ancient Medicine* has a startlingly modern look. A contemporary philosopher of science writes: "it is the methodology of science that defines physical reality."[216]

Thus *The Art* and *Ancient Medicine* emphasize the discovery of new knowledge. The practice of medicine is a "method of inquiry," a method of discovery (*Ancient Medicine,* cap. XII: Jones I, 33). "Medicine has long had all its means to hand, and has discovered both a principle and a method, through which the discoveries made during a long period are many and excellent, while full discovery will be made, if the inquirer be competent, conduct his researches with knowledge of the discoveries already made, and make them his starting point" (cap. II: Jones, I, 15). "To this discovery and research what juster or more appropriate name could be given than medicine?" (cap. III: Jones, I, 21). "Even at the present day those who study gymnastics and athletic exercises are constantly making some fresh discovery by investigating on the same method" (cap. IV: Jones, I, 21). "All this goes to prove that this *tekhne* of medicine, if research be continued on the same method, can all be discovered" (cap. VIII: Jones, I, 27). "To discover what was unknown before, when the discovery of it is better than a state of ignorance, is the ambition and task of intelligence" (*The Art,* cap. I: Jones, II, 191).

Here again the contrast with Group III is very great. In the latter works medicine is not considered to be a technique for making discoveries. Their authors feel that the essential has already been discovered, that (as in *Nature of Man*) the *physis* has been subjected to a thoroughgoing philosophical or scientific analysis. To these physicians the major criterion is logical consistency, not success in practice. This attitude, which will be encountered below in the philosophy of Aristotle, is the opposite of scientific method. It is not a method of investigation at all but a method of philosophical controversy, and as such it is the opposite of the method proposed in Groups I and IV. These are the philosophical physicians castigated by the author of *The Art:* "who have made an art of vilifying the *tekhne's* . . . [and] are making a display of their own knowledge . . . to be eager to bring shame through the art of abuse upon the *discoveries* of others, improving nothing, but disparaging, before those who do not know, the *discoveries* of those who do, seems to me to be not the ambition and work of intelligence, but the sign of a hasty nature or of want of *tekhne* . . . to indulge their malevolence by disparaging what is right in their neighbors' works and by cavilling at what is amiss."[217]

NOTES

[1] Some of the most recent efforts have been: Werner Jaeger, *Paideia: The Ideals of Greek Culture* (Oxford, 1939), Vol. III, Chapter I: Greek Medicine as Paideia; L. Bourgey, *Observation et Experience chez les Medecins de la Collection Hippocratique* (Paris, 1953), which is an expansion of Jaeger's cursory outline; Josef-Hans Kuehn, *System und Methodenprobleme im Corpus Hippocraticum* (Wiesbaden, 1956). Good introductions to the study of the Hippocratic Corpus are L. Edelstein's article "Hippokrates," in *Pauly-Wissowa,* Supplementband VI (1935), Col. 1290-1345 and his "The Genuine Works of Hippocrates," *Bulletin of the History of Medicine* VII (1939), 236-248.

[2] The sources used for the Hippocratic writings are: *Oeuvres Completes d' Hippocrate,* trans. E. Littre, 10 vols. (Paris, 1839-1861); *Hippocrates,* trans. W.H.S. Jones, 4 vols. (Loeb Classical Library); John Chadwick and W. N. Mann, *The Medical Works of Hippocrates* (Springfield, 1950).

All references below to the Littre edition of Hippocrates are in the standard form, e.g., VII, 179, L. The Jones edition will be cited as, e.g., Jones, II, 34.

The works covered by the ensuing analysis are: *Prorrhetic I* (dated at 440 B.C. in Jones, II, xxix); *Coan Prognosis* (dated at 410 in Jones, II, xxix); *Prognosis* (dated at 415 in Jones, II, xxix and at 410 in Bengt Alexanderson, *Die Hippokratische Schrift Prognostikon* [Stockholm, 1963], p. 23); *The Sacred Disease* (dated at 420-410 in Jones, II, 134 and in Albin Lesky, *A History of Greek Literature* [London, 1966], p. 490); *Regimen in Acute Diseases* (not dated but viewed as "genuine" by Jones, II, 59; dated at about 390 in I. M. Lonie, "The Hippocratic Treatise Peri diaites okseon," *Sudhoffs Archiv,* Bd. 49, H. 1 [March, 1965], 50-79, at p. 79); *Aphorisms* (dated at 415 in Jones, II, xxviii-xxix); *Airs Waters Places* (dated at "before 430" in Lesky, p. 490); *Nature of Man* (dated at 400 in Lesky, p. 491, and at 440-400 in Jones, IV, xxvii); *Regimen in Health* (dated at 400 in Lesky, p. 491, and at 440-400 in Jones, IV, xxvii); the *Appendix to Regimen in Acute Diseases* (dated at about 390 in Lonie, "The Hippocratic Treatise Peri diaites okseon," p. 79); *Ancient Medicine* (dated at 430-400 in Lesky, p. 489; at 430-420 in Jones, I, 5; at "before 400" in L. Bourgey, *Observation et Experience chez les Medecins de la Collection Hippocratique,* p. 36); *Breaths* (dated at the end of the fifth century in Jones, II, 221); *The Art* (dated at the end of the fifth century in Jones, II, 188); *Epidemics I* and *III* (dated at about 410 in Lesky, p. 490, at 410 in Alexanderson, p. 23, and at "before 400" in Bourgey, p. 36); *Regimen I-IV* (dated at "400 or later" in Jones, IV, xlvi, and at 400 in Robert Joly, *Recherches sur le traite pseudo-Hippocratique du Regime* [Paris, 1960], p. 209. Joly, however, notes that other writers date it much later); *Affections, Diseases I-III,* and *Internal Diseases* (no attempt has been made to date these works in either of the two authoritative discussions of them: J. Ilberg, "Die Aerzteschule von Knidos," *Berichte ueber die Verhandlungen d. Saechs. Akad. d. Wiss.,* LXXVI, No. 3 [1924] and I. M. Lonie, "The Cnidian Treatises of the Corpus Hippocraticum," *Classical Quarterly,* N.S. XV, No. 1, [1965], 1-30).

Our analysis does not include several works ascribed to this early period of the Corpus, although they are referred to occasionally below. These are the surgical works: *On Fractures-On Joints, Mochlicon, Wounds of the Head,* and *In the Surgery;* they have not been considered because they do not contain a systematic discussion of the therapeutic ideas with which this study is concerned.

Other works not included in the analysis are *Epidemics II, IV,* and *VI* (dated at 399-395 in Lesky, p. 490 and at the early fourth century in Bourgey, p. 38); *Epidemics V and VII* (dated at the early fourth century in Bourgey, p. 38, and at about 350 in Lesky, p. 490); *Diseases IV* (not dated in Ilberg, *op. cit.*); and *The Places in Man* (dated at about 350 in K. Schubring, "Zu Aufbau und Lehre der hippokratischen Schrift De Locis in Homine," *Berl. Med.* [1964], XV, 739-744, at p. 744).

In the discussion below the translation of *Coan Prognosis* is that of Chadwick and Mann; the translations of the *Appendix to Regimen in Acute Diseases, Affections, Diseases I-III,* and *Internal Diseases* are from Littre, *Oeuvres Completes d'Hippocrate;* all others are from the Loeb edition of the Hippocratic writings.

[3] L. Bourgey, *Observation et Experience chez les Medecins de la Collection Hippocratique,* p. 36, note 1, discusses the parallels among *Prognosis, Epidemics I* and *III, On Fractures—On Joints,* and *Regimen in Acute Diseases.* In this he follows Karl Deichgraeber, *Die Epidemien und das Corpus Hippocraticum* (Berlin, 1933), pp. 17-21, 94. Bengt Alexanderson, *Die Hippokratische Schrift Prognostikon* (Stockholm, 1963), pp. 22-23, maintains that *Prognosis* and *Epidemics I* and *III* cannot be by the same writer, since their doctrines of critical days differ. Another scholar, W. C. Wake, on the basis of a statistical study of word frequencies and sentence lengths (unpublished Ph.D. dissertation, London University, summarized recently in *The Listener,* LXXVI [1966] 966-968) states "*Prognostic, Regimen in Acute Diseases, Fractures and Joints* could all have been written by one author (which does not, of course, say that they were) but . . . *Epidemics I* and *III* could not have been written by the same author as the others. The evidence is objective and decisive; if *Prognostic* is by Hippocrates, the *Epidemics* is not."

[4] For example, black bile (*Coan Prognosis,* II: 68: Chadwick and Mann, p. 223), bile and phlegm (*Coan Prognosis,* XXXII: Chadwick and Mann, p. 268), phlegm (*Epidemics III,* Case III of First Series: Jones, I, 227), blood considered as a humor (*Epidemics I,* Third Constitution, cap. XV: Jones, I, 169), bile (*Epidemics I,* Second Constitution, cap. V: Jones, I, 155). Bile and phlegm are by far the most frequently mentioned humors, with blood a poor third. Black bile is mentioned comparatively rarely (*Regimen in Acute Diseases,* cap. LXI: Jones, II, 117; *Epidemics III,* Constitution, cap. XIV: Jones, I, 255; *Aphorisms,* IV: 9, 22-24: Jones, IV, 137, 139, 141).

[5] In *Epidemics III,* Constitution, cap. XIV, there is a famous passage which some have taken to be the first reference in Greek literature to the four-humor doctrine (e.g., Deichgraeber, *Die Epidemien und das Corpus Hippocraticum,* p. 13). The most recent commentator on Greek humoralism, however, denies that this is so, since, although four temperaments are mentioned—bilious, phlegmatic, melancholic, and sanguine—the sanguine temperament is assimilated to the melancholic (Erich Schoener, "Das Viererschema in der antiken Humoral-

pathologie," *Arch. Gesch. Med.* Suppl. 4, [1964], p. 49). The passage in question reads: "as to those with a melancholic or a rather sanguine complexion" (Jones, I, 255). Schoener's treatise presents a very thorough analysis of Hippocratic humoralism.

[6] *Epidemics III,* Constitution, cap. XIII (Jones, I, 253); *RAD I,* cap. LXI (Jones, II, 117).

[7] *Epidemics III,* First Series, Case III (Jones, I, 223).

[8] *Coan Prognosis,* II: 39; XX: 384; XXI; 436; XXIV: 571, 587 (Chadwick and Mann, pp. 221, 251, 257, 271, 273); *Epidemics I,* Second Constitution, cap. V, XI, Cases I, II, V, VII, IX, XIII (Jones, I, 155, 165, 187, 189, 195, 199, 203, 209); *Epidemics III,* Constitution, cap. X, First Series, Cases I, II, III, IX (Jones, I, 251, 219, 221, 223, 233); *Aphorisms,* I: 22 and VII: 6, 23, 69 (Jones, IV, 109, 195, 197, 211).

[9] On ripening, coction, and crisis or critical days see *Coan Prognosis,* I: 15, 24, 28; II: 38, 39, 74, 79, 80; III: 142, 143, 144, 146, 148; VIII: 213; XX: 373, 374, 377 (Chadwick and Mann, pp. 220, 221, 224, 229, 236, 250); *RAD I,* cap. XLII (Jones, II, 99); *Prognosis,* cap. XX (Jones, II, 43); *Epidemics I,* Third Constitution, cap. XXVI (Jones, I, 185); *Aphorisms,* I: 12, 19, 20, 22; II: 40; III: 8, 28 (Jones, IV, 105, 107, 109, 119, 125, 133).

[10] *Epidemics I* and *III passim.*

[11] *Prognosis,* cap. XIV (Jones, II, 29); *Aphorisms,* IV: 47 (Jones, IV, 147).

[12] *Epidemics I,* Cases I, III, IV, V, VIII, X, XI, XII, XIV (Jones, I, 187, 191, 193, 199, 201, 203, 205, 207, 211); *Coan Prognosis,* XXXIV: 564-588, VI: 194 (Chadwick and Mann, pp. 270-273, 234). Contra: *Epidemics I,* Cases II and VII (Jones, I, 189, 199). See also *Prognosis,* cap. XII (Jones, II, 25ff); *Aphorisms,* IV: 69-75; VII: 31-36 (Jones, IV, 153, 155, 199, 201).

[13] *Aphorisms,* IV: 36-38, 41, 42; V: 36; VII: 85 (Jones, IV, 145, 147, 167, 217).

[14] On empyema and abscession see *Coan Prognosis,* II: 112, 135; III: 137, 139, 141; IV: 156; XIX: 359, 370; XX: 384 (Chadwick and Mann, pp. 226, 228, 229, 230, 248, 249, 251); *Prognosis,* cap. XIV, XXIV (Jones, II, 29, 49); *Epidemics I,* Second Constitution, cap. VIII (Jones, I, 159); *Epidemics III,* Constitution, cap. XII, Second Series, Case II (Jones, I, 251, 261). It is possible to have a disease without crisis (*Epidemics I,* Second Constitution, cap. VIII: Jones, I, 161). *Aphorisms,* II: 47; IV: 31-33, 51; V: 8, 15; VII: 36, 44, 45 (Jones, IV, 119, 143, 149, 159, 161, 201, 203).

[15] *Aphorisms,* I: 9 (Jones, IV, 103). See W.H.S. Jones, "Hippocrates and the Corpus Hippocraticum," *Proc. Brit. Acad.* XXXI (1945), p. 8. *Prognosis,* cap. I (Jones, II, 9).

[16] I. M. Lonie, "The Hippocratic Treatise Peri diaites okseon," p. 63.

[17] *RAD I,* cap. II (Jones, II, 63).

[18] Werner Jaeger, *Paideia: the Ideals of Greek Culture,* Volume III, pp. 24, 296 n. 53.

[19] Jaeger, *Paideia,* Volume III, pp. 53, 296.

[20] *Aphorisms,* I: 3, 15; II: 4, 17, 34, 44, 51, *et passim* (Jones, IV, 101, 105, 109, 113, 117, 119, 121).

[21] Hemorrhage: *Coan Prognosis* II: 57, 77, 116, 125, 128; IV: 166. *Aphorisms,* IV: 174 and V: 33. Hemorrhoids: *Coan Prognosis* XXXI: 518.

Aphorisms, VI: 11, 12, 21. Epistaxis: *Aphorisms,* IV: 60 and V: 33. Chadwick and Mann, 222, 224, 227, 231, 266. Jones, IV, 151, 155, 167, 183, 185. See also *Epidemics I,* Third Constitution, cap. XV (Jones, I, 169).

[22] *Coan Prognosis* XVII: 348; XXII: 440; XXV: 465 (Chadwick and Mann, pp. 247, 257, 260). *Aphorisms,* II: 26; IV: 57; VI: 40, 44, 51; VII: 52 (Jones, IV, 115, 151, 189, 191, 205).

[23] *Coan Prognosis* II: 57 (epistaxis); XXI: 429 (Chadwick and Mann, pp. 222, 257). *Epidemics III,* First Series, Case VII (stools and urine) (Jones I, 233).

[24] Max Neuburger, "The Doctrine of the Healing Power of Nature Throughout the Course of Time," *Journal of the American Institute of Homeopathy* XXV (1932), p. 866. See discussion in Arturo Castiglioni, *A History of Medicine* (New York: Knopf, 1941), p. 178.

[25] *Prognosis,* cap. I (Jones, II, 7).

[26] *Prognosis,* cap. XXV (Jones, II, 55).

[27] *Prognosis,* cap. XV (Jones, II, 31).

[28] *Coan Prognosis,* XVI: 304; XXXII: 556, 558, 559 (Chadwick and Mann, pp. 244, 269). *RAD I,* cap. XXIII (Jones, II, 89). *Aphorisms,* IV: 13-16 (Jones, IV, 137, 139).

[29] Chapters XXIII and LXIV (Jones, II, 81, 119). The classic analysis of the use of drugs in the Hippocratic Corpus is J. H. Dierbach, *Die Arzneimittel des Hippokrates* (Heidelberg, 1824).

[30] *RAD I,* cap. V (Jones, II, 67).

[31] *RAD I,* cap. X (Jones II, 71).

[32] *RAD I,* cap. XII (Jones, II, 71).

[33] *RAD I,* cap. XIII (Jones, II, 73).

[34] *RAD I,* cap. XVIII (Jones, II, 77).

[35] *Aphorisms,* VII: 42 (Jones, IV, 203).

[36] *RAD I,* caps. XVI, XXI, XXII, LXV, LXVI (Jones, II, 75, 79, 81, 121, 123). *Epidemics III,* Second Series, Case VIII (Jones, I, 271). *Aphorisms,* V: 22 (Jones, IV, 163).

[37] *Aphorisms,* V: 21 (Jones, IV, 163).

[38] *RAD I,* cap. XIX (Jones, II, 77). *Epidemics I,* Cases I, II, IV, VII, XII (Jones, I, 187, 189, 193, 199, 207).

[39] *RAD I,* cap. L (Jones, II, 105).

[40] *RAD I,* caps. LI, LIII (Jones, II, 107, 109).

[41] *RAD I,* caps. LVIII, LIX (Jones, II, 113, 115).

[42] *RAD I,* cap. LII (Jones, II, 107).

[43] *Aphorisms,* VII: 37 (Jones, IV, 201).

[44] *Aphorisms,* VII: 60 (Jones, IV, 207).

[45] *Aphorisms,* V: 19 (Jones, IV, 163).

[46] *Aphorisms,* V: 23 (Jones, IV, 165).

[47] *Aphorisms,* V: 25 (Jones, IV, 165).

[48] *Aphorisms,* V: 68; VI: 22, 31, 36; VII: 46, 48 (Jones, IV, 179, 185, 187, 203, 205). *Epidemics III,* Second Series, Case VIII (Jones I, 271).

[49] *Epidemics I,* Third Constitution, cap. XXIII (Jones, I, 181).

[50] *Aphorisms,* I: 1 (Jones, IV, 99).

[51] *Epidemics I,* Second Constitution, cap. XI (Jones, I, 165).

[52] *Aphorisms,* II: 52. See, also, II: 27 (Jones, IV, 115, 121).

[53] Caps, 8, 10, 11, 14 (II, 431, 451, 461, 471, L.).

[54] Cap. 15 (VI, 165, L.).

[55] Cap. 19 (VI, 175, L.).

[56] Cap. 27 (VI, 195, L.). Also, caps. 25, 26, 28 (VI, 191, 193, 197, L.); *Diseases III,* cap. 16 (VII, 147, L.).

[57] See also the discussion of cataplasms which mature tumors in *Affections,* cap. 34 (VI, 245, L.).

[58] *Diseases I,* caps. 7, 17, 18 (VI, 153, 171, 173, L.).

[59] *Diseases I,* cap. 7 (VI, 153, L.).

[60] *Diseases III,* caps. 15, 16 (VII, 137, 143, L.).

[61] *Internal Diseases,* caps. 21, 42 (VII, 219, 271, L.).

[62] *Diseases II,* caps. 21, 22, 41, 40 (VII, 37, 57, 59, L.).

[63] *Diseases II,* caps. 4, 14, 16, 17, 27, 47, 64 (VII, 11, 25, 29, 31, 43, 65, 99, L.); *Diseases III,* caps. 2, 5 (VII, 119, 123, L.).

[64] Caps. 18, 13 (II, 469, 491, L.).

[65] Caps. 5, 18 (II, 407, 489, L.).

[66] Caps. 1, 3, 5, 6, 14, 16 (II, 395, 403, 407, 409, 415, 469, 475, L.).

[67] "Sub-bilious phlegm" (*Diseases II,* cap. 2: VII, 9, L.); "thick and thin parts of the bile" (*Diseases I,* cap. 25 and *Diseases II,* cap. 3: VI, 191 and VII, 11, L.); "a certain wet vapor from the bile and the phlegm" (*Diseases I,* cap. 20: VI, 179, L.).

[68] That is, *Diseases I, Affections, Diseases II, Diseases III, Internal Diseases.*

[69] Cap. 3 (VI, 145, L.).

[70] *Ibid.*

[71] Caps. 30, 34 (VI, 201, 205, L.).

[72] Caps. 12, 13, 14 (VI, 159, 161, 163, L.).

[73] Cap. 8 (VI, 155, L.).

[74] Cap. 19 (VI, 173, L.).

[75] Cap. 24 (VI, 189, L.).

[76] Cap. 30 (VI, 201, L.).

[77] Cap. 4 (VI, 211, L.).

[78] Cap. 10 (VI, 219, L.).

[79] Cap. 35 (VI, 247, L.).

[80] Cap. 5 (VI, 215, L.).

[81] Cap. 32 (VI, 245, L.).

[82] Cap. 16 (VI, 225, L.).

[83] Cap. 20 (VI, 229, L.).

[84] Cap. 18 (VI, 227, L.).

[85] *Ibid.*

[86] Cap. 29 (VI, 241, L.).

[87] Cap. 30 (VI, 243, L.).

[88] Cap. 31 (VI, 243, L.).

[89] Cap. 17 (VII, 207, L.).

[90] Caps. 18, 19 (VII, 211, 215, L.).

[91] Cap. 47 (VII, 281, L.).

[92] Black bile in caps. 4, 16, 27, 34, 43 (VII, 179, 205, 237, 253, 273, L.), blood in caps. 7, 15, 32 (VII, 183, 205, 249, L.), phlegm in caps. 10, 14, 20, 21, 22, 24, 33, 38, 49, 50 (VII, 191, 203, 215, 219, 221, 229, 251, 261, 289, 293, L.), bile in caps. 28, 30, 31, 35, 39, 48, 51 (VII, 241, 245, 249, 253, 261, 285,

295, L.). Diseases are also attributed to "blood or salty phlegm" (cap. 3: VII, 175, L.), "blood or black bile" (cap. 5: VII, 179, L.), "phlegm and blood" (cap. 6: VII, 181, L.), "blood and bile" (caps. 12, 41: VII, 193, 267, L.), "bile, phlegm, and blood" (caps. 29, 51: VII, 243, 297, L.). Thus the author's statement in cap. 20 of this work: "I have the same opinion of phlegm as I have of bile, that there are many varieties" (VII, 215, L.) is doubtless only lip-service to the Group I tradition.

[93] Cap. 13 (VI, 161, L.).

[94] Cap. 15 (VI, 165, L.).

[95] Cap. 23 (VI, 189, L.).

[96] Cap. 28 (VI, 197, L.).

[97] Cap. 27 (VI, 195, L.).

[98] *Diseases I,* cap. 18 (VI, 173, L.).

[99] *Diseases I,* cap. 14 (VI, 163, L.).

[100] *Diseases II,* caps. 8, 17, 18 (VII 17, 31, 33, L.).

[101] *RAD II,* cap. 1 (II, 395, L.).

[102] *RAD II,* cap. 6 (II, 409, L.). Also, cap. 5 (II, 407, L.).

[103] *Internal Diseases,* cap. 29 (VII, 243, L.).

[104] *Internal Diseases,* cap. 4 (VII, 179, L.).

[105] *Internal Diseases,* cap. 12 (VII, 193, L.).

[106] *Affections,* cap. 22 (VI, 233, L.).

[107] *Affections,* cap. 21 (VI, 231, L.).

[108] *Diseases III,* cap. 14 (VII, 135, L.).

[109] *Internal Diseases,* cap. 10 (VII, 191, L.).

[110] *Internal Diseases,* cap. 22 (VII, 221, L.).

[111] *Internal Diseases,* cap. 24 (VII, 229, L.).

[112] *Internal Diseases,* cap. 23 (VII, 225, L.). Also, caps. 18, 26, 28, 29, 33, 42 (VII, 211, 233, 241, 243, 251, 271, L.).

[113] *Epidemics I,* First Constitution, cap. 1 (Jones, I, 147); Second Constitution, cap. 5 (Jones, I, 155); Third Constitution, cap. XIV (Jones, I, 167), etc. *Epidemics III,* First Series, Case III (Jones, I, 223). *Aphorisms,* III: 2, 3, 5, 6, 7, 15, 17-24 (Jones, IV, 123, 127, 129, 131).

[114] *Diseases I,* cap. 2 (VI, 143, L.).

[115] *Affections,* cap. 1 (VI, 209, L.). Also, *Diseases I,* cap. 23 (VI, 189, L.).

[116] *Diseases I,* cap. 18 (VI, 173, L.).

[117] *Diseases I,* cap. 13 (VI, 161, L.), cap. 11 (VI, 159, L.).

[118] *Diseases II,* cap. 6 (VII, 15, L.).

[119] *Diseases II,* cap. 11 (VII, 19, L.).

[120] *Internal Diseases,* cap. 6 (VII, 181, L.). Also, *Diseases II,* cap. 55 (VII, 85, L.).

[121] Carolus Gottlob Kuehn, *Medicorum Graecorum Opera Quae Exstant: Claudii Galeni Opera Omnia,* Twenty Volumes, Leipzig, 1821-1833. Volume XV, pp. 420-421. Henceforth references to the Kuehn edition of Galen will be in the abbreviated form, e.g., K XV 420-421.

[122] K XV 419ff., 731.

[123] II, 403, L.

[124] II, 417-425, L.

[125] II, 507-509, L.

[126] *Diseases II*, caps. 1, 12, 13 (VII, 9, 19-25, L.).

[127] *Diseases II*, cap. 47 (VII, 65, L.).

[128] *Affections*, cap. 7 (VI, 215, L.).

[129] *Diseases III*, cap. 6 (VII, 123, L.).

[130] *Diseases III*, cap. 9 (VII, 129, L.).

[131] *Internal Diseases*, cap. 7. Also, Chapters 6, 12, 14, 16, 17, 52 (VII, 183, 181, 193, 203, 204, 207, 299, L.).

[132] *Diseases I*, cap. 6 (VI, 153, L.).

[133] *Diseases I*, cap. 17 (VI, 163, L.).

[134] *Diseases I*, cap. 14 (VI, 163, L.).

[135] *Diseases II*, cap. 68 (VII, 105, L.).

[136] *Diseases II*, cap. 71 (VII, 109, L.). Also, *Affections*, cap. 19 (VI, 229, L.).

[137] *Internal Diseases*, cap. 20 (VII, 215, L.).

[138] *Internal Diseases*, cap. 22 (VII, 221, L.).

[139] *Diseases II*, caps. 8, 25 (VII, 17, 39, L.).

[140] *Diseases III*, cap. 14 (VII, 135, L.).

[141] *Diseases III*, cap. 1 (VII, 119, L.).

[142] *Affections*, cap. 38 (VI, 249, L.).

[143] *Affections*, cap. 22 (VI, 233, L.).

[144] *Affections*, cap. 20 (VI, 229, L.).

[145] *Affections*, cap. 11 (VI, 219, L.).

[146] *Affections*, cap. 4 (VI, 211, L.).

[147] For examples see *Diseases II*, cap. 60 (VII, 93, L.); *Internal Diseases*, caps. 9, 14, 15, 17 (VII, 187, 203, 205, 207, L.).

[148] *Diseases II*, cap. 47 (VII, 69, L.).

[149] *RAD II*, caps. 11, 18, 25 (II, 465, 481, 511, L.); *Affections*, caps. 40, 43 (VI, 251, 253, L.); *Internal Diseases*, cap. 27 (VII, 239, L.).

[150] *Affections*, caps. 43, 54 (VI, 253, 265, L.).

[151] Lonie, "The Cnidian Treatises of the Corpus Hippocraticum," p. 3.

[152] *Affections*, caps. 45, 48, 49, 54 (VI, 259, 265, L.).

[153] *Affections*, cap. 45 (VI, 255, L.).

[154] *Affections*, cap. 47 (VI, 255, L.).

[155] *Affections*, cap. 45 (VI, 255, L.).

[156] *Affections*, cap. 59 (VI, 269, L.).

[157] *Affections*, cap. 55 (VI, 265, L.).

[158] *Affections*, cap. 54 (VI, 265, L.).

[159] *Affections*, cap. 55 (VI, 265, L.).

[160] *Affections*, cap. 39 (VI, 249, L.).

[161] *Aphorisms*, I: 16; II: 49, 50 (Jones, IV, 107, 121). See, also *RAD II*, cap. 18 (II, 479, L.) and *Affections*, cap. 44 (VI, 255, L.).

[162] *Diseases I*, cap. 28 (VI, 197, L.).

[163] *Diseases III*, cap. 7 (VII, 125, L.).

[164] *Diseases II*, cap. 19 (VII, 33, L.).

[165] *Diseases II*, cap. 27 (VII, 41-45, L.). Also, cap. 26.

[166] *Affections*, cap. 19 (VI, 229, L.).

[167] *Affections*, cap. 20 (VI, 231, L.).

[168] *Affections*, cap. 34 (VI, 245, L.).

[169] *Aphorisms* II: 34 and VII: 82 (Jones, IV, 117, 215).

[170] *Prognosis,* cap. I (Jones, II, 9) and *Aphorisms,* I: 9 (Jones, IV, 103).

[171] *Epidemics I,* Third Constitution, cap. XV (Jones, I, 169).

[172] On the use of *prophasis* in *Epidemics III* and *Coan Prognosis* see Karl Deichgraeber, " 'Profasis,' eine terminologische Studie," *Quellen und Studien zur Geschichte der Naturwissenschaften und der Medizin,* III (1933), 1-17.

[173] On *aition* see caps. II, III, and IV. On *prophasis* see caps. I, II, V, and VI (Jones, II, 139-153).

[174] *Sacred Disease,* cap. V (Jones, II, 151).

[175] *Ibid.,* cap. XVI (Jones, II, 173).

[176] *Ibid.,* cap. XXI (Jones, II, 183).

[177] *Ibid.,* cap. XVIII (Jones, II, 177).

[178] *Ibid.,* caps. VI and VII (Jones, II, 153, 155).

[179] *Ibid.,* cap. X (Jones, II, 159).

[180] *Breaths,* caps. I-VI, X, XII, XV (Jones, II, 227-253).

[181] *Ibid.,* cap. III (Jones, II, 229).

[182] *Ibid.,* cap. VII (Jones, II, 235).

[183] *Ibid.,* cap. XIV (Jones, II, 249).

[184] *Sacred Disease,* cap. IX: palpitation, difficult breathing, diarrhoea. *Breaths,* cap. IX: ileus, tormina; cap. XI: lacerations; cap. XII: dropsy; cap. XIII: apoplexy (Jones, II, 157, 241, 245, 247).

[185] *Aphorisms,* III: 2, 3 (Jones, IV, 123).

[186] *Ibid.,* III: 19 (Jones, IV, 129).

[187] *Ibid.,* III: 8 (Jones, IV, 125).

[188] *Epidemics I,* Constitution, cap. I, and Second Constitution, cap. V; *Epidemics III,* cap. II; *Aphorisms,* III: 1 (Jones, I, 147, 155, 241 and IV, 123).

[189] *Epidemics I,* Second Constitution, cap. V; *Epidemics III,* cap. XV; *Aphorisms,* II: 45 (Jones, I, 155, 255 and IV, 119).

[190] *Aphorisms,* III: 7 (Jones, IV, 123).

[191] *Ibid.,* III: 14 (Jones, IV, 127).

[192] *Internal Diseases,* cap. 7 (VII, 185, L.).

[193] *Ibid.,* cap. 27 (VII, 237, L.).

[194] *Ibid.,* cap. 30 (VII, 245, L.).

[195] *Ibid.,* cap. 32 (VII, 249, L.).

[196] *Internal Diseases,* cap. 34 (VII, 253, L.).

[197] *Internal Diseases,* cap. 35 (VII, 253, L.).

[198] *Internal Diseases,* cap. 38 (VII, 261, L.).

[199] *Internal Diseases,* cap. 39 (VII, 261, L.).

[200] *RAD II,* cap. 6 (II, 417, L.).

[201] *Diseases I,* cap. 24 (VI, 189, L.).

[202] *Diseases I,* cap. 5 (VI, 151, L.).

[203] *Diseases II,* cap. 8 (VII, 17, L.). Also *Diseases I,* caps. 23 and 27 (VI, 189, 195, L.).

[204] *Diseases II,* cap. 3 (VII, 11, L.).

[205] *Diseases I,* cap. 26 (VI, 193, L.).

[206] *Nature of Man,* cap. VIII (Jones, IV, 25). See, also, *ibid.,* cap. XV (Jones, IV, 41).

[207] See Gert Plamboeck, *Dynamis im Corpus Hippocraticum.* Academie der

Wissenschaften und der Literatur (Mainz), Abhandlungen der Geistes– und Sozialwissenschaftlichen Klasse, 1964, No. 2, pp. 63-109.

[208] *Nature of Man,* cap. XV (Jones, IV, 39).

[209] *Breaths,* cap. IX (Jones, II, 241).

[210] *Regimen I,* cap. II (Jones, IV, 231).

[211] *Regimen III,* cap. LXIX (Jones, IV, 383).

[212] *Regimen IV* (Jones, IV, 420-447).

[213] See Benjamin Farrington, *Head and Hand in Ancient Greece* (London: Watts, 1947), pp. 34ff.; G. Bratescu, "L'Hippocratisme et sa Revision dans l'Antiquite," *Studii Clasice* V (1963), 43-67 (in Rumanian).

[214] August Comte, *Cours de Philosophie Positive* (3rd ed.; Paris, 1869), I, 8-9.

[215] F.S.C. Northrop reduces induction to a relatively unimportant stage of investigation, the sorting-out of facts prior to the elaboration of a hypothesis (*The Logic of the Sciences and the Humanities* [New York, 1959], p. 37). Karl Popper writes "a theory of induction is superfluous. It has no function in a logic of science" (*The Logic of Scientific Discovery* [New York, 1959], p. 315).

[216] Henry Margenau, *The Nature of Physical Reality* (New York, 1950), p. 13.

[217] *The Art,* cap. I (Jones, II, 191).

CHAPTER II

THE HIPPOCRATIC CORPUS: ORIGINS

In the sixth and fifth centuries B.C. two important schools of medicine existed in Italy: that of Agrigentum on the southern coast of Sicily and that of Croton on the west coast of the Gulf of Taranto.

Agrigentum was the home of Empedocles, while Croton was the birthplace of the Pythagorean sect. The medical views of the Group III Hippocratic works owe much to the school of Agrigentum, and the writings of Groups I and IV were influenced by the school of Croton.

Plato, who was on intimate terms with the Sicilian physicians, helped propagate their views.

Another important source of ideas for the Hippocratic authors, especially those of the Group II writings, was the Egyptian school of medicine which held that most diseases start with the putrefaction of food residues in the large intestine.

Empedocles and Alcmaeon

Pythagoras established the school of Croton late in the sixth century, and its first medical philosopher, Alcmaeon of Croton, flourished about 500. Alcmaeon's physiological theory has been preserved by a later Greek compiler in the following words:

> Alcmaeon maintains that the bond of health is the "equal balance" of the powers [*dynameis*], moist and dry, cold and hot, bitter and sweet, and the rest, while the "supremacy" of one of them is the cause of disease; for

> the supremacy of either is destructive. Illness comes about directly through excess of heat or cold, indirectly through surfeit or deficiency of nourishment; and its center is either the blood or the marrow or the brain. It sometimes arises in these centers from external causes, moisture of some sort or environment or exhaustion or hardship or similar causes. Health, on the other hand, is the proportionate admixture [*krasis*] of the qualities [*poiotetes*].[1]

This simile is apparently taken from the political realm. As democracy is maintained by equality among the citizens, so is health maintained by a balance among the forces making up the organism.[2]

The second school, that of Empedocles, harks back to the Ionian philosophers who, a hundred years before the birth of Hippocrates, had turned their attention to interpretation of the physical world. In the middle of the fifth century their tradition was taken up by Empedocles who hypothesized that the universe was made from four elements—earth, water, air, and fire—and attempted to explain the origin of matter by generation out of these four elements and their mutual attraction and repulsion by love and hatred (the two dynamic qualities of the Empedoclean system).

The conflict between these two systems of thought is profound, and in the opposition between them we see the Group I-Group III polarity. Alcmaeon proposes an indefinite number of abstractly conceived qualities (*poiotetes* or *dynameis*) as the components of the organism, while Empedocles posits four concrete and substantial elements. Empedocles is the inspiration for the humoral doctrine of *Nature of Man*, and Alcmaeon's theory is the forerunner of the therapeutic doctrine of Groups I and IV.[a]

[a]Jones states ("Philosophy and Medicine," p. 4) that "*Ancient Medicine* . . . is little more than an essay in defense of Alcmaeon's theory."

Furthermore, Alcmaeon's assumption that the internal mechanisms of disease are infinite in number and may not be defined too closely by the physician or philosopher—the basic operating assumption of Empirical medicine—seems to have as its corollary the other typically Empirical doctrine that mortal man is not capable of seeing into the organism:

> These are the words of Alcmaeon of Croton . . . "Of things invisible, as of mortal things, only the gods have certain knowledge; but to us, as men, only inference from evidence is possible," and so on.[3]

A passage from the *Phaedo* is likewise taken by some scholars to reflect the sense-based epistemology of Alcmaeon: Socrates states that he once examined the theory whether "it is the brain that gives the sensations of hearing, seeing, and smelling, and from these come memory and opinion, and from memory and opinion, when it has reached a state of stability, comes knowledge." (96B)

The teachings of Empedocles were developed by the Sicilian school of medicine whose most famous representative was Philistion of Locri, a contemporary of Plato. Philistion's physiology is given in the Menon Papyrus:

> Philistion thinks that we are composed of four "forms," that is, of four elements—fire, water, air, earth. Each of these too has its own power [*dynamis*]; of fire the *dynamis* is the hot, of air it is the cold, of water the moist, and of earth the dry. According to him diseases occur in many ways, but speaking quite generally and in outline we may call them three: (1) because of the elements, (2) because of the condition of our bodies, (3) because of external causes. The elements cause disease when the hot and the moist are in excess, or when the hot becomes less and weak. External causes are of three kinds: (1) wounds and sores; or (2) excess of heat, cold, and so on, or change of heat to cold or of cold to heat; or (3) of nutriment to what is unsuitable or corrupt. The

> condition of the body is a cause of disease in the following way. When, he says, the whole body breathes well and the breath passes through unhindered, health is the result. For breathing takes place not only by way of mouth and nostrils, but also all over the body. When the body does not breathe well, diseases occur, and in different ways.[4]

It can be seen that Philistion attaches a *dynamis* to each of the four Empedoclean elements, and "thus Empedocles' theory of the elements was reconciled with Alcmaeon's theory of the qualities (*dynameis*), with the result that the elements lost their uncompromisingly material nature, while the number of qualities, which Alcmaeon had left indefinite, was now reduced to a tetrad."[b] The similarity of Philistion's medical doctrine to that of *Nature of Man* is striking and was pointed out in ancient times by Galen.[5]

The above passage also shows that Philistion was the first to introduce the *pneuma* into medicine.[6] Hence *Breaths* and *Sacred Disease* may also be ascribed to the Sicilian influence.

The Influence of Plato on Medicine

Plato is known to have visited Syracuse three times, in the years 388-387, 367, and 361-360, and one of the (possibly spurious) epistles indicates that he was in contact with Philistion.[7] Plato's medical views, as given in the *Timaeus,* reveal a strong input from the Sicilian School.

> Now everyone can see whence diseases arise. There are four natures out of which the body is compacted, earth and fire and water and air, and the unnatural excess or defect of these, or the change of any of them from its own natural place into another, or—since there are more kinds than one of fire and of the other elements—the

[b] Raymond Klibansky *et al., Saturn and Melancholy* (London, 1934), pp. 13-15. This work contains an excellent description of the origins of humoralism.

> assumption by any of these of a wrong kind, or any similar irregularity, produces disorders and diseases; for when any of them is produced or changed in a manner contrary to nature, the parts which were previously cool grow warm, and those which were dry become moist, and the light become heavy, and the heavy light; all sorts of changes occur. (82A)

> When the constitution is disordered by excess of fire, continuous heat and fever are the result; when excess of air is the cause, then the fever is quotidian; when of water, which is a more sluggish element than either fire or air, then the fever is a tertian; when of earth, which is the most sluggish of the four, and is only purged away in a fourfold period, the result is a quartan fever, which can with difficulty be shaken off. (86A)

The historically recorded contacts between Plato and Philistion may explain the considerable parallels between the medical doctrines of the *Timaeus* and those of the works of Group III. Since Plato's name is not mentioned in the Hippocratic Corpus, we have no direct evidence of his influence, and it is equally possible that Plato derived his own ideas from the Hippocratic writers. In any case, there are striking similarities between the ideas of the *Timaeus* and those we have discussed as characteristic of the works of Group III.

The first of the above quotations indicates a relationship with the quadripartite humoral doctrine of Philistion and *Nature of Man.*

The second suggests the identification of humors with specific diseases which is characteristic of Group III.[8]

In the *Timaeus* Plato ascribes many diseases to the movement of air in the organism, in a manner very reminiscent of *Sacred Disease* and *Breaths:* "the parts which are unrefreshed by air corrode, while in other parts the excess of air forcing its way through the veins distorts them and, decomposing the body, is enclosed in the midst of it and occupies the midriff; thus numberless painful diseases are produced, accompanied by copious sweats." (84C and D)

The *Timaeus* contains a great deal of physiological explanation of disease: "the white phlegm, though dangerous when detained within by reason of the air-bubbles, yet if it can communicate with the outside air, is less severe, and only discolors the body, generating leprous eruptions and similar diseases. When it is mingled with black bile and dispersed about the courses of the head, which are the divinest parts of us, the attack, if coming on in sleep, is not so severe . . . an acid and salt phlegm, again, is the source of all those diseases which take the form of catarrh, but they have many names because the places into which they flow are manifold." (85A *et passim*)

The view expressed in the *Timaeus* that "all kindred substances are drawn toward one another . . . like to like" resembles the explanation, given in *Nature of Man,* of the operation of purgative medicines by the similarity between these medicines and the elements in the body which they purge.[9]

Platonic philosophy in general is characterized by the idea that perception is not by the senses but by the soul directly. And we find the physicians of Group III assuming that the reasoning power is capable of perceiving physiological mechanisms which are invisible to sight.

Finally, we find in the *Timaeus* the very novel idea that a process occurring within the organism may be "unnatural" or "contrary to nature" (*para physin*). In the first quotation above the "unnatural excess or defect" of an element or its change "from its own natural place into another" are given as causes of disease. This view is developed at length in another passage of the *Timaeus,* where Plato indicates what happens when the generation of substances in the body occurs in the wrong order:

> Now when each process takes place in this order, health commonly results; when in the opposite order, disease.

> For when the flesh becomes decomposed and sends back the wasting substance into the veins, then an over-supply of blood of diverse kinds, mingling with air in the veins . . . contains all sorts of bile and serum and phlegm. For all things go the wrong way, and having become corrupted, first they taint the blood itself, and then ceasing to give nourishment to the body they are carried along the veins in all directions, no longer preserving the order of their natural courses, but at war with themselves, because they receive no good from one another, and are hostile to the abiding constitution of the body, which they corrupt and dissolve. (82D-83A)

The concept of the "unnatural" physiological process appears in both Group II[10] and Group III,[11] the *locus classicus* being in *Nature of Man:* "in the body are many constituents which, by heating or cooling, by drying or by wetting one another contrary to nature engender diseases."[12] *Para physin* is not used in this way in Group I or Group IV.[13]

That the physician should presume to know better than the *physis* what is "natural" and what is "unnatural" is an important development in therapeutic theory, whether introduced by Plato or borrowed by him from the physicians of Group III.[c] This is in the sharpest possible contrast to the physiological doctrine of Group I, which is based on the assumption that all the processes of the *physis* are by definition "natural." The physician now felt entitled to substitute his own judgment for that of the *physis.* This reflects the claim of philosophy to be able to establish *a priori* standards against which the very physiology of the human body can be measured.

[c]Cornford writes (*Plato's Cosmology,* p. 336): "I cannot find evidence that any medical writer had formulated this notion of a reversal of the normal course of nutrition as the cause of a special class of diseases beyond the testimony . . . that Philolaus regarded bile, blood and phlegm as sources of disease and bile (if present at all) as a 'useless' substance." On Philolaus of Croton see Jones, *Medical Writings of Anonymus Londinensis,* cap. XVIII).

Egyptian Influences in the Hippocratic Corpus

A major influence on the Hippocratic writers was the food-residues doctrine underlying the system of medicine obtaining in Egypt. The Egyptians discovered from their practice of embalming that after death putrefaction starts in the large intestine, and they reasoned from this that disease in the healthy is caused by the rotting of food in the same place.[14] They maintained that noxious agents from the bowels then enter the bloodstream, causing corruption and coagulation of the blood and the formation of pus. Hence, they utilized two forms of therapy—cathartics and blood-letting—which they viewed as more or less equivalent.[15]

Herodotos in the middle of the fifth century knew of this doctrine, noting that the Egyptians took enemas, emetics, and cathartics three days in every month to purge their intestines of substances which might generate disease.[16][d] The Menon Papyrus describes a certain Ninyas the Egyptian as:

> dividing affections into congenital and acquired, the congenital, he says, being innate in our bodies. He holds that there is another cause by which diseases are produced in the following way. Whenever nutriment is taken that is not absorbed into the body, but remains in the organs, the warmth in us generates out of this nutriment residues [*perittomata*].[17]

The influence of the Egyptian doctrine of putrefaction is strongest in the Cnidian works, and it seems probable that

[d]One ancient chronicler states that the ibis, an Egyptian bird with a long neck and a curved beak, suggested to mankind the enema: "for this bird is gluttonous and scrounges his food from the seashore; and when constipated he arouses his *physis* to defend himself against what is paining him; and having filled his beak with water, he discharges it into himself from the rear; then, relieved of these food-residues, he takes his fill of the next meal. And thus was this remedy made known to man." Karl Deichgraeber, *Die Griechische Empirikerschule* (Berlin/ Zurich: Weidmann, 1965), Fr. 43b.

this doctrine penetrated Greek medicine through the school of Cnidos. This is indicated both by internal evidence in the works of Group II and by the historical record.

The founder of the Cnidian School and the author of the earliest book of this school, the Cnidian Sentences, was Euryphon of Cnidos who lived about 450 B.C.[18] His pathological views are given in the Menon Papyrus:

> Euryphon of Cnidos for example thinks that diseases are caused in the following manner. "When the belly does not discharge the nutriment that has been taken, residues are produced, which then rise to the regions about the head and cause diseases. When however the belly is empty and clean, digestion takes place as it should . . ."[19]

His pupil, Herodicos of Cnidos, who was a contemporary of Plato (*Gorgias* 448B, 456A), expanded this doctrine:

> [Herodicos] himself is partly in agreement with Euryphon but partly in disagreement. Insofar as he himself too says that residues are the cause of disease, he is in agreement. Insofar as he says that proper digestion is not due to the bowels being clean or empty, he differs, having recourse to the following explanation. When men take in nutriment without previous exercise, the result is that the nutriment is not assimilated, but, lying in the belly undigested and unaltered, it is broken up into residues. From the residues, however, are produced two liquids, one acid, the other bitter, and the affections turn out different according to the predominance of one or the other. And he says that according to the strength or weakness of these the affections resulting are different; what I mean is, if the acid be on the weak side, and not unblended, and correspondingly, if the bitter be not too bitter but on the weaker side, or if both be strong, the affections also will differ according to the blendings of the liquids. . . . Affections will turn out different accord-

ing as the fluids are carried to head, liver, or spleen.[20][e]

There is historical evidence of contact between the Cnidians and the Egyptians. The head of the Cnidian School in the middle of the fourth century, Eudoxos of Cnidos (c. 407-357), studied medicine in Egypt, as did his associate, Chrysippos of Cnidos; furthermore, both Eudoxos and Chrysippos studied with Philistion of Locri.[21]

As we have mentioned, the concept of "food-residues" (*perittomata*) lies at the basis of the Egyptian therapeutic doctrine. This involved the idea of plethora and putrefaction within the organism. The word, *perittomata,* does not appear in the Hippocratic Corpus,[22] but the Egyptian influence seems clearly manifested in the concepts of "impure" or "impurities" (*akathartos, akatharsies*—literally, "unpurged remnent") and putrefaction *(sepomenon)* which figure in all the works of Group II as etiological factors.

Affections has a series of cases in which the concept of the "unpurged remnent" is combined with that of fecal matter in the intestines and the vitiation of the blood as etiological factors in disease. Chapter 18 of this work ascribes tertian and quartan fevers to the body's impure (*akathartos*) state; the remedy is an evacuant. Chapter 19 states that leucophlegmasy arises when, the patient being phlegmatic after a long series of fevers, the body becomes impure (*akathartos*), and the phlegm settles in the flesh; treatment is through evacuation. Chapter 20 discusses a disease caused when bile-and-phlegm settle in the spleen; if the patient appears unpurged (*akathartos*), he should be purged. Chapter 21 takes up a case of ileus characterized by the heating and

[e]In this connection note the criticism of the Cnidian School in *Regimen in Acute Diseases,* cap. II: "the remedies they used were few in number; for most of their prescriptions, except in the case of acute diseases, were to administer purges, and to give to drink, at the proper season, whey and milk" (Jones, II, 63). This sort of therapy would precisely reflect Herodicos' physiology—purges to evacuate the residues and the two bland liquids to counteract the acid and bitter liquids produced by the residues.

drying of fecal matter in the intestine; phlegm accumulates around it, the intestines swell up, and the outcome is a case of ileus. Chapter 22 describes a case of dropsy which arises when the patient remains a long time with an "impure" (*akathartos*) body after a disease; the flesh is consumed and melts into water. Chapter 23 discusses a case of dysentery caused when the blood is infected *(noseei)* and overheated by bile-and-phlegm in the veins and the stomach and is then passed out with the stools.[23]

This series of cases, with their combination of "impurities," fecal matter, and diseased blood, apparently reflects the Egyptian doctrine. The doctrine appears again in Chapters 30 and 31. The former mentions a case of arthritis caused when bile-and-phlegm are set in motion by the contents of the stomach. Cure is through purging the patient and giving him various milk drinks. Chapter 31 ascribes gout to corruption (*ephtharmenon*) of the blood in the veins by the action of the bile-and-phlegm. Cure is through purgation and, if this is ineffective, by cauterizing the veins.[24] This last case, especially, suggests a connection between the contents of the stomach and the circulatory system in a manner analogous to the assumed relationship in Egyptian medicine between the feces and the circulatory system.

Diseases II and *Diseases III* also discuss "impurities" as morbific causes.[25] This concept does not appear in *Diseases I* or *Internal Diseases*.

Parallel to the "impurities" concept in Group II is the idea that "pus," "corruption," or "putridity" of elements of the organism are etiological factors in disease. *Diseases I* contains much discussion of the rotting or putrefaction (*sepesthai* and cognates) of bile, blood, and phlegm,[26] and there are similar passages in *Diseases II* and *Internal Diseases*.[27] "Pus" as an etiological agent is mentioned frequently throughout the works of Group II.[28]

It is easy to see how the Egyptian therapeutic theory could have fused with the coction theory. The doctrinal lines were not so rigidly drawn that a physician could easily avoid confusing, for example, the coction of food with its putrefaction in the intestine; or the pus caused by some septic process in the organism with pus (*empyema*) which was the outcome of an incomplete coction; or the humor which is pathogenic because it is "crude" with blood which is pathogenic because tainted by food residues. The structure of the coction theory was sufficiently similar to that of the food-residues doctrine to permit of their confusion and ultimate fusion.[29]

The food-residues doctrine left its imprint not only on Cnidian medicine. We have noted that Philistion of Locri attributed some diseases to the alteration of nutriment into what is unsuitable or corrupt.[30] Plato himself was influenced by it: the *Timaeus* mentions, as one of the causes of disease, the corruption of the flesh and consequent tainting of the blood,[31] and the Menon Papyrus also ascribes a food-residues doctrine to this philosopher.[32]

The concept of "impurity" (*akathartos*) as an etiological factor figures in Group III in *Airs Waters Places,* but here it is the atmosphere which is "impure" or unpurged.[33f]

It is possible that the concept of plethora (*plesmone*), which is invoked as an etiological factor in Group III, is an extension of the Egyptian doctrine. The Menon Papyrus mentions the view of a certain Aegimius of Elis that plethora arises when fresh nutriment is introduced into the stomach before the older food has been digested.[34] In *Regimen III* there is a detailed discussion of plethora as a causal agent.[35]

Historical and Doctrinal Development of the Hippocratic Corpus

The works examined by us above, which are the oldest of the Hippocratic collection, can hardly have formed a unitary tradition. Not only do we have historical testimony to the

[f]This treatment of *akathartos* resembles the externalization of "coction" in the same work (cap. VIII. See above, p. 51).

existence of at least two different schools, Cos and Cnidos, but such a complex doctrinal development could hardly have occurred within the few decades during which these writings were produced.

They more probably reflect parallel and contemporaneous traditions whose representatives were familiar with each other's ideas and literature.

Thus we would propose the following theory of the rise of the Hippocratic Corpus.

From its inception up through the mid-fifth century Greek medicine was based upon the assumption of two humors or principles: bile and phlegm. The remnents of this early view, which probably originated in folk medicine, are seen in all of the Group II works and all of the Group III works except *Nature of Man.* There is even a passage in *Prognosis* which suggests this dualistic view (cap. XIII: Jones II, 29).

In the Group I writings, which must be ascribed to the school of Cos, the two-humor theory yielded at an early date to the theory of coction with its assumption of an infinite or indefinite number of humors. Coction is mentioned in *Prorrhetic I,* which Jones dates at 440 B.C.[36] And the author of *Ancient Medicine,* as we have seen, attributes the theory of coction to "the ancients" and "the first discoverers."[37]

This development was perhaps caused by contact between Cos and the school of Croton. It doubtless owes something also to Heracleitus (*fl. circa* 500 B.C.)—who defined reality as a process and stated that "all things are one."[g] These works propose a holistic philosophy of the organism and view disease and health as a continuum or process. To use the language of Comte, they represent the transition from metaphysical speculation to a scientific

[g]Windelband writes (*History of Philosophy,* I, p. 28): "Heracleitus . . . analyzed destructively the presupposition of an abiding substance, and allowed only a law of change to stand as the ultimate content of knowledge." The above quotation from Heracleitus is Fragment I (Jones, IV, 471). For further discussion of Heracleitus see below, pp. 136-137.

attitude toward the analysis of physical reality—from speculation about causes to a doctrine which rejects causal analysis and only seeks the patterns and regularities in the succession of events.

Whatever the origin of this doctrine, and it may have arisen in isolation from these philosophical influences, we regard it as the conscious formulation, by one or several physicians, of the prototypical Empirical medical ideology, identical in all important respects with that of the later Empirical School.

The theory of coction appears as a minor theme also in the writings of Group II, together with basic reliance on the primitive bile-phlegm humoralism. These, together with *ad hoc* drug therapeutics, must have been the doctrine of the earliest work of this school, the *Cnidian Sentences*.[38] The authors of these works, however, were eventually subjected to the influence of Philistion and the Sicilian School (Eudoxos and Chrysippos studied with Philistion) which led to the introduction of etiological speculation into this school and a more differentiated and elaborate humoral theory.[39] This trend was furthered by incorporation of the Egyptian food-residues doctrine with its implied knowledge of the hidden physiological processes of the human body.

In Group III the influence of the Sicilian school is very marked indeed. Here the original bipartite humoralism conflicts (in *Nature of Man*) with a quadripartite humoralism clearly inspired by the views of Philistion, which assigns two *dynameis* to each of the four humors. The balance between these two formulations was unstable, and it has been pointed out that the four elements of Empedocles and Philistion can be reduced to a dualistic system in which fire is opposed to earth, water, and air (perhaps accounting for the ambiguous position of blood in later Rationalist humoralism).[40][h] Plato's physiol-

[h]It was sometimes regarded as the fourth humor and sometimes as a mixture of all the humors. See below, p. 217.

ogy in the *Timaeus* also reflects this tension, as he discusses two etiological theories: (1) through bile and phlegm, and (2) through the four elements:

> There are four natures out of which the body is compacted, earth and fire and water and air, and the unnatural excess or defect of these, or the change of any of them from its own natural place into another . . . or any similar irregularity, produces disorders and diseases . . . (82A)

> There is a third class of diseases which may be conceived of as arising in three ways; for they are produced sometimes by wind, and sometimes by phlegm and sometimes by bile. (84B)

The second of these passages reminds us that Philistion's *pneuma*—a recognizable and identifiable etiological agent—contributed to the analytical orientation, the search for proximate causes, which distinguishes the works of Group III.

To invoke Comte's analysis once again, the works of Group III represent the stage in man's intellectual development in which divine intervention (*Sacred Disease*) is rejected in favor of metaphysical theories of causation.

As we have suggested above, the theory of coction set forth in the Group I writings appears to be somewhat senior to the analytical theory (based on contraries) of Group III. It also had the support of a majority of physicians if we are to believe the author of *Nature of Man* who states that "most physicians" of his day adhered to a holistic therapeutic doctrine.[41]

Thus the Group III writings represent an effort to convert the profession to an analytical medicine derived from Philistion and the Sicilian School via Plato. This is associated with the desire of this reforming group to break with the tradition that the physician is only a craftsman who relies on sense-perception and experience, and to convert him into a philosopher.

Finally, the two writings of Group IV, which attack those "who prosecute their researches in the art after the novel fashion, building on a postulate" and who "abandon the old method to rest the art on a postulate," are a reaction to the Group III doctrine and a call for return to the Group I theory of coction as the foundation of medical practice.[42]

We feel that the works of Groups I and IV reflect the ideas of Hippocrates himself and that some of these writings are from his hand. One reason for this view is that these works call for a holistic medicine, and we know from Plato that Hippocrates called for a holistic medicine. In the *Charmides* he writes:

> I dare say you have heard eminent physicians say to a patient who comes to them with bad eyes, that they cannot cure his eyes by themselves but that if his eyes are to be cured, his head must be treated; and then again they say that to think of curing the head alone, and not the rest of the body also, is the height of folly. And arguing in this way they apply their methods to the whole body, and try to treat and heal the whole and the part together. (156B-157A)

and in the *Phaedrus* (270C) he ascribes this view to Hippocrates.

Additional evidence for this is found in the remark of Celsus that Hippocrates was "the first, of all those worthy of commemoration, who separated this branch of learning from the study of philosophy."[43] Pliny also stresses the practical aspect of the Hippocratic teachings, stating that Hippocrates was "the first to put together rules for medical practice."[44]

Hippocrates and his disciples sought a scientific approach to therapeutics. This meant combining a set of rules for medical practice with a holistic doctrine of the organism. They avoided speculation about causes which they viewed as unreliable. They rejected philosophical analysis of the body as alien to the aim and purpose of medicine.

Thus we may assume that Plato felt no affection for Hippocrates–a man who stood for the opposite of the emerging Platonic teachings. W.H.S. Jones has pointed out that the discussion of Hippocrates in the *Protagoras* (311B), where he is said to give instruction for fees, actually classes him with the "despised sophists."[45] Jones notes further that for Plato to call him "Hippocrates of Cos, the Asclepiad," is mildly sarcastic, equivalent to calling someone "the learned doctor."[46] Jones goes on to remark that the discussion of Hippocrates in the *Phaedrus* (270C) is also derogatory:

Soc. And do you think that you can know the nature of the soul intelligently without knowing the nature *(physis)* of the whole?

Phaedr. Hippocrates the Asclepiad says that the *physis* even of the body can only be understood as a whole.

Soc. Yes, friend, and he was right:–still, we ought not to be content with the name of Hippocrates, but to examine and see whether his argument agrees with his conception of the *physis*.

Phaedr. I agree.

Soc. Then consider what truth as well as Hippocrates says about this or about any other *physis*. Ought we not to consider first whether that which we wish to learn and to teach is a simple or multiform thing, and if simple, then to enquire what power it has of acting or being acted upon in relation to other things, and if multiform, then to number the forms; and see first in the case of one of them, and then in the case of all of them, what is that power of acting or being acted upon which makes each and all of them to be what they are?

Phaedr. You may very likely be right, Socrates.

Socrates first notes that Hippocrates' opinion must be compared with the *logos* before it can be accepted and then proceeds to outline a view which runs entirely counter to that of Hippocrates.[47] The opposition between the holistic view ascribed by Socrates to Hippocrates and the analytical view which Socrates himself then proposes is a precise formulation of the opposition between the therapeutic doctrines of Groups I and III. And this is in fact the fundamental conflict within the Hippocratic Corpus. In the past, attention has been distracted from this point by historical awareness of the existence of the competing schools of Cos and Cnidos. As we have brought out, however, the Cnidian School actually represents an eclectic combination of the Empirical and Rationalist elements found in purer form in Groups I and III, while the significant opposition within the Corpus is between the Empirical and Rationalist ideologies themselves.

Regimen in Acute Diseases and its Appendix

Although we have classified *RAD I* and *RAD II* in Groups I and II, respectively, there is evidence that they represent two parts of the same work and were written by the same person. This is the opinion of I. M. Lonie, the most recent commentator,[48] and much may be said in its favor. Our own view is not far from Lonie's, since, although we have classified the two works in different Groups and do not regard them as by the same author, we have noted that *RAD I* differs in some important respects from the other works of Group I,[49] as *RAD II* differs in important respects from the other works of Group II,[50] and these points are precisely the points of similarity between the two works. But, on the other hand, there are powerful resemblances between *RAD I* and the other works of Group I, as between *RAD II* and the other works of Group II,[i] and with respect to several important

[i]These, of course, have been discussed extensively above.

points there is very considerable divergence between *RAD I* and *RAD II*—a divergence which, in our opinion, makes it impossible to consider them as parts of the same writing.[51]

NOTES

[1] G. S. Kirk and J. E. Raven, *The Presocratic Philosophers* (Cambridge, 1962), p. 234 (Aetios of Amida V, 30, 1). Jones, "Philosophy and Medicine in Ancient Greece," Supplement No. 8 to the *Bulletin of the History of Medicine* (Baltimore, 1946), p. 4, states that Alcmaeon was connected with those Pythagoreans who, early in the history of the brotherhood, substituted a doctrine of opposites for the Pythagorean doctrine of numbers. It is possible, however, that Alcmaeon was not a Pythagorean at all. Aristotle contrasts him with the Pythagoreans (*Metaphysics* 986a 22ff.).

[2] F. M. Cornford, *Plato's Cosmology* (London, 1956), p. 333.

[3] Diogenes Laertius, *Lives of the Philosophers,* VIII, 83.

[4] Jones, *Medical Writings of Anonymus Londinensis,* cap. XX: 24.

[5] K II 110. Wellmann, *Die Fragmente der Sykelischen Aerzte,* p. 75.

[6] *Ibid.,* pp. 69ff.

[7] *Ibid.,* Philistion Fr. 2 (Epist. II, 314D)

[8] See, in particular, *Nature of Man,* cap. XV (Jones, IV, 39).

[9] *Nature of Man,* cap. VI (Jones, IV, 17).

[10] *Affections,* cap. 18 (VI, 229, L.): the body is abnormally hot or cold. *Affections,* cap. 24 (VI, 237, L.): the food in the stomach is unnaturally heated by the stomach.

[11] *Sacred Disease,* caps. XIV and XVII (Jones, II, 169, 175): the brain is unnaturally moist. *Regimen I,* cap. XXXV (Jones, IV, 283): the physician can prescribe a regimen which will make a man "more intelligent and sharper than natural endowment warrants."

[12] *Nature of Man,* cap. II (Jones, IV, 7). The Menon Papyrus also alludes to this concept: "of psychic affections some are according to nature and others are contrary to nature." The editor views this as a reference to the Cnidian School (Jones, *Medical Writings of Anonymus Londinensis,* p. 27).

[13] In the works, *On Joints* and *On Fractures,* which we would assign to Group I and would have discussed in this connection if they contained any therapeutic theory, the term, *para physin,* is used for dislocations, broken bones, and torn muscles (*On Joints,* cap. 31: Jones, III, 257; *On Fractures,* cap. 42: Jones, III, 189). In the *Aphorisms para physin* is used twice in the sense of "unnaturally" thin or fat (V: 44, 46: Jones, IV, 169, 171) and once with the apparent meaning of internal "unnatural" bleeding from a wound (VI: 20: Jones, IV, 185). The contrast is fundamental between these uses of *para physin* and its use to describe an invisible physiological process.

[14] The sources for the Egyptian doctrine of medicine are: Robert O. Steuer, "Whdw: Aetiological Principle of Pyaemia in Ancient Egyptian Medicine," Supplement No. 10 to *Bulletin of the History of Medicine* (Baltimore, 1948); J. B. de C.M. Saunders, *The Transition from Ancient Egyptian to Greek Medicine* (Lawrence, Kansas, 1963); J.B. de C.M. Saunders and Robert O. Steuer, *Ancient*

Egyptian and Cnidian Medicine: the Relationship of their Aetiological Concepts of Disease (Berkeley, California, 1959).

[15] Steuer and Saunders, *Ancient Egyptian and Cnidian Medicine,* pp. 18, 25.

[16] Herodotos, II, 77.

[17] Jones, *Medical Writings of Anonymus Londinensis,* cap. IX: 12.

[18] K XVIIA 886.

[19] Jones, *Medical Writings of Anonymus Londinensis,* cap. IV: 3.

[20] *Ibid.,* cap. V: 4.

[21] Wellmann, Philistion Fr. 3 (Diogenes Laertius, VIII, 86-91).

[22] Steuer and Saunders, *Ancient Egyptian and Cnidian Medicine,* p. 16.

[23] *Affections* (VI, 227, 229, 231, 233, 235, L.). Chapter 21 of *Affections* (VI, 231, L.), a parallel passage from *Diseases III,* cap. 14 (VII, 135, L.), and one from *RAD II,* cap. VII (II, 419, L.) are the only references to fecal matter as an etiological agent in the works of Groups I, II, III, or IV.

[24] *Affections,* cap. 31 (VI, 243, L.).

[25] *Diseases II,* caps. 16, 41, 43 (VII, 31, 59, 61, L.). *Diseases III,* caps, 2, 3 (VII, 119, 121, L.).

[26] *Diseases I,* caps. 12, 13, 14, 15, 17, *et passim* (VI, 161, 163, 165, 171, L.).

[27] *Diseases II,* caps 2, 32, 64 (VII, 9, 49, 99, L.). *Internal Diseases,* cap. 10: corrupted phlegm (*sussepetai to phlegma*), cap. 41: corrupted bile (*chole sapiesa*), cap. 49: corrupted phlegm *(phlegmatos sapentos)* (VII, 191, 267, 289, L.).

[28] *Internal Diseases,* caps. 4, 9, 10 (VII, 179, 187, 191, L.). *Diseases II, passim.*

[29] The Cnidian work, *Diseases IV,* is heavily influenced by the Egyptian doctrine.

[30] Jones, *Medical Writings of Anonymus Londinensis,* cap. XX: 24.

[31] *Timaeus,* 83A and B: *diephtharmena.*

[32] Jones, *Medical Writings of Anonymus Londinensis*, caps. XVII and XVIII.

[33] Cap. VI (Jones, I, 83).

[34] Jones, *Medical Writings of Anonymus Londinensis,* cap. XIII: 18. Also, Steuer and Saunders, *Ancient Egyptian and Cnidian Medicine,* p. 30.

[35] *Regimen III,* caps. 69-85 (Jones, IV, 381-419).

[36] Jones, II, xxix. *Prorrhetic I,* sec. 59, 102, 133, 153 (V, 524ff., L.).

[37] *Ancient Medicine,* caps. III, XIV (Jones, I, 19, 37).

[38] J. Ilberg maintains that the Cnidian Sentences were based on a bile-phlegm physiology ("Die Aerzteschule von Cnidos," p. 16).

[39] It will be seen that our interpretation of the development of Cnidian medicine differs from that of the most recent writer on this school (I.M. Lonie, "The Cnidian Treatises of the Corpus Hippocraticum," *Classical Quarterly,* N.S. XV [1965], No. 1, 1-30). Lonie points out with insight that the Cnidian works combine two inconsistent doctrines: "it is significant that bile and phlegm in the Cnidian treatises show distinct signs of a double and inconsistent use: on the one hand they are treated as *dynameis,* while on the other they are opposed to the *dynameis* which act upon them" (pp. 4-5, note 3). Lonie, however, maintains that the latter–etiological–formulation of Cnidian humoralism is the original doctrine of the Cnidian Sentences, and that the development within this school was from an etiologically oriented approach to one which was non-etiological and therapeutically pragmatic. We maintain the opposite. Lonie's views are based

upon a very different reading of the Cnidian works themselves. For instance, he regards *Internal Diseases* as characterized by a "comparative indifference to aetiology" (p. 3), while we regard it as the Cnidian work most characterized by etiological speculation.

[40] Schoener, "Das Viererschema in der antiken Humoralpathologie," p. 6.

[41] *Nature of Man*, cap. II (Jones, IV, 7).

[42] *Ancient Medicine*, caps. XIII, XV (Jones, I, 35, 41).

[43] Celsus, *De Medicina, Prooemium*, 8. Our translation differs slightly from that of the Loeb edition and relies on a variant reading in one of the manuscripts: *"Hippocrates Cous, primus ex omnibus memoria dignis . . .* " (Friedrich Marx, CML, Vol. I: *A. Cornelii Celsi Quae Supersunt*, Leipzig, 1915, p. 18). Marx and W.G. Spencer prefer *dignus* which deprives Hippocrates of credit as the "first" to separate medicine from philosophy.

[44] Pliny, *Natural History*, XXVI, vi.

[45] Jones, *Hippocrates and the Corpus Hippocraticum*, p. 16.

[46] *Loc. cit.*

[47] *Ibid.*, p. 16.

[48] Lonie, "The Hippocratic Treatise *Peri Diaites Okseon*," pp. 50-79.

[49] Note its very involved discussion of compound medicines, its tendency to adduce physiological explanations and rationalizations for the use of such medicines (caps. LIX, LXI, LXII, etc.: Jones, II, 115-119), and the use of the word, *dynamis*, to mean the power of a remedy (cap. XXXVII)–the only such use of the word in Group I.

[50] Particularly in the relatively greater prominence of the theory of coction (caps. 8, 10, 11, 14: II, 431, 451, 461, 471, L.) and the unstructured humoralism of the whole work.

[51] We have in mind the physiological speculation of *RAD II*. In our view, a passage such as "*causus* is produced, most of the time, by a forced march and by a prolonged thirst, which causes the small veins to dry up and attract sharp and hot fluxes" (cap. 1) could never have been written by the author of *RAD I*. See also *RAD II*, caps, 4, 5, 6 (II, 403-417, L.). Lonie notes the resemblance between *RAD II*, cap. I, and the Cnidian doctrines ("The Hippocratic Treatise Peri Diaites Okseon," p. 65).

CHAPTER III

ARISTOTLE

After the Hippocratic Corpus itself the most important influence on Western medical thought, ancient and modern, has been the philosophy of Aristotle. In the ancient world this influence was manifested in the Rationalist ideology, and, to the extent that Rationalist elements have remained embedded in the medical speculation of more modern times, Aristotle's influence remains potent to this day.

Aristotelian philosophy is hence of primordial importance for the history of therapeutic method. Since he was not primarily a medical thinker, however, and since whole libraries have been written on all aspects of his thought, we can only indicate briefly the general outline of this philosophy, emphasizing the elements which are of particular significance for medicine.

Our first task is to trace the parallels between Aristotelianism and Rationalist medical thought. These parallels are found in two areas: (1) the observation and analysis of the phenomena of health and disease, and (2) the structure of the medical *tekhne.* In both of these areas the Rationalist physicians leaned heavily on Aristotle.

In a sense our task will be complete when we have indicated Aristotle's influence on the Rationalists, since this medical tradition was the vehicle of his influence on later generations. However, this would not be doing justice to Aristotle himself, since his own views on medical subjects differ considerably from those of the Rationalists. To summarize a great part of the ensuing discussion, we may note that Rationalist medicine stems primarily from

Aristotle's metaphysical analysis of reality but that Aristotle's specifically medical views have little in common with his metaphysics (and are, in fact, closer to Empiricism).

Like any philosophy, that of Aristotle is an effort to reconcile *logos* and experience. The polarity seen in the Hippocratic Corpus—the stress on experience in Groups I and IV vs. emphasis on the *logos* in group III—is fundamental also to Aristotelianism. In his early writings, when he was still under the influence of Plato, he gravitated toward the pole of *logos,* while the works of his maturity reveal an increasingly high evaluation of experience.[1] But the conflict is inherent in all of his writings.

It is particularly significant for his discussion of medicine. For he was the son of a physician and had himself received medical training. Therefore, although his medical doctrine contains a large theoretical component, he is fully aware of the importance of experience for medical practice. This awareness leads him to support the therapeutic principles of the Hippocratic works of Groups I and IV. The concept of coction is fundamental to his medical views, and he even broadens it to cover new areas of physiology.

Since his analytical and metaphysical doctrines are in the tradition of Plato and Greek Idealism, and thus continue the trends reflected in the Hippocratic works of Group III, we may state that there is a dichotomy between Aristotle's metaphysics and his views on the practice of medicine.

We will discuss this dichotomy in connection with Aristotle's physiology, his theory of disease and health, and his doctrine of the medical *tekhne.*

Aspects of Aristotle's Philosophical System

The starting-point of Aristotle's philosophy is the conviction, inherited from Plato, that the visible world is merely the reflection and the evanescent embodiment of another world. Like his great predecessor he takes a dualistic view of physical reality, and in the light of this assumption of a division between the visible external world and another world lying above or beyond it we may understand both his principal philosophical doctrines and the relevance of his philosophy to Rationalist medicine.[a]

Plato had called this other world the abode of the Ideas. To him the Ideas were eternal and unchanging, while the visible world represented their shifting and distorted reflection. Plato's philosophy, however, failed to explain how the Ideas were able to generate matter, and this was the problem which Aristotle set out to resolve.

How was a connection to be established between the Idea and the visible object? Aristotle's solution was to abolish the separate world of the Ideas and to convert the Ideas into "forms" potentially present beneath the visible surface of matter. The sense-perceptible was thereby hypothesized as a battlefield between "form" and matter. The "forms" endeavor to assert or realize themselves against the drag and inertia of matter, and Aristotle's philosophy is an analysis of this interaction.

The components of Aristotle's metaphysical universe are bound together by cause-and-effect relations. The physical objects are "caused" or produced by the underlying forms. Within the hierarchy of forms—running from the more universal to the less universal, the particular—there are relations of cause and effect, as the more universal generate the less universal. And, finally, knowing itself is a causal process: the forms or causes operating behind the sense-perceptible surface of the physical world generate or cause

[a]It will be noted that, although we hope to give Aristotle's "intellectual love for the objects of experience" its due, we nonetheless take the position that the effect of his thought on medicine was to strengthen the existing Platonic tendencies. The dualism which he shares with Plato is the most significant aspect of his philosophy for medical thought. Thus we follow those authors who take a somewhat "platonizing" view of Aristotle. Glenn Morrow writes in *Journal of Philosophy*, LIX (1962), p. 151: "Call it a remnent of Platonism or what you will, we find Aristotle eventually asserting that Being is more fundamental than Becoming and grounding his naturalism in a higher order of eternals and unchangeables".

their reflections in the human mind. "Men do not think that they know a thing till they have grasped the 'why' of it (which is to grasp its primary cause)."[2] In the mind the forms are reflected as "concepts" linked together by judgments—the judgment being defined as the assertion of a relationship or absence of relationship between two concepts. As there is a hierarchy of forms, from the more universal to the less universal, so there is also a hierarchy of judgments, those of lesser universality being deduced syllogistically from those of greater universality.

The movement of thought therefore parallels the movement of reality. As external reality consists of a hierarchy of causally related forms, so knowledge consists of a hierarchy of judgments about causes. "Just as *in rerum natura* the universal or conceptually defined essence is the cause or ground of definition of the particular, so also the ultimate task of an explanatory science consists in deriving the single from the universal and thereby in attaining the conceptual necessity of the empirically actual. Scientific explanation consists in understanding the perceptually known from its causes. It is the reproduction by the process of knowledge—in the relationship of ground and consequent—of the real relationship of the universal cause to its particular result."[b]

The variety of relationships and modes of being in nature is thus limited to what can be encompassed by formal logic: "The kinds of essential being are precisely those that are indicated by the figures of predication; for the senses of 'being' are just as many as these figures."[c]

[b]Wilhelm Windelband, *A History of Ancient Philosophy* (New York, 1956), pp. 249-250. Jaeger states that Aristotle "had broken up the old ontologic—the only form of logic known to Pre-Aristotelian philosophy—once and for all into the elements Word (*logos*) and Thing (*on*). The bond between them had to be restored somehow, and this was done by means of the conception of formal cause, which was at once conception and thing, ground of knowing and ground of being" (*Aristotle*, p. 370).

[c]*Metaphysics* 1017a 23-25. Windelband writes: "The highest presupposition, even if not expressly formulated by Aristotle, is the identity of the forms of apprehending thought with the forms of relationship belonging to actuality"

Another corollary of Aristotle's dualism is the relative unimportance of sense-perception. The senses perceive only the external visible world, and thus they take in only a mixed conglomerate of matter and form.[3] This is not the reality of the forms. The world of the forms is the "real" world in that it is the permanent and rational world, the world which is significant for philosophical and scientific discourse. Since sense-perception is only of matter, it cannot be a direct source of scientific or philosophical knowledge.[d]

Knowledge of the universal forms, i.e., the implanting of the concepts in the mind, is through a mediated sense-perception. Aristotle writes in a famous passage:

> So out of sense-perception comes to be what we call memory, and out of frequently repeated memories of the same thing develops experience; for a number of memories constitute a single experience. From experience again—i.e., from the universal now stabilized in its entirety in the soul, the one beside the many which is a single identity within them all—originate the skill of the craftsman and the knowledge of the man of science, skill

(*History of Ancient Philosophy,* p. 250). John Herman Randall states: "The Greek language . . . is a perfect expression of the world's intelligibility. The structure of the Greek language and the structure of the world are ultimately the same, because the Greek language is a natural instrument for knowing and expressing the world's structure" (*Aristotle* [New York, 1960], p. 7). Ernst Kapp notes that Greek logic developed out of techniques of oral instruction; thus the subject-matter of this philosophy reflects such pedagogical techniques as definition, syllogism, and induction. From there it was only a step to assuming that the reality described by these techniques was identical with the subject-matter of the philosophy (Ernst Kapp, *Greek Foundations of Traditional Logic* [New York, 1942]). Also, George Boas, *Some Assumptions of Aristotle,* Transactions of the American Philosophical Society, New Series, Part 6 (Philadelphia, 1959), p. 23.

[d]Scientific knowledge is not possible through the act of perception. Even if perception as a faculty is of 'the such' and not merely of a 'this somewhat', yet one must at any rate actually perceive a 'this somewhat', and at a definite present place and time: but that which is commensurately universal and true in all cases one cannot perceive, since it is not 'this' and it is not 'now'; if it were, it would not be commensurately universal . . ." *Posterior Analytics* 87b 27-33.

> in the sphere of coming to be and science in the sphere of being.
>
> We conclude that these states of knowledge are neither innate in a determinate form, nor developed from other higher states of knowledge, but from sense-perception. It is like a rout in battle stopped by first one man making a stand and then another, until the original formation has been restored. The soul is so constituted as to be capable of this process.
>
> (*Posterior Analytics* 100a 4-14)

The soul is capable of this process because there is a super-sense or common sense in the heart—"the common sensorium belonging to all the sense organs"—which can in some mysterious way filter the universal form out of the series of percepts.[4][e] Once grasped, these concepts can be manipulated by the intellect (*nous*), defined as "the part of the soul with which the soul knows and thinks."[5] It is possession of the *nous* which distinguishes man from animal, and by superior development of the *nous* the educated man is distinguished from the uneducated, the natural aristocrat from the slave.[6]

Thus, although the senses yield information which enables the observer to attain to knowledge of the world of the forms, sense-perception alone cannot do this. Scientific knowledge is obtained from the operations of the intellect. Repeated observation can only reinforce a conclusion of the intellect—and cannot take its place.

An important corollary of Aristotle's dualism is the unimportance of the accidental. Only the regular—that which happens all of the time or for the most part—has reality and rationality. Events and phenomena which are unpredictable, which happen only sporadically and without any pattern, are

[e]As Boas (*Some Assumptions of Aristotle,* p. 18) has pointed out, this doctrine is illogical. If the universal is present in each percept, why are several percepts needed? The universal is not, after all, a statistical average of the individual percepts.

due to chance—which Aristotle posits as a separate category of causation. Chance is outside the four classes of causes (material, efficient, formal, and final) upon which his philosophy draws and is thus relegated to a sort of limbo.[7] Chance happenings are due to the capacity of matter to distort and inhibit the development of the forms, and it is the logical processes of the forms which are of philosophical and scientific interest.

The dichotomy between what is rational and what is accidental is paralleled by the distinction between the "natural" and the "unnatural." Whatever occurs all of the time or most of the time, i.e., whatever conforms to an underlying logical pattern, is natural, and chance events are unnatural.[f]

As the one general principle underlying the whole of his logic and method Aristotle posits the principle of contradiction—meaning that a concept or combination of concepts cannot be both affirmed and denied at the same time, or, in the metaphysical realm, that "it is impossible for anyone to believe the same thing to be and not to be."[8] This principle is the point of departure of all proof and explanation and as such is itself unprovable.

Implications of Aristotelianism for the Rationalist Observation and Interpretation of Disease

The purpose of any philosophy is to simplify the meaning of experience—to make experience intelligible. The danger of such an undertaking, however, is that experience will be thereby oversimplified:

> We have to distinguish here between the needs of cognition and the needs of that which is cognized.

[f]Nature leaves nothing to chance" (*De Coelo* 290a 31). "Nature is no wanton or random creator" (*De Coelo* 291b 14). "No natural fact can originate in chance" (*De Coelo* 301a 11). See Boas, *Some Assumptions of Aristotle*, pp. 16, 35.

> Apparently the latter can tolerate so great a diversity of kinds and manners that imprecise writers often call it infinite. It need not be infinite in any literal sense to be highly bewildering to the lovers of simplicity. But it is, regardless of that, very great. Knowledge itself is the simplifier, not God or nature. They are the complicators.
>
> As long as we think of cognition as a reflection of the objective order, then our cognitive simplifications will be thought of as the uncovering of an underlying arrangement of things. But that arrangement may be nothing more than a projection of our technique of classification into our subject-matter.[9]
>
> Aristotle's methodological assumptions were bound to end in a distinction between the rational and the surd, just as any others would. The rational became whatever his method could handle; the surd all the rest.[10]
>
> Subject matters will take on a character which is inevitably determined by the method used to study them . . .[11]

By imposing a logical order upon the diversity and variety of the physician's experience Aristotle greatly simplified this experience. And the Rationalist physicians followed in his footsteps.

As we noted in the Introduction, the elemental data of the physician's experience are the patient's symptoms. We noted also that the Empirical tradition has stressed symptomatic knowledge while the Rationalists seek the entity assumed to lie hidden behind the "veil" of the symptoms.

This instinctive urge of medical Rationalism was supported and encouraged by the Aristotelian philosophy.

The fundamental dichotomy in Aristotelianism between the world of sense-perception and the underlying reality of the forms became in medicine a dichotomy between the organism (with its sense-perceptible symptoms) and the disease conceived as an entity inhering in the organism. The *aition*, the (material) proximate cause of disease whose emergence we have traced above—especially in *Breaths, Sacred Disease*, and *Nature of Man*—took on an added dimension under the impact of the Aristotelian fusion of "form" and "cause." The result was identification of the proximate cause with the disease "form" or "entity." Just as the forms beneath the surface of objects have a reality in some ways superior to that of the objects themselves, so the invisible disease forms or entities became more real to the physician than the sick body of the patient.

Thus, depicting the disease as an entity within the patient's body led inexorably to a preference for physiological or pathological knowledge over symptomatic—a tendency which was strengthened by Aristotle's own copious biological investigations. The symptoms suffered a bizarre fate. No longer were all of the patient's symptoms worthy of consideration (for what they revealed about the process of coction)—only those regarded as causally linked to the disease entity.[g] These were the "genuine" symptoms, while the others possessed a lesser degree of legitimacy.

Although this development cannot be justified logically—since who can say that one symptom is more or less important than another? who can justify the proposition that some symptoms have no causal relation to the patient's illness?—it is psychologically quite comprehendable: the idea that "disease" is an entity leads the physician to seek this entity in every case presenting similar symptoms. Eventually certain symptoms come to be accepted as those most frequently associated with the given disease entity, and this provides the basis for relegating to oblivion the symptoms which appear less frequently. The decision to reject the "unimportant" symptoms is made easier by the Aristotelian distinction between the "form" and the visible reality, and the consequent denigration of sense-perception as a path to

[g]The idea that "chance" is a separate causal category may have contributed to the physician's willingness to disregard some of the symptoms.

knowledge. Just as in philosophy the *nous* can apprehend the "form" beneath the surface, so in medicine can the physician's *nous* perceive the disease "form" beneath the changing pattern of the symptoms.

A doctrine of signs—whereby the symptoms might be connected with the underlying disease reality—was required for the full development of this trend in medical thought, and such a doctrine seems to have been supplied by Stoicism. While Aristotle confined his discussion of signs to those of the "commemorative" variety (i.e., indicating that which in itself is potentially visible),[12] the Stoics extended the doctrine of signs to include "indicative" signs—i.e., those indicating something which is not in itself potentially visible but is known and discovered only through the *logos*.[h]

The outcome was heightened emphasis on the disease entity, i.e., on pathology, at the expense of the symptoms, and neglect of the peculiar features of the individual case in favor of the idea that diseases fall into logically discriminable classes. Aristotle states quite forthrightly that medicine does not deal with individual cases but with classes of disease: "the physician does not prescribe what is healthy for a single eye, but for all eyes, or for a determinate species of eye."[13] "None of the arts theorize about individual cases. Medicine, for instance, does not theorize about what will help to cure Socrates or Callias, but only about what will help to cure any or all of a given class of patients; this alone is its business. Individual cases are so infinitely varied that no systematic knowledge of them is possible."[14] Only the symptoms which were recognized as forming part of a disease "form" or entity

[h]The only source for this Stoic doctrine is Sextus Empiricus who states (*Against the Mathematicians,* VIII, 143ff.): "the indicative signal, on the contrary, can never be observed in connection with the object signified, since what is not observable is *a fortiori* not observable in connection with something else. The soul is an example of something that is naturally nonevident, for it never presents itself to our clear perception. Nevertheless, it is indicated, or signified indicatively, by the bodily motions. For we 'reason' that the body has a kind of internal power to manifest such motions." On this see Benson Mates, *Stoic Logic* (Berkeley, 1953), pp. 13-14; R. F. Hicks, *Stoic and Epicurean* (New York, 1962), p. 392.

had a right to recognition, to reality; these symptoms, and the diseases of which they formed a part, were "real," and all others were accidental—due to chance.[i]

The infinite symptoms were thereby reduced to a logically ordered classification of disease entities. The Rationalist physician no longer observed all the symptoms. He saw only those which were logically significant in the light of his preconceived disease categories. Aristotelianism provided him with a path through the thicket of the symptoms straight to the underlying disease entity.

This same Aristotelian analysis also yields the key to therapy. As the principle of contradiction governs Aristotle's analysis of the physical world, so the doctrine of contraries is the key to Rationalist therapeutics.

The metaphysical significance of the doctrine of contraries becomes readily apparent if one recalls the dualism of Aristotle's philosophy.

This philosophy aims to reconcile in a higher synthesis the contradictions of sense-perception. The physician follows the same procedure. He reduces the complexity of disease to a finite set of logical categories: heat, cold, wetness, and dryness. He abstracts the very same qualities from the medicines and foods which he uses for treatment. When the disease is acted upon by the medicine of opposite quality, it

[i]The concepts, "natural" and "unnatural", also figure here. In several passages Aristotle suggests that health is "natural" and disease is "unnatural" (*Metaphysics* 1044b 34: *Physics* 230b 5-6; *Generation of Animals* 777a 12-22). Jaeger suggests that in his later writings Aristotle altered the meaning of "natural." Instead of denoting the Platonic ideal of health, it came to encompass certain settled disease categories, "pathological phenomena which occur with a certain regularity." Thus, perhaps, "patients alter naturally or unnaturally according as they throw off fevers on the critical days or not" (*Physics* 230b 5-6). If Jaeger is correct, it means that the Rationalist urge to classify symptoms into disease classes was strengthened by the decision to characterize these categories as "natural." See Jaeger, *Aristotle, Fundamentals of the History of His Development*, p. 415.

Aristotle's use of "natural" in both senses is, in any case, to be contrasted with the idea of "natural" in the Group I Hippocratic works—where disease and health are equally "natural" in being two ends of the same continuum.

disappears, since "it is impossible that contrary attributes should belong at the same time to the same subject."[15]

An illustration of the importance of the principle of contradiction to Aristotle, and a further illustration of the doctrinal opposition between the works of Group I and Group III, is provided by the contrast between Aristotle and Heracleitus. Heracleitus who, as we have noted, seems to have provided the philosophical inspiration for the Hippocratic works of Groups I and IV, took the opposite approach to the analysis of physical reality—asserting the possibility of coexistence of opposed qualities and attributes. "They understand not how that which is at variance with itself agrees with itself; there is attunement of opposite tensions, like that of the bow and the harp."[16] "The road up and the road down is one and the same."[17] "The beginning and the end are common."[18] "Living and dead are the same, and so are awake and asleep, young and old. The former when shifted are the latter, and again the latter when shifted are the former."[19] His holistic philosophy glories in the contradictions of sense-perception instead of trying to synthesize them. Thus Heracleitus asserts an opposition between formal and scientific truth. This is the point of his famous statement: "you could not step twice into the same river; for other waters are ever flowing onto you."[20] By the same token he claims that the sun is new every day.[21] The categories, "river" and "sun," have an ever-changing content.

Aristotle's reaction to Heracleitus is what we might expect. He maintains the identity of logical and scientific truth; thus the sun is not new every day but is always the same since the category, "sun," is unchanging. Aristotle even denies that Heracleitus could have rejected the principle of contradiction: "it is impossible for any one to believe the same thing to be and not to be, as some think Heracleitus says. For what a man says, he does not necessarily believe . . . obviously it is impossible for the same man at the same time to believe the same thing to be and not to be."[22]

Elsewhere he suggests that the Heracleitean thesis is advanced merely "for the sake of argument."[23]

In the Hippocratic works of Group I the parallel to Heracleitus' conviction that reality is internally contradictory is the physician's conviction that the organism is not knowable in itself and can be known only through its external sense-perceptible manifestations.[j] The view that disease is a process involving the whole organism reflects the holism of Heracleitus and his interpretation of physical reality as a process.[k]

This contrasts with the Group III doctrine that the physician's task is to analyze the holism of the organism and resolve its contradictions.

Physiology and Therapeutics

Aristotle's philosophical analysis of physical reality—the search for the causes producing the visible phenomena—has as its medical corollary the physiological analysis of the organism, and his successors did indeed apply themselves to physiological and anatomical research.[24] Aristotle himself, however, is ambiguous. For while his writings encourage logical analysis of the organism and by implication favor such logical analysis as the basis for medical practice, his actual discussion of medical practice has little or nothing in common with his own logical analysis. In fact, Aristotle reverts to the Group I tradition of the Hippocratic Corpus—the theory of coction—for his discussion of therapeutics. The two sides of his intellect are thus reflected in his medical writings: the Empirical side in his emphasis on the theory of

[j] Heracleitus also observed: "Nature [the *physis*] is wont to hide herself." "The Lord whose is the oracle in Delphi neither declares nor hides, but sets forth by signs" (Jones, *Hippocrates,* IV, 473).

[k] G. S. Kirk seems to conclude that Heracleitus regarded the world as explicable because it is "essentially one," but this is hardly acceptable. All holistic philosophies maintain that physical reality is not knowable or explicable directly, only indirectly or allegorically (see G. S. Kirk, *Heracleitus: The Cosmic Fragments* [Cambridge, 1962], p. 402).

coction, the logical side in his willingness to investigate and analyze human and animal physiology.

* * * *

An examination of Aristotle's physiology shows that—consonant with his habit of doing justice to the views of his predecessors—he mixes together the Empedoclean postulate that the organism is composed of substantive elements and the teaching of Alcmaeon that the organism consists of insubstantial *dynameis,* in a way which is very reminiscent of Philistion's treatment of the same themes.[25]

> Now there are three degrees of composition; and of these the first in order, as all will allow, is composition out of what some call the elements such as earth, air, water, fire. Perhaps, however, it would be more accurate to say composition out of the elementary forces [*dynameis*]; nor indeed out of all of them, but out of a limited number of them, as defined in previous treatises. For fluid and solid, hot and cold, form the material of all composite bodies; and all other differences are secondary to these, such differences, that is, as heaviness or lightness, density or rarity, roughness or smoothness, and any other such properties of matter as there may be . . .
> (*Parts of Animals* 646a 13-20)

Interestingly, while Aristotle is willing to agree with Alcmaeon that the components of the organism are immaterial, he will not agree that they are unlimited in number. In fact, the *dynameis* are reduced also to a mere four, and these are associated logically with the four Empedoclean elements: "for fire is hot and dry, whereas air is hot and moist (air being a sort of aqueous vapor); and water is cold and moist, while earth is cold and dry. Thus the differences are reasonably distributed among the primary bodies, and the number of the latter is consonant with theory."[26] Aristotle is not willing to accept the full Empirical physiology—that the components of the organism are both immaterial *and* infinite in number.[1]

Aristotle draws general parallels between these four elements and the four traditional humors: blood is "essentially hot"[27] or hot and fluid;[28] phlegm is cold[29] and moist;[30] dark bile is naturally cold;[31] bile possesses some heat;[32] yellow bile is hot.[33] He also analyzes the various organs of the body in terms of these elements: the brain is the coldest organ;[34] it is also dry;[35] the bone marrow is hot.[36] The youthful organism is more hot and wet, while the older organism is more cold and dry.[37] Health is "a blending of hot and cold elements within the body in due proportion, in relation either to one another or to the surrounding atmosphere."[38]

This sort of analysis is not a very pronounced feature of his physiological writings, however. And he guards against the excessive abstraction of later Rationalist thought by his doctrine of the three levels of composition of the body: the first level consisting of the four elements, the second level being the homogeneous parts, and the third level being the heterogeneous parts. The homogeneous parts are made up of combinations of the four elements: thus blood and milk are composed of earth and water,[39] while fat contains a good deal of air.[40] The heterogeneous parts—the face, the hands,

[1]He criticizes this very tendency in Alcmaeon: "Certain others of the Pythagoreans assert that the principles are ten, namely those of the parallel series of opposites: limit, unlimited; odd, even; one and multitude; right and left; male and female; rest and motion; straight and curved; light and darkness; good and bad; square and oblong. A similar view was apparently adopted by Alcmaeon of Croton. He either took this doctrine from the Pythagoreans or they took it from him. For Alcmaeon was a young man when Pythagoras was old, and his doctrine was similar to that of the Pythagoreans. For he says that most human matters go in pairs, not referring to opposites that were *limited,* like the Pythagorean opposites, but to *any that he happened to observe,* e.g., white, black, sweet, bitter, good, bad, great, small. About the other opposites Alcmaeon made only random suggestions, but the Pythagoreans clearly defined the *number* and nature of them. By both, however, we are told that the opposites are the first principles of existence" (*Metaphysics* 986a 23-986b 1). The translation of this passage is from Jones, "Philosophy and Medicine in Ancient Greece." p. 4.

the feet—are, in turn, composed of mixtures of the homogeneous parts. Knowledge of the four elements alone is not enough:

> But if men and animals and their several parts are natural phenomena, then the natural philosopher must take into consideration not merely the ultimate substances of which they are made, but also flesh, bone, blood, and all the other homogeneous parts; not only these, but also the heterogeneous parts, such as face, hand, foot; and must examine how each of these comes to be what it is, and in virtue of what force. For to say what are the ultimate substances out of which an animal is formed, to state, for instance, that it is made of fire or earth, is no more sufficient than would be a similar account in the case of a couch or the like.
>
> (*Parts of Animals* 640b 18-23)

Pneumatism is an important element of Aristotle's philosophy,[41] and his discussion of the generation of diseases contains passages reminiscent of *Breaths* or *Sacred Disease:*

> Tetanus and spasms are motions of wind, and their force is such that the united efforts of many men do not succeed in overcoming the movements of the patients.
>
> (*Meteorologica* 366b 25-28)

> Sleep is like epilepsy, and, in a sense, actually is a seizure of this sort. Accordingly, the beginning of this malady takes place with many during sleep, and their subsequent habitual seizures occur in sleep, not in waking hours. For when the spirit moves upwards in a volume, on its return downwards it distends the veins, and forcibly compresses the passage through which respiration is effected.
>
> (*De Somno et Vigilia* 457a 9-14)

But his writings contain none of the exaggerated humoralism characteristic of the later Rationalist tradition and such as is found even in the Group III Hippocratic works. He even warns that man does not possess extensive knowledge of physiology and must investigate the anatomy of animals in order to acquire it.[42]

Furthermore, his humoralism is subordinated to a general and pervasive theory of coction. The analytical dimension of his physiological thinking is held in check by the empirical.

In terms of the four elements, coction is defined as the process through which the two active qualities—heat and cold, act upon the two passive qualities—the dry and the moist, drying and ripening the substance and making it denser.[43]

> True becoming, that is, natural change, is always the work of these powers, and so is the corresponding natural destruction . . . When the hot and the cold are masters of the matter, they generate a thing; but if they are not, and the failure is partial, the object is imperfectly boiled or otherwise unconcocted.
>
> (*Meteorologica* 378b 29-379a 3)

Coction is a general process of nature, producing plants, animals, and even stones and metals.[44] In plants it is the equivalent of ripening "for we call it ripening when there is a concoction of the nutriment in fruit."[45] In man and the sanguineous animals the heart is the source of heat, and it is also the residence of the sensitive soul.[46] Aristotle thus posits the heart as the source of life, because it is the source of heat and the residence of the sensitive soul. Death occurs through loss of this heat, either through the natural aging process or artificially—the cause of death from wounds is the escape of the heat.[47]

In one major respect Aristotle adds to the Hippocratic theory of coction. While the Hippocratic works had not distinguished between the coction of morbific causes and the digestion of food in the stomach, Aristotle defines digestion as one form of coction (a proposition which generates ambiguity in the later development of Greek medicine):

> Now broiling and boiling are artificial processes, but the same general kind of thing, as we said, is found in the

> *physis* too. The affections produced are similar though they lack a name, for art imitates the *physis*. For instance, the concoction of food in the body is like boiling, for it takes place in a hot and moist medium and the agent is the heat of the body. So, too, certain forms of indigestion are like imperfect boiling.
> (*Meteorologica* 381b 3-9)

In fact, coction becomes a general principle of physiology, and the whole growth of the body is viewed by Aristotle as an extension of the digestive process. The embryo becomes male if the seed is properly concocted—otherwise female: "for when the first principle does not bear sway and cannot concoct the nourishment through lack of heat nor bring it into its proper form, but is defeated in this respect, then must needs the material which it works on change into its opposite. Now the female is opposite to the male."[48] And the development of the embryo and of the organism is also conditioned by digestion. The food is taken into the mouth where it is cut up into little bits to facilitate coction; thence it passes to the upper and lower abdominal cavities where the first stage of coction takes place—the food becomes ichor and then blood.[49] "In sanguineous animals the homogeneous or uniform part most universally found is the blood, and its habitat the vein."[50] By further coction of blood—in the liver, spleen, and kidneys—the lymph, fiber, flesh, bone, skin, membranes, fat, sinew, hair, nails, and the "excretions"—are formed.[51][m] "Each of the other parts is formed out of the nutriment, those most honorable and participating in the sovereign principle from the nutriment which is first and purest and fully concocted, those which are only necessary for the sake of the former parts from the inferior nutriment and the residues left over from the other."[52] "It is from the

[m] "By being fat [the kidneys] are the better enabled to secrete and concoct their fluid; for fat is hot, and it is heat that effects concoction" (*Parts of Animals* 672a 21-22). The liver and spleen are hot organs "owing to the blood which they contain" (*Ibid.*, 670a 22).

blood, when concocted and somehow divided up, that each part of the body is made."[53]

The "excretions" [*perittomata*], which are the end product of the whole process of coction, are dung, phlegm, yellow bile, and black bile.[54] Aristotle alters the humoralism of *Nature of Man* by assigning the blood a more noble place than the other three humors—a distinction which also causes confusion in the later Rationalist tradition.[n]

By examining the body's secreta and excreta the physician can tell whether or not coction has been successful—"that the proper heat has got the better of the indeterminate matter."[55] "The liquid and solid excreta and catarrhs are called raw . . . for in every case the word is applied to things because their heat has not got the mastery in them and compacted them."[56]

Diarrhoea is caused by insufficient coction of blood in the bowels.[57] "In the case of boils and phlegm, and the like, the process of ripening is the concoction of the moisture in them by their natural heat, for only that which gets the better of the matter can determine it."[58] "The spleen attracts the residual humors from the stomach and, owing to its bloodlike character, is enabled to assist in their concoction. Should, however, this residual fluid be too abundant, or the heat of the spleen too scanty, the body becomes sickly from over-repletion with nutriment. Often, too, when the spleen is affected by disease, the belly becomes hard owing to the reflux into it of the fluid."[59]

Aristotle is thus aware of the Egyptian doctrine, making a place for the "excretions" as the end product of coction. He elaborates on this elsewhere: "Concoction goes on in the upper belly, but the excretion putrefies in the lower."[60] Putrefaction is the "destruction of the peculiar and natural heat in any moist subject by external heat, that is, by the heat of the environment."[61] "Putrefaction and the thing putrefied is only a residue of that which is concocted."[62] He

[n]See below, p. 217; above, p. 116.

criticizes Empedocles who "either mistook the fact or made a bad metaphor when he composed the line: 'On the tenth day of the eighth month the milk comes into being, a white pus,' for putrefaction and coction are opposite things, and pus is a kind of putrefaction, but milk is concocted."[63]

This last passage, however, reveals a possible confusion in Aristotle's mind between the Egyptian doctrine and the Hippocratic doctrine of empyema (pus formation resulting from incomplete coction), as also the following: "blood, if it corrupt in the body, has a tendency to turn into pus, and pus may turn into a solid concretion."[64]

Consonant with his general view that disease is a disturbance of the process of coction, Aristotle posits as the principal remedy the production of warmth:

> The healthy subject is produced as a result of the following train of thought—since *this* is health, if the subject is to be healthy, *this* must first be present, e.g., a uniform state of body, and if this is to be present, there must be heat; and the physician goes on thinking thus until he reduces the matter to a final something which he himself can produce. Then the process from this point onward, i.e., the process toward health, is called a 'making'. . . . Of the productions or processes one part is called thinking and other making—that which proceeds from the starting-point and the form is thinking, and that which proceeds from the final step of the thinking is making. And each of the other, intermediate, things is produced in the same way. I mean, for instance, if the subject is to be healthy his bodily state must be made uniform. What then does being made uniform imply? This or that. And this depends on his being made warm. What does this imply? Something else. And this something is present potentially; and what is present potentially is already in the physician's power.
>
> (*Metaphysics* 1032b 6-22)

This warmth can be produced by rubbing or by means of hot baths.[65] Aristotle also mentions barley gruel as a suitable remedy in fever; presumably he follows the view of *Regimen in Acute Diseases* that this serves to promote coction.[66] Along the same lines is his prescription of rennet in diarrhoea. As we have noted, diarrhoea is due to unconcocted blood: "rennet . . . consists of milk *with an admixture of fire,* which comes from the natural heat of the animal as the milk is concocted . . . Rennet improves in quality the longer it is kept; and cow's rennet, after being kept a good while, and also hare's rennet, is good for diarrhoea, and the best of all rennet is that of the young deer."[67] For diarrhoea in elephants Aristotle prescribes "draughts of lukewarm water" or dipping their fodder in honey (in ancient times honey was classified as a hot and dry food).[68] White honey is a good salve for sore eyes and wounds (i.e., which require coction).[69]

Aristotle's writings also contain considerable discussion of the purely ad hoc ("empirical") remedies used by his contemporaries in diseases of humans and animals. Stall-reared horses have a disease in which they trail their hind legs under the belly so far as almost to fall back on the haunches; it may be useful to draw blood or castrate the male.[70] Walks are recommended for evacuating the bowels.[71] Bloodletting is advocated as a general procedure for alleviating pain.[72] [o] Powdered sea-urchin is a good remedy in strangury.[73] A certain disease in swine is treated by applying wine fomentations to the snout and by rinsing the nostrils with wine.[74] In a hoof disease in cattle the horny parts are smeared with warm pitch.[75] Tapeworm in swine is cured by feeding them spelt.[76]

What is interesting is that no logical justification is given by Aristotle for the use of these remedies. While occasionally

[o] Venesection for relief of pain is mentioned in *Diseases I,* cap. 28; *Affections,* cap. 2; *Diseases II,* caps. 16, 17, 26, 27; and *Diseases III,* caps. 1 and 8 (VI, 197, 211, L.; VII, 31, 41, 45, L.).

such an explanation can be devised by the reader, Aristotle does not give one himself; he seems to base his advocacy of these remedies on empirical experience and not on the doctrine of contraries.

This is odd, since his writings do contain occasional statements to the effect that the doctrine of contraries is the basis of therapeutics: "punishment . . . is a kind of cure, and it is the nature of cures to be effected by contraries."[77]

Nonetheless, Aristotle did not propose the doctrine of contraries as the basis of medical practice. This was the invention of his followers. His writings contain no discussion of therapeutics in terms of opposition between the *dynamis* of the remedy and the *dynamis* of the disease. His pupil, Theophrastus, who wrote a famous treatise on plants describing, among other things, their medicinal uses, also refrains from rationalizing these uses in terms of contraries.[78]

Aristotle thus occupies an unstable position between the views of Group I and those of Group III. While accepting, in principle, that the physician's duty was to conduct biological investigation, when it came to medical practice he supported the theory of coction. He did not base therapeutics on "opposition" to the disease cause but on the promotion of coction.[p]

The Structure of the Medical Tekhne

Aristotle's theory of the medical *tekhne* embodies the same conflict between an analytical and an experiential dimension that has been noted in connection with his physiology.

We may first examine his view that medicine is based upon the *logos,* as this was the interpretation of therapeutic method which the Rationalist tradition inherited from Aristotle.

[p]This may be why he calls Hippocrates "the Great" (*Politics* 1326a 15), in an apparent contrast to Plato's attitude.

Aristotle distinguishes pure science (*episteme*) from applied science or art (*tekhne*). The former is the reflection in the observer's mind of the causal processes of nature—of the way in which nature produces form out of undifferentiated matter. *Tekhne* is the body of knowledge governing the manner in which *man* produces.[79]

In their logical structure the *episteme* and the *tekhne* are identical.[q] The component principles of both are derived from experience and take the form of universal judgments.[80] Since the universal judgment embodies knowledge of causes, the *tekhne* is a body of knowledge about causes and effects in the sphere of human production.[81]

Aristotle distinguishes the *tekhne* which is carried on for its own sake from the one which is carried on for the sake of its product. Medicine falls in the latter category as it is carried on for the sake of producing health.[82] The production of health is in two stages: a mental one (*noesis*) and a physical one (*poiesis*), and the latter is based entirely on the former.[83] The idea or form in the mind of the artisan is the cause of the thing produced: "*tekhne* indeed consists in the conception of the result to be produced before its realization in the material."[84] To produce health the physician must have prior knowledge of the body and its mechanisms:

> The doctor has a knowledge of health and also of bile and phlegm in which health is realized.
>
> (*Physics* 194a 23-24)

> Physicians of culture and refinement make some mention of natural science and claim to derive their principles from it.
>
> (*De Respiratione* 480b 26-28)

> We may say of most physical inquirers, and of those physicians who study their art philosophically, that while the former complete their works with a disquisition on

[q]Thus, although Aristotle usually calls medicine a *tekhne*, he sometimes calls it an *episteme* (*Topics* 101b 10; *Eudemean Ethics* 1226a 35).

medicine, the latter usually base their medical theories on principles derived from physics.

(*De Sensu* 436a 20-436b 1)

. . . consider how the physician, or how the builder, sets about his work. He starts by forming for himself a definite picture, in one case perceptible to mind, in the other to sense, of his end—the physician of health, the builder of a house—and this he holds forward as the reason and explanation of each subsequent step that he takes . . . For if a house or other such final object is to be realized, it is necessary that such and such material shall exist; and it is necessary that first this and then that shall be produced, and first this and then that set in motion, and so on in continuous succession until the end and final result is reached, for the sake of which each prior thing is produced and exists. . . . For it is that which is yet to be—health, let us say, or a man—that, owing to its being of such and such characters, necessitates the preexistence or previous production of this and that antecedent and not this or that antecedent which, because it exists or has been generated, makes it necessary that health or a man is in, or shall come into, existence.

(*Parts of Animals* 639b 16-640a 8)

Such knowledge is obtained from biological investigation, and in this area Aristotle was a pioneer.[r]

Possessing this knowledge is not sufficient, however, as the physician must still be able to produce health. Aristotle

[r]We have not discussed the problem of whether or not Aristotle's method of biological and anatomical investigation is itself scientific (on this see W. H. Whewell, *The Philosophy of the Inductive Sciences: On the Philosophy of Discovery* [London, 1860], pp. 202-204). Ingemar Duering writes: "his reasoning is based on *a priori* principles and book-learning more than observation . . . he was perhaps to a far greater extent than we are sometimes inclined to believe a desk-work scholar . . . Everywhere in his biological writings we can see how he adapts his observations or his knowledge about various things to certain sets of preconceived ideas" ("Aristotle's Method in Biology," *Aristote et les Problemes de Methode* [Louvain and Paris, 1961], pp. 218-219).

notes that difficulties may arise with the production of health even though the physician has all the requisite knowledge:

> There are two things in which all well-being consists: one of them is the choice of a right end and aim of action, and the other the discovery of the actions which are means towards it; for the means and the end may agree or disagree. Sometimes the right end is set before men, but in practice they fail to attain it; in other cases they are successful in all the means, but they propose to themselves a bad end; and sometimes they fail in both. Take, for example, the art of medicine; physicians do not always understand the nature of health, and also the means which they use may not always effect the desired end. In all arts and sciences both the end and the means should be equally under our control.
> (*Politics* 1331b 26-37)

> Why do doctors deliberate about matters within their *episteme* but not grammarians? The reason is that error may occur in two ways (either in reasoning or in perception, when we are engaged in the very act), and in medicine one may go wrong in both ways, but in grammar one can do so only in respect of the perception and action.
> (*Eudemean Ethics* 1226a 34-38)

This question is discussed frequently by Aristotle, and, as the following passages indicate, he accepts the idea that "experience" is the guide to the production of health:

> And generally we observe that the possessor of medical knowledge is not necessarily healing, which shows that something else is required to produce action in accordance with knowledge: the knowledge alone is not the cause.
> (*De Anima* 433a 3-5)

> Even among doctors the best educated spend much labor on acquiring knowledge of the body.
> (*Nicomachean Ethics* 1102a 20-22)

> Even medical men do not seem to be made by a study of textbooks. Yet people try, at any rate, to state not only the treatments, but also how particular classes of people can be cured and should be treated—distinguishing the various habits of body; but while this seems useful to experienced people, to the inexperienced it is valueless.
> (*Nicomachean Ethics* 1181b 2-7)

> With a view to action experience seems in no respect inferior to art, and men of experience succeed even better than those who have theory without experience. (The reason is that experience is knowledge of individuals, art of universals, and actions and productions are all concerned with the individual; for the physician does not cure *man,* except in an incidental way, but Callias or Socrates or some other called by some such individual name, who happens to be a man. If then a man has the theory without the experience, and recognizes the universal but does not know the individual included in this, he will often fail to cure; for it is the individual that is to be cured).
> (*Metaphysics* 981a 13-24)

As is seen from the last passage, the concomitant of Aristotle's stress on the value of experience is emphasis on the individual patient. See further:

> Private education has an advantage over public, as private medical treatment has; for while in general rest and abstinence from food are good for a man in a fever, for a particular man they may not be; and a boxer presumably does not prescribe the same style of fighting to all his pupils.
> (*Nicomachean Ethics* 1180b 8-11)

> It is hard to see how a weaver or a carpenter will be benefited in regard to his own craft by knowing this "good itself," or how a man who has viewed the Idea itself will be a better doctor or general thereby. For a doctor seems not even to study health in this way, but the health of man or perhaps the health of a particular man; it is individuals that he is healing.
> (*Nicomachean Ethics* 1097a 8-14)

> In matters of medicine we all know what is absolutely wholesome and what is productive of health, that hellebore and an aperient and surgery and cautery are wholesome and productive of health and yet we do not possess the *episteme* of medicine, for without it we no longer know what is good in particular cases, just as the doctor knows for whom a given thing is good and when and in what disposition; for herein the *episteme* of medicine displays itself.
> (*Magna Moralia* 1199a 31-37)

Thus Aristotle's discussion of the medical *tekhne* reveals the polarity in his mind; the *logos* is important for the physician's knowledge of the end or purpose of his treatment, and experience is necessary in order to produce this end. While knowledge is of classes of patients or diseases, practice is concerned with individuals; while knowledge is developed analytically, practical skill is the fruit of time and experience.[s]

[s]In this connection one topic worthy of investigation is the precise methodological implication of *phronesis* for the medical *tekhne*. "Practical wisdom," which in Plato and the early Aristotle had been assimilated to theoretical knowledge, assumed a more important and independent role in the later Aristotle, especially the *Nicomachean Ethics* (see 1140a 24-1140b 30 and Jaeger, *Aristotle,* pp. 81-84). Jaeger notes that it means "a habitual disposition of the mind to deliberate about practically everything concerning human weal and woe . . . concerned not with the universal but with the fleeting details of life" (p. 83), and Sir David Ross states that one variety of practical reason "knows the right thing to do without arriving at it by a process of deliberate analysis—a wisdom about details which is found in those who have had a certain experience of life, even if they cannot formulate general principles" (*Aristotle* [London, 1966], p. 219).

Even when due allowance is made for the practical experiential component, however, Aristotle's method remains opposed to that set forth in *Ancient Medicine.* Although for Aristotle the mechanism of coction is obscure, and experience is required to produce it, medical practice for him is based on theory. Production by means of the *tekhne* is *imitation* of reality, the reproduction of some preexisting thing of which the artist has knowledge. The artist does not create something new but only imitates what already exists. Thus theory still precedes practice, even though the practice is itself important and is based upon experience.

The Hippocratic author had maintained precisely the opposite—that medical theory rises out of practice, and thus he transformed medicine into a theory of investigation. In this sense he is proposing a scientific method for medicine—the unification of theory and practice.

Aristotle discusses practical reason in connection with ethics and politics; he notes that it is a faculty of the mind concerned with the ultimate individual fact, not with "reasoned facts," and that it is developed through experience (so that young men do not have it, as a rule: *Nicomachean Ethics* 1142a 12-20). Most importantly, "practical wisdom" is not a set of rules governing behavior; the rules are themselves derived from the behavior of the man possessing *phronesis* (see the analysis in Emmanuel M. Michelakis, *Aristotle's Theory of Practical Principles* [Athens, 1961], p. 8 *et passim*). Thus practice precedes theory.

Phronesis and *tekhne* are similar in that both deal with the variable, i.e., things which are not of necessity; the former is concerned with doing, while the latter is concerned with making (*Nicomachean Ethics* 1140a 1-10). But the precise significance of *phronesis* for the activity involved in the *tekhne* is not clear. Much of what Aristotle states with respect to the role of *phronesis* in ethics and politics would be equally applicable to medicine, and he does seem to assimilate *phronesis* and medicine in occasional passages (see, for instance, *Nicomachean Ethics* 1141b 15-20). The fact that *phronesis* is developed by experience, that it deals with ultimate unanalyzable facts and not with classes of facts, and that it takes its starting-point in the practitioner rather than in an externalized set of rules or norms make it very similar to the Empirical theory of therapeutics. Max Neuburger writes: "As Socrates individualized abstractions, as Thucydides placed personality in the foreground, so does Hippocratic medicine find its starting-point in the physician as exponent of an art. . . ." (*History of Medicine* [London, 1910], p. 133).

Hence Aristotle's doctrine of *phronesis* must be considered highly relevant to his attempted reconciliation of *logos* and experience in medicine.

The conflict between these two approaches would not have been less acute if Aristotle's method of biological investigation had been more scientifically accurate and less a matter of "*a priori* principles and book-learning," since it is a conflict between *physiological knowledge derived from the practice of medicine* and physiological knowledge derived from *any* other source. For the latter knowledge—obtained from a source other than medical practice (regardless of how scientific the method of investigation)—must be viewed as *a priori* in comparison with the former.

Aristotle was doubtless aware of the conflict between his own method and that proposed in *Ancient Medicine*.[t] He seems to contest the definition of medicine given in this Hippocratic work when he writes:

> Suppose someone to have defined "medicine" as a "science of reality." For if medicine be not a science of anything that is real, the definition is clearly altogether false . . . for not only medicine, but the majority of the other sciences, too, have for their object some real thing, so that each will be a science of reality. Clearly, then, such a definition does not define any science at all, for a definition ought to be peculiar to its own terms, not general.
>
> (*Topics* 149b 7-24)

Although Aristotle is willing to accept a large experiential component in medical practice, he refuses to base medical theory on medical practice in the way advocated by the Hippocratic author. He wants to define and analyze the organism and base practice upon this definition and analysis.

The Empirical School would inherit the tradition that medical practice itself is the most appropriate method of investigating and elucidating the physiology of the organism. Hence this school continued the tradition of the Group I and IV Hippocratic writings.

[t]See above, pp. 92-93.

The Rise of Medical Rationalism

Aristotle's metaphysics is an unending search for causes, and its integrating principle is the principle of contradiction. In his medical thought, however, the theory of coction occupies a central place. Although he proposes an analysis of coction in terms of the hot and the cold overcoming the wet and the dry, the tone and content of his writings on medicine reveal that for him coction is ultimately a mystery. The physician does not heal by manipulating the four qualities; he heals by producing coction. And this is learned only through experience.

Thus his thought contains in suspension the dichotomy of the Group I and III Hippocratic writings.

His followers, however, were unable to live with this tension. The principle of contradiction (in its medical avatar: of contraries) was too strong for them, and they resolved Aristotle's ambiguity by reducing coction to a clash of opposed qualities.

The physicians, Diocles of Carystos, Praxagoras of Cos, and Mnesitheos of Athens, developed Rationalist medicine in the period between 350 and 250 B.C.[85] Their solution to the problem of coction was: 1) to assimilate it entirely to digestion and 2) to shift attention from the digestive process to its products—the varieties of humors which could be treated as hot, cold, wet, or dry.

The pseudo-Aristotelian *Problemata,* probably given their ultimate formulation in the first century B.C., also reflect the progress of medical thought in the Rationalist tradition.[86] The Empirical side of Aristotle's medical thought is completely eclipsed by the metaphysical, as this work places major stress on theories of disease etiology; coction is usually identified with digestion, and cure, in any case, is through contraries.

The theory of coction imposed a certain discipline on the practicing physician, and these efforts to evade the theory of coction were at the same time efforts to evade the associated discipline. Instead of being bound to a rigorous therapeutic method, he could escape into the abstract world of the clash among invisible principles. Where the criterion of sensory observation had been abolished, one physician's opinion was as good as another's.

* * * * * * * * *

While we know very little of the thinking of Diocles, Praxagoras, and Mnesitheos (merely some dozens of fragments of what must have been an equal number of books), they were clearly preoccupied with the digestive process and the selection and preparation of food. Diocles wrote a work on *pepsis* and one on cooking; Praxagoras was an authority on dietetics; his colleague, Phylotimos, wrote on foods and cookery, as did Mnesitheos.[87]

Diocles limits himself to observing and noting the effects of various foods on the whole organism: sweet wine induces salivation; water is useful for digestion, does not cause flatulence, and stimulates activity of mind and body; beans of a certain type are less flatulent than others, etc.[88] Galen notes that while some of his writings mention the "powers" (*dynameis*) of foods, others refer only to their "uses."[89]

Indeed, Diocles seems to fall in the Group I tradition in renouncing the analysis of foods in terms of abstract powers, as his longest fragment indicates:

> Who, therefore, thinks that all things with the same juice, smell, heat, or other things of this sort will have the same *dynameis,* will hardly be correct, for anyone can point out many things different from these even though, as regards the above characteristics, they agree with them. Nor indeed, if anything is cathartic or diuretic or has some other *dynamis,* is it to be regarded as being such because it is hot or cold or salty; since not all sweet things, or bitter, or salty, or others have the same *dynameis,* but it is to be considered that the whole nature is the cause of whatever happens. Whoever indeed thinks that the causes why certain things are nutritive or

cathartic or diuretic or anything else are to be ascertained, is seen to be unaware, in the first place, that such inquiries are hardly needed for the practice of medicine, and, in the second place, that there are many natural things which are similar in certain principles of their nature, so that they do not admit of any reason of the cause of their action. Certain people go very far astray when, laying hold of unknown and controversial, and even quite improbable things, they seek to assign causes to everything. Therefore, pay no attention to those who produce causes of this sort nor to those who feel that causes of everything are to be assigned, but rather stand by those things which have been confirmed by daily experience. We can assign causes when we hope to make the things we are talking about more credible.[90u]

Mnesitheos is like Diocles, observing only that such-and-such foods have such-and-such effects on the body and the digestive process: salt and sweet foods move the bowels, acid and pungent juices stimulate urination, astringent juices check the excretions, etc.[91]

Praxagoras, however, alters the problem in an important way by analyzing foods in terms of their capacity to produce a particular humor: "When the nutriment becomes altered in the veins by the innate heat, blood is produced when the heat is in moderation, and the other humors when it is not in proper proportion . . ."[92v] Thus fish with hard flesh, and hard foods in general, yield salty humors,[93] barley cake

[u]Jaeger discusses this passage in terms of *phronesis* (*Diokles von Karystos*, pp. 37-45), but this seems a forced interpretation in view of the perfectly good precedents for this attitude in the Hippocratic Corpus. The fragment shows that Diocles had much sympathy for the Group I doctrines and that the conflict discussed above (pp. 48 and 64) over the two approaches to the analysis of foods and medicines was still alive in Diocles' time.

Galen himself was surprised by these sentiments of Diocles, prefacing his quotation with the words: "Diocles, even though he was a Dogmatist, wrote the following" (K VI 455).

[v]Cf. Aristotle, *History of Animals* 511b 1-10 (*supra*, p. 142).

produces a thick, cold, and glutinous humor,[94] overeating gives rise to a crude, cold, and phlegmatic humor, etc.[95]

He postulates the existence of ten humors, not including the blood, but this was not a departure from the quadripartite arrangement (as in *Nature of Man*) "for Praxagoras divides into species and varieties the humors which Hippocrates first mentioned, with the demonstration proper to each."[96][w] The "crude" humor of the Group I writings "falls under the species phlegm, being less liquid than what is commonly called phlegm; Praxagoras calls such a humor vitreous."[97]

> [Praxagoras] named the humors in a peculiar way, calling them sweet, equally mixed, and vitreous. These belong to the genus of the phlegm. The names of others are acid, sodic, salty, and bitter. These are differentiated according to taste. Others are called leek-green because of their color, others yolk-like because of their thick consistency. Another kind is given the name, corrosive humor, because they have the quality of corrosiveness.[98]

Praxagoras thus directs the physician's attention to the humors resulting from various diets, rather than to the diets themselves. "The physicians associated with Pleistonikos, Praxagoras, and Phylotimos . . . worked out very extensively the theory of the humors . . ."[99] "Praxagoras . . . attributed to the humors the establishment of all that is according to the *physis* and the cause of all that is contrary to the *physis*."[100]

In this way medicine moved further in the direction of an analytical therapeutics: diseases were viewed as "entities" and subjected to classification, precise humoral causes were associated with such entities, and treatment was by contraries.

[w]Diocles and Mnesitheos adhered to the quadripartite humoral theory (Diocles Fr. 8 and 9; Mnesitheos Fr. 4 and 6).

Praxagoras makes a distinction between the disease entity and the sense-perceptible symptoms,[101] calls diseases deviations from the body's "natural state,"[102] and classifies them: Galen observes that he was "most powerful in his analysis of the phenomena of the *physis*" and knew "what diseases there are, how many, and of what kind."[103]

Mnesitheos, however, carried nosological classification to its ultimate, starting from the first and highest genera and subdividing them into other genera, species, and subspecies until he reached an indivisible unit.[104]

This classification was in terms of humoral causes;[105] Diocles and Praxagoras also wrote works on disease causes.[106] And the pathological fragments of these physicians show that the trend of early Rationalism was toward increasing identification of diseases with individual humors. The vitreous humor causes strong spasmodic pains when it breaks through the intestinal walls.[107] Melancholy is due to black bile gathering around the heart.[108] Violent chills are due to very cold phlegm.[109] Apoplexy and paralysis are due to blockage of the arteries by cold phlegm, thus inhibiting passage of the *pneuma*.[110x]

Consequently, treatment must be by contraries. The best theoretical discussion of this is by Mnesitheos:

> The physician either preserves the health of the healthy or cures the diseases of the sick; but health he preserves through the like, while disease he rids by contraries, and all the while he eradicates the causes [*aitia*] of diseases. And these causes are excessive either in quantity or in quality: and quantity is observed either in *pneuma* or in fluid, while quality is pungent or salty or acid or acrid or warm or cold . . .[111]

[x]Pneumatism is a very important element in the pathology of these early Rationalists (Mnesitheos Fr. 4. Pleistonikos Fr. 4. K XIX 344). Praxagoras, in particular, made a major contribution to this by his hypothesis that the arteries contain *pneuma* (instead of blood). See Harris, *The Heart and the Vascular System in Ancient Greek Medicine*, pp. 108-109. This theory of Praxagoras is discussed below, pp. 176-177.

The division of causes into those which harm quantitatively and those which harm qualitatively is a logical device justifying employment of the two alternative modes of therapy discussed in the Hippocratic writings. When the peccant humor was quantitatively in excess, it was to be removed by diuretics, vomitives, venesection, clysters, sweating, or purgatives.[112] If the excess was qualitative, a medicine of the "opposite" quality was employed: cooling substances in mania,[113] a dry and cold diet in sciatica,[114] wine, steam-bath, and highly seasoned food in diseases due to cold,[115] sharp potions in lethargy,[116] etc.

The fragments do not discuss how the physician was to distinguish between the two classes of disease. Indeed, the distinction must have been entirely arbitrary—reflecting the physician's preference for a particular medicine or therapeutic technique.

The logical restructuring of medical theory is seen even in Diocles who, in other respects, was close to the holistic tradition of Coan medicine. Because he accepts a limitation of the body's humors to four, he disputes the division of fevers (in the Hippocratic Corpus) into those which are continuous and those with periods every 3, 4, 5, 7, and 9 days, claiming that there are not enough humors in the body to account for such a large number of fevers.[117] He claims that the male foetus develops more rapidly than the female foetus.[118][y] Noting that acute diseases sometimes exceed the fourteen days allotted them by Hippocrates, he explains this in two ways: either the period of the acute disease is 21 days (i.e., a multiple of seven) or else the first days of the onset of the acute disease do not count, being a sort of dormant period, and the disease runs its course in fourteen days from the point at which it actually becomes acute.[119] These views manifest a tendency to subordinate the data of disease and therapy to logical rules, and it is not surprising that Galen

[y]I.e., because formed in the right (warmer) side of the uterus (Cornford, *Plato's Cosmology*, p. 336).

eulogizes him as a "physician and rhetorician" and notes that he put Hippocratic medicine into a more logical form.[120]

A final theme which crops up in the fragments of these physicians (and which recurs in the later Rationalist tradition) is the willingness to employ painful, and even cruel modes of therapy. It is a parallel to the Rationalist advocacy of vivisection[121] and has the same psychological roots: the idea that the disease is an entity separate and apart from the patient himself, perhaps bolstered by the doctrine that the disease is "unnatural", make for a certain psychological distance between the physician and the patient. And the former's confidence in the logical structure of his art emboldens him to attempt radical and far-reaching procedures.

Diocles treated prolapsed uterus by blowing air in through the vagina with a blacksmith's bellows and then inserting pomegranates soaked in vinegar,[122z] but Praxagoras' treatment of constipation was even more violent:

> Praxagoras, giving medicaments of a purgative effect, orders the application of a clyster and desiccation of the body by vomiting. He further prescribes as a drink honey-vinegar with pepper and natron, and fresh milk which has been mixed with honey and water. Then he gives radishes at evening, oil being administered before or afterwards. Besides, he puts collyrium at the anus and inserts a clyster, having before given the patients wormwood with vinegar and pure wine and iris-oil. He makes them vomit until the excrement is ejected. He also phlebotomizes some patients after vomiting and, like Hippocrates, fills them with air through the anus. . . . He only aims at tearing the intestines apart and tries to achieve that by giving sharp medicaments and drinks of flatulent effect and clysters of similar power which, if

[z] The ancients regarded the uterus as possessing a life of its own and thus withdrawing spontaneously from contact with the acidity of vinegar.

> held back, cause on account of the morbid tension and inflammation of the intestines, a breaking through or a putrefaction; and which if given off in a mass, bring about death in another way. Then, every excrement evacuated through vomiting is a proof of inflammation of the intestines, since this cannot happen if there is not a very strong inflammation. For the excrement pressed out from the intestines passes through the stomach and hurled into the esophagus is ejected through this part. From this can be seen that Praxagoras intended to describe rather a magnificent death than a therapy. Furthermore, compressing the intestines with the hands, he shakes them vehemently, and this in the case of those patients whose caecum . . . has slipped down into the scrotum, filled with much excrement. Moreover, he approves of cutting the abdomens of some patients, treated by the above-mentioned means, down to the pubes. The rectum also is to be divided, and then to be sewn together after the excrement has been removed. Reckless surgeon that he is![123]

The maxim, *primum non nocere,* was often ignored in the Rationalist tradition.[a]

* * * * * * * * *

The *Problemata,* which set forth the medical thinking of the Peripatos down to the first century B.C., show graphically the confusion to which an infatuation with abstract etiological theories can lead. This work contains no consistent pathological or therapeutic doctrine but is a self-contradictory mixture of nearly all the themes of medical speculation discussed above.

The doctrine of food residues (which also figures in the fragments of Diocles, Praxagoras, and Mnesitheos[124]) plays

[a]The origin of this maxim is unclear, but it is close to the following from *Epidemics I*: "As to diseases, make a habit of two things—to help, or at least to do no harm" (Second Constitution, cap. XI: Jones, I, 165).

an important role. The harm which such residues could cause was almost limitless. They could interfere with coction/digestion.[125] They could be carried up and down the body, causing external sores, internal pains, and diseases of all kinds.[126] They could liquefy and have the same effect.[127] Or they could deposit sediments which also had a morbific potential.[128]

Coction in this work seems generally the equivalent of digestion, but sometimes it has its pristine meaning.[129]

Pneumatism also appears, but in a minor role.[130]

These three etiological theories are mixed together in a way which must have been endlessly confusing to the practitioner.

Some examples: disease is due to an excess of one quality, and health to their equality; disease is brought to a crisis by the opposite quality.[131] Acute diseases due to bile are more severe in the winter when the body is moist, since the excess excretions (*perittomata*) inhibit coction.[132] Ophthalmia in the summer is caused by alien humors in the body; the excretion in the head liquefies, and fever ensues.[133] Dry weather is unhealthy for the bilious; the bile becomes overheated, and as the contrary humors are dried up black bile comes to the surface causing madness.[134] If excretions in the upper part of the body do not kill the patient at once, they descend unconcocted to the stomach and cause dysentery; if the dysentery ceases, quartan fevers arise, as the sediment of the unconcocted moisture remains in the body and becomes active like black bile.[135] The sick die more easily in the winter because the hot matter, due to its density, has become collected in the body, and we suffer from the excretions which solidify in us if we cannot concoct them.[136]

These kinds of etiological theories are nothing more than *ad hoc* explanations dreamt up by armchair philosophers knowing little of medicine. They are evidence of a triumph of the *logos* over power of observation in the later Rationalist tradition.

Cure is generally through contraries.[137] "Some diseases are caused by heat, others by moisture; those which are caused by heat are cured by moisture, and those which are due to moisture are cured by heat, for heat dries up moisture."[138] "The causes of diseases are opposites of one another, so that each reduces the other to the mean."[139] Similars are viewed as exacerbating the disease.[140]

The rationale of cure through contraries, however, is as confused and inconsistent as the etiologies of this work. Remedies for stanching blood have a drying effect and stop the discharge of excretions (*perittosis*).[141] Barley-gruel is suitable for sick persons because, although more difficult of concoction than wheat, due to its moistness, it is also cooler, and feverish patients require cooling foods.[142b] Drugs are purgative because of their excess heat or cold which prevents them from being concocted; foods are purgative not through their qualities but through quantity.[143] Sweet-smelling seeds and plants are diuretic due to their heat which makes them easily concocted.[144] Hot drugs are carried upwards in the body, melting alien substances and carrying them, together with the excretions (*perittomata*), to the upper stomach and stirring up the *pneuma* which causes vomiting.[145] Cold drugs do the same in the downward direction.[146]

* * * * * * * * *

Stress on coction signifies stress on experience. The breakdown of the theory of coction signifies the encroachment of logic into the area of experience. The social reasons for this trend, as discussed above, are: (1) to absolve the physician of the discipline imposed by the theory of coction and grant him more latitude in diagnosis and treatment (once sensory observation is abandoned, each person's opinion is equally valid), (2) to raise medicine from a craft in which lay

[b] In *RAD I,* caps. X-XIII barley-gruel is advocated because it is *easy* of coction. In the *Problemata* it is still viewed as beneficial but given a rationale based upon contraries. See the discussion of this passage above, pp. 28-29.

knowledge is qualitatively identical with professional (the only difference between the two being relative skill, i.e., experience) to an arcane doctrine from which the uninitiated layman is barred.

The rationalization of medical theory thus served to oppress society at the same time as it liberated the physician. The freedom of the former was curtailed as that of the latter was extended.

NOTES

[1] This is the theme of Werner Jaeger's seminal work, *Aristotle: Fundamentals of the History of His Development* (2nd ed.; Oxford, 1962).

[2] *Physics* 194b 18-20.

[3] *Physics,* 184a 22-26.

[4] *De Iuventute et Senectute* 469a 10-14.

[5] *De Anima* 429a 10. The *nous* is divine and enters the body after conception (*Generation of Animals* 736b 27-30).

[6] *Politics* 1254a 17-1255a 2.

[7] *Physics* 196b 10-16.

[8] *Metaphysics* 1005b 23.

[9] Boas, *Some Assumptions of Aristotle,* p. 24.

[10] *Ibid.,* p. 29.

[11] *Ibid.,* p. 30.

[12] Signs are discussed in *History of Animals* 491b 15, *Physiognomica* 805a-814b, *Meteorologica* 380a 1, *Politics* 1340a 33 and 1381a 6, *Rhetoric* 1357a 34-1357b 20 and 1403a 10, *Prior Analytics* 70a 10.

[13] *Posterior Analytics* 97b 27-28.

[14] *Rhetoric* 1356b 29-32. Also, *Metaphysics* 981a 5-10.

[15] *Metaphysics,* 1005b 25-26.

[16] Jones, *Hippocrates,* IV, 485.

[17] *Ibid.,* p. 493.

[18] *Loc. cit.*

[19] *Ibid.,* p. 495.

[20] *Ibid.,* p. 483.

[21] *Meteorologica* 355a 14.

[22] *Metaphysics* 1005b 23-30.

[23] *Physics* 185a 6-7.

[24] O. Temkin, "Greek Medicine as Science and Craft," *Isis* XLIV (1953), p. 218. An excellent discussion of anatomical research in antiquity can be found in L. Edelstein, "Die Geschichte der Sektion in der Antike," *Quellen und Studien zur Geschichte der Naturwissenschaft und der Medizin* III (1932), 50-106.

[25] Aristotle was in contact with the Sicilian physicians (Jaeger, *Diokles von Karystos* [Berlin: Gruyter, 1938], pp. 7-10).

[26] *On Generation and Corruption* 330b 4-8. See also *Physics* 192b 8-11.

[27] *Parts of Animals* 649b 26.

[28] *Ibid.,* 650a 1-5.

[29] *De Somno et Vigilia* 458a 4.

[30] *History of Animals* 487a 6.

[31] *De Somno et Vigilia* 457a 31.

[32] *Parts of Animals* 649a 26.

[33] *Ibid.*, 649b 33. Good sources of information on Aristotle's physiology are Paul Kalthoff, *Das Gesundheitswesen bei Aristoteles* (Berlin, 1934), and Erich Schoener, "Das Viererschema in der antiken Humoralpathologie."

[34] *De Somno et Vigilia* 457b 30.

[35] *Parts of Animals* 652a 35.

[36] *Ibid.*, 33.

[37] *De Longitudine et Brevitate Vitae* 466a 20-23; *Generation of Animals* 784a 34-35.

[38] *Physics* 246b 5-6. See, also, *De Anima* 408a 1 and *Posterior Analytics* 78b 21.

[39] *Meteorologica* 384a 17.

[40] *De Longitudine et Brevitate Vitae* 466a 24.

[41] C.R.S. Harris, *The Heart and the Vascular System in Ancient Greek Medicine*, pp. 165-167.

[42] *Historia Animalium* 494b 22-24.

[43] *Meteorologica* 378b 10-13 and 380a 11-25.

[44] *De Plantis* 822a 27-29.

[45] *Meteorologica* 380a 12.

[46] *De Iuventute et Senectute* 469b 4-20. *De Anima* 416a 15.

[47] *De Respiratione* 474b 12-24.

[48] *Generation of Animals* 766a 17-22. Note this use of the principle of contradiction.

[49] *Parts of Animals* 650a 3-650b 13. *History of Animals* 521a 18.

[50] *History of Animals* 511b 1-3.

[51] *History of Animals* 511b 4-10, 521a 18. *Parts of Animals* 672a 1-6.

[52] *Generation of Animals* 744b 12-15.

[53] *Ibid.*, 726b 5-6.

[54] *History of Animals* 511b 8-10.

[55] *Meteorologica* 380a 1-3.

[56] *Ibid.*, 380b 5-6. Concocted substances are dense and heavy (*Ibid.*, 380a 4-5).

[57] *Generation of Animals* 728a 22-24.

[58] *Meteorologica* 380a 20-23.

[59] *Parts of Animals* 670b 5-9. This is a reinterpretation of the following passage from *Airs Waters Places*, cap. IV (Jones, I, 85): "Those who drink [stagnant water] have always large stiff spleens and hard, thin, hot stomachs, while their shoulders, collar-bones, and faces are emaciated."

[60] *Meteorologica* 381b 12-13 and 389b 7-9.

[61] *Ibid.*, 379a 16-18.

[62] *Generation of Animals* 762a 15-16.

[63] *Ibid.*, 777a 8-12.

[64] *History of Animals* 521a 21-23.

[65] *Metaphysics* 1032b 25-28. *Meteorologica* 379b 22-24.

[66] *Magna Moralia* 1208a 23-25.

[67] *History of Animals* 522b 6-12

[68] *Ibid.*, 605a 27-28.

[69] *Ibid.*, 627a 3-4.

[70] *Ibid.*, 604b 1-5.

[71] *Physics* 197b 23.

[72] *Historia Animalium* 512a 32, 514b 3.

[73] *Generation of Animals* 783a 20.

[74] *History of Animals* 603b 9-10.

[75] *Ibid.*, 604a 16-17.

[76] *Ibid.*, 603b 18-27.

[77] *Nicomachean Ethics* 1104b 16-18. In the *Eudemean Ethics* he defines medicine as a "correction" similar to the corrective measures, such as whipping, used against recalcitrant citizens (1214b 33).

[78] *Enquiry into Plants* (Loeb Edition): tithymallos purges phlegm downwards (IX xi 9), one kind of poppy purges the belly downwards, and another kind purges upwards (IX xii 3, 4), madder has diuretic properties (IX xiii 6). Theophrastus only notes the facts and does not explain them.

[79] *Physics* 199a 9-19.

[80] *Prior Analytics* 46a 17-22. *Posterior Analytics* 100a 7-8. *Metaphysics* 981a 5-12.

[81] *Posterior Analytics* 71b 6-13, 88a 5-8, 100a 7-8.

[82] *Nicomachean Ethics* 1094a 8-9.

[83] J. M. Leblond, *Logique et Methode chez Aristote* (Paris, 1939), p. 334.

[84] *Parts of Animals* 640a 32-33.

[85] The dating of Diocles is a much-controverted issue. Because of his obvious affinities with the Sicilian School Wellmann placed his *floruit* at between 400 and 350 (*Die Fragmente der Sykelischen Aerzte*, p. 67). Werner Jaeger, on the other hand, makes Diocles a pupil of Aristotle and thus prefers a later date—about the year 300 (*Diokles von Karystos*, pp. 16-59; *Aristotle: Fundamentals of the History of His Development*, p. 413). See Harris, *The Heart and the Vascular System* etc., pp. 103-104.

Jaeger places Praxagoras' *floruit* at about 300 or slightly later ("Vergessene Fragmente des Peripatetikers Diokles von Karystos," *Abhandlungen der Preussischen Akademie der Wissenschaften*, Philosophisch-Historische Klasse, No. 4 [1938], p. 40).

The first scholarly treatment of Mnesitheos dates him at between 350 and 300 (Hans Hohenstein, "Der Arzt Mnesitheos aus Athen," Unpublished Doctoral Dissertation, Jena, 1935, p. 6), but Jaeger later altered this to 270 ("Vergessene Fragmente," p. 45). Sterling Dow wrote that Mnesitheos was born about 320, studied under Diocles from 300 to 295, and made his contribution to medicine in the 260's and 250's ("Two Families of Athenian Physicians," *Bulletin of the History of Medicine* XII [1942], 18-26, at p. 24).

[86] On the dating of the *Problemata* see E.D. Forster, "The Pseudo-Aristotelian Problems, Their Nature and Composition," *Classical Quarterly* XXII (1928).

[87] Wellmann, *Die Fragmente der Sykelischen Aerzte*, Diocles Fr. 21, 137, 138. Fritz Steckerl, *The Fragments of Praxagoras of Cos and His School* (Leyden: Brill, 1958): Praxagoras Fr. 36, 78; Phylotimos Fr. 4, 20. Hohenstein, *op. cit.*, Mnesitheos Fr. 19, 32.

One of the Diocles fragments mentions coction of disease causes (Fr. 107), but others indicate an assimilation of coction to the digestion of food (Fr. 12, 22). Praxagoras and Mnesitheos also view coction as digestion (Praxagoras Fr. 76, 90; Mnesitheos Fr. 23, 25, 26).

[88] Diocles Fr. 117, 121, 128, 130.

[89] Diocles Fr. 113.

[90] Diocles Fr. 112 (K VI 455-456).

[91] Mnesitheos Fr. 19, 25, 27, 36, 46.

[92] Praxagoras, Fr. 18 (K II 117-118).

[93] Praxagoras Fr. 24, 25.

[94] Phylotimos Fr. 5.

[95] Praxagoras Fr. 51. See, also, Fr. 50, 52, 54, 55, 56, 59.

[96] Praxagoras Fr. 21 (K II 140-141).

[97] Praxagoras Fr. 53 (K XVI 10). See also Fr. 95.

[98] Praxagoras Fr. 22.

[99] Praxagoras Fr. 16 (K V 105-106).

[100] Praxagoras, Fr. 46 (K XIV 698).

[101] Steckerl, *The Fragments of Praxagoras of Cos,* p. 29. Praxagoras Fr. 96.

[102] Praxagoras Fr. 27 and 46. Plistonikos Fr. 3.

[103] Praxagoras Fr. 47 (K XVI 40).

[104] Mnesitheos Fr. 3, 4.

[105] *Loc. cit.*

[106] Diocles Fr. 39. Praxagoras Fr. 109.

[107] Praxagoras Fr. 55 and 56.

[108] Praxagoras Fr. 69.

[109] Praxagoras Fr. 51 and 52.

[110] Diocles Fr. 55 and 57.

[111] Mnesitheos Fr. 4.

[112] Diocles Fr. 39, 65, 71. Praxagoras Fr. 107, 111, 112.

[113] Diocles Fr. 41.

[114] Diocles Fr. 76.

[115] Praxagoras Fr. 78.

[116] Diocles Fr. 45.

[117] Diocles Fr. 97.

[118] Diocles Fr. 175.

[119] Diocles Fr. 110.

[120] Diocles Fr. 99.

[121] Celsus, *Prooemium,* 24. The Empirics opposed vivisection because of its cruelty (*ibid.,* 40).

[122] Diocles Fr. 182.

[123] Praxagoras Fr. 109 (Caelius Aurelianus, *a.m.* III 17 163).

[124] Diocles Fr. 22, 107. Praxagoras Fr. 7, 60, 68, 79. Plistonikos Fr. 1.

[125] *Problemata* 859b 14; 861b 16, 34; 862a 37.

[126] 861b 10-15, 25-30.

[127] 864b 24.

[128] 861b 18.

[129] 859b 6-18; 861a 5-10, 14; 862b 3-5, 16-24; 863b 3-10; 864b 7-11; 865a 3-24; 865b 6-18.

[130] 862a 29; 864a 14.

[131] 859a 9-14.

[132] 859b 5-14.

[133] 859b 21-29.

[134] 860b 20-25.

[135] 861b 10-20.

[136] 862a 34 - 862b 1.

[137] 859a 9-18.

[138] 866b 4-6.
[139] 859a 6-8.
[140] 859a 14-15; 861a 25-30; 864b 28-31; 866a 1-8.
[141] 863a 13-19.
[142] 863b 1-10.
[143] 864b 1-12.
[144] 865a 18-24.
[145] 864a 6-14.
[146] 864a 14-20.

PART TWO

GREEK MEDICINE IN ALEXANDRIA

PART TWO

GREEK MEDICINE IN ALEXANDRIA

The ancient world was conquered and unified by Alexander the Great (356-323 B.C.), and the city which he founded became the center of Hellenistic culture.

The intellectual ferment which marked Alexandria in the Hellenistic Age affected every area of life, and medicine not least of all. The Rationalist tradition, already a century old, was now challenged by two other approaches to the problems of health and disease: the mechanical and atomistic formulation of Erasistratos of Julis and the Empirical School which first emerged as a self-conscious tradition in the third century B.C.

The doctrines of Erasistratos, influenced by the philosophical ideas of Democritus and Epicurus, represent the inherent impulse of medical Rationalism to seek the ultimate causes of health and disease in the atom. This process was repeated two hundred years later with the rise of Methodism.

The Empirical School, for its part, drew upon the ideas of the Group I and IV Hippocratic writings but added to them the philosophical techniques of the Sceptics. The outcome was the transformation of the sometimes inchoate and unstructured concepts of these Hippocratic writings into a philosophically finished and self-confident therapeutic doctrine which was to serve as the platform of the Empirical School for the next 500 years and leave its imprint on medical thought for many centuries thereafter.

CHAPTER IV

ERASISTRATOS OF JULIS

Erasistratos, born about 300 B.C., was one of the most prominent Alexandrian physicians of his time and fathered a school which remained active for almost five hundred years after his death.

He studied with Praxagoras of Cos and Chrysippos of Cnidos and spent some time as well at the Peripatos in Athens.[1] Hence his early training was in the Rationalist tenets and doctrines. The mature Erasistratean theory, however, departed sharply from Rationalism in postulating the movement of atoms as the ultimate determinant of physiological and pathological processes and seeking to base treatment upon this postulate.

In so doing Erasistratos was only following one of the more powerful philosophical currents of his era. For Aristotelianism at this time was being reformulated by Theophrastus and Strato—who headed the Peripatos after the Master's death.[2] They continued the trend noticeable in Aristotle's later works toward an increased emphasis on the material world of nature, subordinating the formal and final causes (the Platonic element in Aristotelianism) to the material and efficient causes (the Democritic element).

This was significant for physiology and medicine in suggesting a new relationship between matter and cause. For Aristotle the formal and final causes were fundamental and culminated in an Unmoved Mover entirely outside the material world. By abolishing the Unmoved Mover Strato brought to the fore Aristotle's material and efficient causes. He saw the efficient causes of movement and change in the qualities (*poiotetes*) and powers (*dynameis*) which he posited as attributes of matter although themselves immaterial.

The Stoic school, founded by Zeno of Citium in the last decade of the fourth century, brought this doctrine to a culmination by hypostatizing the very qualities and powers themselves, defining them as substances inhering spatially in other substances.[3] The Unmoved Mover was, hence, identified with the world of nature.

While the Stoics in this way reached a standpoint of teleological materialism, the Epicureans went back to Democritus directly and attributed all change and movement to the motion of invisible atoms. The Epicurean doctrine, which arose in Athens in the very end of the fourth century, was thus one of mechanistic materialism. Cause was entirely subordinated to matter—that is, to the atoms—and disappeared almost completely as a separate category.[a]

The *pneuma* plays the same role in Stoic philosophy as does the atom in Epicureanism. Aristotle had identified *pneuma* with the innate heat which effects coction, the life principle of the organism which distinguishes man from a stone or a piece of metal, and at the same time made it the substance of sense perception and the instrument of the body's movements.[4] The Stoics materialized this concept by reviving the Hippocratic (Group III) identification of the *pneuma* with the ambient air; at the same time they greatly expanded its scope by positing the *pneuma* not only as the life-principle of all living beings but also as the instrument of God's rule over the universe.[5][b] In this way the Stoics explained how God, who is immanent in nature and identified with it, could govern nature and cause its movement and development.

[a]Epicurus was compelled to admit that the first motions of the atoms were not mechanically determined, and he decided that they were voluntary. Thus a non-material and indeterminate causation was introduced into his system at a point where it could have no consequences for physiology.

[b]Windelband describes it (jokingly?) as "an extraordinarily condensed conception, full of relations" (*History of Philosophy,* p. 187). Note the parallels with *Breaths* and *Sacred Disease.*

Physiology

The Alexandrian physicians were the first to pursue anatomical investigation on a broad scale, and Erasistratos was a leader of this movement. He described the structure of the brain.[6] By discovering the valves of the heart he came near to understanding the circulation of the blood.[7] He performed vivisection on condemned criminals[8] and is recorded as having carried out the first biological experiment, so to speak, *in vitro:* desirous of proving that part of the body's substance is exhaled with the *pneuma,* he placed a bird in a glass jar for a time without feeding it; upon removal, the bird and its excrements were found to weigh less than the bird alone at the outset of the experiment.[9]

His physiological learning enabled Erasistratos to carry out a fundamental reconstruction of certain of the Hippocratic doctrines.

It will be recalled that the Hippocratic writings (of all Groups) discuss the relations between the organism and the environment—the principal environmental factors examined being food and climatic conditions. The physiology of Erasistratos is an attempt to reinterpret these traditional medical views on the significance of food and air for the support of life.[10] He interprets the former in terms of the atomic-mechanistic hypothesis of Democritus and Epicurus and the latter in terms of the *pneuma.*[11]

His basic doctrine is that the body is a porous solid through which matter and air can flow freely in corpuscular form. Thus the ambient air enters the lungs and passes from there to the arteries.[12] It flows through the arteries and is then exhaled through the body's pores.[13] The food also enters the body and passes to the stomach. There, however, it is not digested but is ground up mechanically by peristalsis aided by the *pneuma.*[14] It is transformed into juice and then into blood which circulates through the veins, supplying nutriment to all the parts.[15]

Thus the veins contain blood, and the arteries contain air (which Erasistratos identified with *pneuma*).[16] This latter proposition, first advanced by Praxagoras, was essential for doctrinal completeness. If the existence of *pneuma* was accepted, a place for it had to be found in the body: logic took precedence over observation.[17]

The other Hippocratic doctrines are reinterpreted in terms of these two physiological processes. The external (procatarctic) caused is abolished, being incorporated in the *pneuma* and transformed into a proximate cause. Erasistratos thus denies the etiological significance of the external cause: "diseases were not produced by such causes, since other persons, and even the same person at different times, were not rendered feverish by them."[18]

The concept of coction is transvalued by Erasistratos in a way which leaves a permanent mark on all later medical speculation.

It will be recalled that the early Rationalists had assimilated coction to the digestion of food in the stomach, thus analyzing out of existence the theory of coction which was the key to the therapeutic doctrine of the Group I Hippocratic writings. Erasistratos develops this line of thought with the further postulate that the digestion itself is not the product of innate heat or of any purposeful activity by the organism but is a purely mechanical process.

Thus the body has no innate heat but takes it in from the outside with the *pneuma,* and the digestion itself is nothing more than the trituration or grinding of food by peristaltic action assisted by this same *pneuma.*[19]

Furthermore, he accounts for the nutrition of the body from the stomach by postulating another aspect of digestion, namely, the delivery (*anadosis*) of the contents of the stomach through the veins to the places where they are needed.[20] The assimilation of this food-mixture by the appropriate parts of the body is called by him *diadosis.*[21]

The processes of *anadosis* and *diadosis* are ascribed to *horror vacui,* the tendency of an empty space to attract liquid from its surroundings.[22] This principle had been originally postulated by Democritus and Strato.[23]

Thus Erasistratos rejects the concept of bodily "function" as implying a teleological view of the organism.[24] The various organs do not possess any vital power of "attracting" humors.[25] It is just that any liquids flowing out of the organs are immediately replaced by others.

In this way he overcomes the contradiction between his own doctrine that the arterial system is filled with *pneuma* and the observed fact that blood flows out of a wounded artery: when the artery is cut the *pneuma* escapes instantaneously, and the resulting vacuum is filled with blood from the veins.[26]

He restructured the Rationalist four humors. Although he admitted the existence of several humors, the only one of significance for therapy was the blood. Erasistratos "was afraid to call any humor either hot or cold, wet or dry," and he rejected the possibility of black bile entirely.[27] His followers doubtless reflected his views in stating that, although these various humors may exist, knowledge of them is not necessary for medical practice.[28]

The outcome was removal of the *physis* from medical speculation.[29] The body possesses no innate heat or life, as both come in from the outside with the *pneuma.*[30] The *pneuma* takes the place of the *physis,* moving about through the arteries and stimulating the body's various mechanisms.[31] The organism does not grow organically, but by simple addition of similar parts.[32] Coction is reduced to the mechanical grinding of food in the stomach and its subsequent mechanical distribution through the body.

He gave a similar non-functional explanation of the feeling of hunger. It is not due to any innate need of the organism for food but only to the mechanical grinding of the empty stomach; the proof of this is that hunger can be relieved, as the Scythians do, by tightening the belt.[33]

The same assumption is responsible for his denial that women are subject to different diseases than men[34] and for his claim that many of the body's organs are superfluous: "For according to him the spleen was made for no purpose, as also the omentum; similarly, too, the arteries which are inserted into the kidneys–although these are practically the largest of all those that spring from the great artery. And to judge by the Erasistratean argument there are countless other useless structures; for . . . he clearly imagines that they were made for no purpose, like the spleen."[35]

Erasistratos' teachings are only a logical extension of Rationalist views on the proximate cause, the *physis,* and the process of coction. His epistemological assumptions themselves remain completely Rationalist. Like the Rationalists, he subordinates sense-perception and experience to the *logos,* practice to theory. He regarded physiology and etiology as the scientific parts of medicine, while semeiotics and therapeutics were conjectural.[36] Therapy was based upon knowledge of causes.[37] The ultimate causes of everything in the organism are the atoms which are not sense-perceptible.[38] Thus the fundamental mechanisms of the body cannot be perceived by the senses but are knowable by the *logos.* Erasistratos did not base his argument in favor of *pneuma* in the arteries on sense-perception, and sensory evidence against it did not lead him to revise his view.[39] In therapy the physician was supposed to use the *logos* to distinguish one disease from another and to determine which part of the body is affected.[40] The disease was recognized by looking beneath the symptoms.[41] He wrote a book against the Empirics who denied the value of causal knowledge for therapy.[42] He maintained that compound remedies can be made up by the logical manipulation of simples.[43]

Pathology and Therapeutics

His pathology is a function of his physiology. The principal cause of disease is excess blood, and this is due to overeating.[44][c] The veins become too full, some of the excess is discharged into the arteries, and there it blocks the movement of the *pneuma* or, in turn, is forced by the latter into unsuitable parts of the body (*error loci*), causing inflammation of the liver, spleen, and stomach, or other disorders such as coughing of blood, epilepsy, phrenitis, pleuritis, peripneumonia, angina, tonsillitis, pharyngitis, and tracheitis.[45]

[c]One can imagine that Erasistratos' fashionable clientele in Alexandria suffered mainly from gluttony.

Inflammations, in turn, give rise to other diseases. Dropsy is caused by a "chronic and scirrhous inflammation of the liver or spleen, which prevents the assimilation of the food in the bowels and its distribution throughout the body, but changes it to water, which, being refrigerated, is deposited between the intestines and the peritoneum."[46]

The *pneuma* could also interact with the other humors of the body, although this etiological process seems to have been less significant. Apoplexy is a brain disease giving rise to excessive secretion of mucus which prevents the psychic *pneuma* from passing into the nerves located at the ends of the arteries. When tough and glutinous humors pass from the veins into some of the nerve passages, this blocks the *pneuma* and causes paralysis. Malnutrition is caused by thick humors in the veins of the stomach which block the *pneuma* and impede the digestion.[47d]

Erasistratos stressed prevention more than cure.[48] The best remedy was to reduce the intake of food.[49e] "The veins when emptied will more easily receive back the blood which has invaded the arteries."[50] He condemned blood-letting on the ground that it deprives the body of nutriment and thus makes it weaker.[51] He advocated exercise and the steam bath—to ensure that the atoms in the body are moving properly in their courses.[52]

He was opposed to strong purges and medications.[53] Some of his prescriptions (such as warm drinks to overcome an acrid bilious condition) seem to be humoral in origin and probably reflect his early Rationalist training.[54] Others (such as astringent medicines in dysentery to constrict and block the pores in the solid parts of the body) have an atomistic basis.[55]

He urges the physician to take the patient's habits into account but does not explain how this is reconciled with his atomism.[56]

* * * * * * * * *

[d]Many of Erasistratos' pneumatic views are identical with those of Praxagoras (his teacher) and the other early Rationalists (Diocles Fr. 55, 57; Praxagoras Fr. 11, 69, 78; Pleistonikos Fr. 4; Mnesitheos Fr. 4).

[e]Galen observes that Erasistratos "obviously does not know for what purpose fasting is employed" (K XI 177).

Galen wrote, on the contrast between Rationalism and the doctrine of Erasistratos: "If the Peripatetics were correct in their contemplation of the *physis* . . . then nothing is more ridiculous than Erasistratos"[57]; the Peripatetics "approve of none of the ideas of Erasistratos"[58]; there is "an opposition between the two doctrines"[59]; Erasistratos "turned . . . completely from the teachings of Hippocrates"[60]; Erasistratos has in common with Rationalism only the postulate that "the *physis* does everything for some purpose and nothing in vain," but this agreement is only verbal, and Erasistratos in practice "makes havoc of it a thousand times over."[61]

At the same time, this doctrine developed organically out of the theses of medical Rationalism—just as would the Methodist doctrine two centuries later.

Hence the rise of Erasistrateanism and Methodism reveal the logical compulsion inherent in medical Rationalism to pass into a mechanistic-atomistic formulation. The atom is the last refuge of the proximate cause, the ultimate stronghold of all indefatigable seekers of causal knowledge in physiology.

And, once attained, the mechanistic-atomistic standpoint compels a reconstruction of all the postulates and assumptions of Rationalism.

Erasistratos' reworking of Rationalist medicine along atomistic lines has a modern ring. Modern, also, is his preference for research in physiology over the practice of medicine; toward the end of his life he retired from practice altogether.[62]

His ideas suffered an ironic fate. The Erasistrateans of Galen's time, anxious to avoid identification with the Methodists, resolved that their master had been an Aristotelian all along.[63][f]

[f]See below, Chapter VIII, for the parallels between Erasistratos and the later Methodist School.

NOTES

[1] Werner Jaeger, "Vergessene Fragmente des Peripatetikers Diokles von Karystos," pp. 38-39. Werner Jaeger, "Das Pneuma im Lykeion," *Hermes* XLVIII (1913), pp. 62-63.

[2] Jaeger, "Das Pneuma im Lykeion," p. 62. I. M. Lonie, "Erasistratos, the Erasistrateans, and Aristotle," *Bulletin of the History of Medicine* XXXVIII (1964) 426-443, p. 441.

[3] K II 92.

[4] Jaeger, "Das Pneuma im Lykeion," pp. 43ff.

[5] *Ibid.*, p. 56ff.

[6] K III 673.

[7] Lonie, "Erasistratos," p. 426.

[8] Celsus, *Prooemium,* 24.

[9] Jones, *Medical Writings of Anonymus Londinensis,* XXXIII: 30.

[10] *Ibid.*, XXII-XXIII.

[11] On Erasistratos' atomism see K XIV 699 and K II 95-106.

[12] K II 114; K IV 473, 706-707; K V 166, 185, 206, 548, 563; K VIII 429; K XV 248. Also, J. F. Dobson, "Erasistratos," *Proc. Royal Society of Medicine* (1927), XX, 825-832.

[13] Jones, *Medical Works of Anonymus Londinensis,* cap. XXIII.

[14] K II 119-120; K XV 247; K XIX 372. Celsus, *Prooemium,* 20.

[15] Lonie, "Erasistratos," p. 439. Also, Jones, *Medical Works of Anonymus Londinensis,* caps. XXV-XXVI, XXXVI.

[16] Praxagoras Fr. 9 and 31.

[17] K IV 706.

[18] Celsus, *Prooemium,* 54. See also K II 126.

[19] K II 119-120, 166. K VII 614. K XV 247. K XIX 372.

[20] K II 104. He wrote works on coction (*pepsis*) and *anadosis* (K II 111).

[21] K II 104.

[22] K II 104.

[23] K II 105.

[24] K II 107-108, 110.

[25] K II 93.

[26] K IV 706. K VIII 950. Jaeger, "Das Pneuma im Lykeion," p. 65.

[27] K V 123, 685.

[28] K II 126.

[29] *Loc. cit.* At the same time, Erasistratos professed admiration for the *physis*. Galen notes that this is incompatible with his medical views generally (K II 78, 81, 87).

[30] K VII 614.

[31] K IV 706. K V 185. K VIII 429. K II 97, 105, 120-121.

[32] K II 87.

[33] Aulus Gellius, *Attic Nights,* XVI, 3.

[34] Wellmann, Diocles Fr. 169.

[35] K II 91-92.

[36] Ludwig Englert, "Untersuchungen zu Galens Schrift Thrasybulos," *Studien zur Geschichte der Medizin,* Heft 18 (1929), p. 23. K XIV 684.

[37] K XIV 692, 699. Deichgraeber, *Die Griechische Empirikerschule,* Fr. 25.

[38] K XIV 699. Jones, *Medical Works of Anonymous Londinensis,* cap. XXI.

[39] K VIII 950.

[40] K VIII 14; K V 138.

[41] K X 101; K V 138.

[42] Deichgraeber, *Die Griechische Empirikerschule,* Fr. 25 and p. 255.

[43] K I 75; K XI 433.

[44] K VII 537-539.

[45] K VII 537-539; K X 101, 461; Celsus, *Prooemium,* 15-16, 60-61; Dobson, "Erasistratus," p. 830.

[46] K XIV 746; Dobson, "Erasistratus," p. 830.

[47] Dobson, "Erasistratus," p. 831.

[48] K XIV 692.

[49] K XI 176, 228.

[50] K XI 228.

[51] K XI 187-249.

[52] K XI 237.

[53] K X 377-379. K XI 239, 245, 324. K XIV 692. K. F. H. Marx, *De Herophili celeberrimi medici, vita scriptis, atque in medicina meritis* (Goettingen, 1840), p. 49.

[54] Caelius Aurelianus, *m.a.* III 213 (I. E. Drabkin, *Caelius Aurelianus on Acute Diseases and on Chronic Diseases,* Chicago: University of Chicago Press, 1950). Celsus, V, 1.

[55] Caelius Aurelianus, *m. chr.,* II 187 and IV 90.

[56] Galen, *Scripta Minora* (ed. Marquardt, Leipzig, 1893), Vol. II, p. 16.

[57] K XV 307.

[58] K II 90.

[59] K II 91.

[60] K II 93.

[61] K II 91.

[62] Deichgraeber, *Die Griechische Empirikerschule,* p. 279. K V 602.

[63] K II 88-90. K XI 222. Lonie, "Erasistratos," p. 441, note 53.

CHAPTER V

THE ORIGINS OF EMPIRICISM

While Erasistratos was inspired by Stoicism, the Empirical School, which enters history as an autonomous medical tradition in the middle of the third century B.C., looked to the Sceptics.

This philosophical school was engaged in developing a method for ensuring success in the affairs of daily life, and the Empirics applied their method to medicine. Just as the Sceptics derived rules of practical conduct by inference from day-to-day experience, so the Empirics used medical experience as the source of rules for medical practice.

Scepticism also provided Empiricism with a technique for analyzing and criticizing the doctrines of Rationalism.

In this chapter we first discuss the significance of Scepticism for Empirical therapeutic theory and the Empirical critique of Rationalism. Then we examine the medical views of Herophilos of Chalcedon—the first physician to apply the Sceptical doctrines to medicine. And finally we will mention some of the Empirics whose names have come down to us from the pre-Christian and early Christian era—indicating their significance for the emergence of Empiricism as a conscious tradition in therapeutics and, in particular, for the Empirical interpretation of the Hippocratic Corpus.

Scepticism: The Search for a Reliable Guide to Action

Scepticism was the culmination of a long-term shift in the focus of philosophical interest. While Plato and Aristotle had concentrated on developing knowledge for its own sake, Stoicism and Epicureanism sought to apply knowledge to the practical affairs of life and thus evolved philosophically based ethical doctrines. Scepticism took the final step of separating action (practice) from knowledge (theory) and establishing practice on a new basis. Greek thought thus proceeds from the preeminence of theory in Platonism to the preeminence of practice in Scepticism.

Sceptical thought has two aspects. The first task of these philosophers was to disprove the claims of the other schools to provide a valid theoretical guide to action. Then they had to develop a substitute for this theoretical guide, and here they made a new and revolutionary contribution to Greek speculation.

Both aspects of the Sceptical philosophical effort are of significance to medicine. Their critique of Rationalist theory and the Rationalist analysis of physical reality affected the physician's interpretation of the phenomena of health and disease, while their formulation of a reliable guide to action helped lay the basis for the Empirical interpretation of the medical *tekhne*.

The Sceptical tradition has six principal figures.[1] The founder, Pyrrho of Elis (*c.* 360-270), left no writings, and we know of him mainly through those of his pupil, Timon of Phlius (*c.* 320-230). After Timon came Arcesilaus of Pitane (*c.* 315-240), the founder of the Middle Academy, who concerned himself mainly with refutation of the Stoic doctrine of the "irresistible impression" (*phantasia kataleptike*). He was the first Sceptic to suggest probability as a basis for action. Carneades of Cyrene (*c.* 213-129), the founder of the New Academy and perhaps the greatest of the Sceptical thinkers, continued the arguments against the Stoic theory of knowledge and also worked on the doctrine of probability. Aenesidemos, who lived in the first century B.C., to a certain extent rejected the views of his two Academic predecessors and revived those of Pyrrho and Timon, emphasizing the epistemological side of Scepticism and its criticism of causality and sense-perception. Finally, in the third century A.D., the physician, Sextus Empiricus, gathered together the views of his predecessors in a series of writings which provide most of our knowledge of the Sceptical tradition.

Since we are not attempting a history of Scepticism but are interested only in its relevance for medicine, we will not enter into the details of the differences among the above thinkers but will rather present this philosophy as a unified outlook, noting the contributions of each of the important Sceptical philosophers.

The Critique of Rationalism

Pyrrho and Timon criticized the claim of the Stoic and Peripatetic philosophers to provide a reliable guide to action.[a] This attack on Rationalist theory was two-pronged: the Sceptics denied the possibility both of unambiguous perception and of unambiguous judgment. "From two deceivers combined it is only right to expect no truth."

In attacking perception they hypothesized a radical distinction between the object and its appearance. Appearance could be accepted, but there was no assurance that this actually represented the object.[2] For a number of reasons appearance may differ from the underlying reality. Appearance may be affected by the conditions under which it appears. Observers also differ, as do their sense organs. The observer may be misled by customs, prejudices, or preconceived ideas. For these and other reasons the Sceptics doubted the certainty of sense perception.[3]

They also attacked the Stoic doctrine of signs, that is, they distinguished between commemorative and indicative signs and rejected the latter.[4] The commemorative sign, such as that smoke indicates fire or a scar a preceding wound—revealing that which is occasionally non-evident but inherently evident—was accepted by the Sceptics.[5] The reason for accepting it, however, was not its visibility, as such a line of reasoning would have been vulnerable to their own critique of appearance. They accepted the commemorative sign because it is accepted by everyone and means the same to every observer.[6] For the same reason they rejected the

[a]Sextus Empiricus uses the word, "Dogmatist," to denote Stoic, Platonic, and Peripatetic thought.

indicative sign: it points to something "naturally non-evident" and has a different meaning for every observer.[7]

In their attack on judgment the Sceptics criticized causes, definitions, the syllogism, and induction. Aenesidemos developed eight arguments against the Rationalist theory of causation.[8] He pointed out that etiology deals with the non-apparent and thus cannot be confirmed by any data apparent to the senses. Most things are caused by a variety of causes, while Rationalist theories usually ascribe them to a single cause. The Rationalists, when they have understood the manner in which apparent things are produced, assume that non-apparent things are produced in the same way. Actually they may well be produced in quite different ways. Each Rationalist assigns causes according to his own particular theory, and they do not agree on a single theory of causation. They frequently admit only those facts which can be explained by their theories.[9][b] Furthermore, the Sceptics produced arguments against material causes[10] and efficient causes.[11] These arguments can be reduced to a denial of the Stoic doctrine that cause is a thing in itself and causality some sort of objective quality inherent in it.

Turning their fire against the idea of "definition," the Sceptics argued that apprehension precedes definition, rather than the other way around (as the Rationalists maintained). Hence, the definition cannot tell a person more about the object than he already knows.[12] Sextus Empiricus gives the following example:

> . . . suppose that one wished to ask someone whether he had met a man riding a horse and leading a dog and put the questions in this form—"O, rational, mortal animal, receptive of intelligence and science, have you met with an animal capable of laughter, with broad nails and receptive of political science, with his [posterior] hemispheres seated on a mortal animal capable of neighing, and leading a four-footed animal capable of barking?"—how would one be otherwise than ridiculous, in thus

[b]Note the relevance of this argument for the Empirical critique of the Rationalist selection of "important" symptoms.

> reducing the man to speechlessness concerning so familiar an object, because of one's definitions?[13c]

The Sceptics were thus nominalists.[d] They rejected the process of logical division (*dieresis*), since, as they claimed, names are conventional and not based on nature. All nouns are proper nouns, and nature cannot be investigated by the logical analysis of word meanings.[14]

They attacked induction with the argument that it is valid only when all possible instances of an event have been assembled. Since this is impossible, induction from a series of particulars is never justified.[15]

Finally, the Sceptics attacked the syllogism based on indicative signs, of the sort:

> All men with redness of skin suffer from surfeit of blood.
> Socrates has a red skin.
> Therefore, Socrates suffers from surfeit of blood.

The attack was on two levels. First they denied that the indicative sign (redness of skin) reveals its consequent (surfeit of blood). Either the consequent must be evident in itself, in which case the sign is not necessary, or it is non-evident, in which case there is no agreement among men as to which signs serve to make it evident.[16] Then the Sceptics went on to attack the major premise ("All men with redness of skin suffer from surfeit of blood") on logical grounds. They pointed out that such a major premise, far from being self-evident, is actually based on induction from a series of particular instances ("Socrates has a red skin and therefore suffers from surfeit of blood"). Thus it is circular reasoning to deduce from the universal proposition the same particular instances upon which the universal proposition was initially based. "They are establishing the universal proposition inductively by means of each of the particulars and deducing the particular proposition from the universal syllogisti-

[c]This same definition of "man" is given in the pseudo-Galenic work, *Medical Definitions* (K XIX 355).

[d]Galen and the Rationalists, of course, were essentialists: "We utter a noun for the thing" (K VIII 720).

cally."[17] Furthermore, in this case the particular instances themselves are unreliable, being founded upon indicative signs.[e]

A Methodical Basis for Action

The effect of this destructive critique of knowledge was initially to deprive the Sceptics of any grounds for action. Hence, the founder of the school opted for total passivity, advocating suspension of judgment (*epokhe*) and imperturbability (*ataraksia*). Diogenes Laertius describes this attitude:

> The Sceptics, then, were constantly engaged in overthrowing the dogmas of all schools, but enuntiated none themselves; and though they would go so far as to bring forward and expound the dogmas of the others, they themselves laid down nothing definitely, not even the laying down of nothing. So much so, that they even refuted their laying down of nothing, saying, for instance, "We determine nothing," since otherwise they would have been betrayed into determining . . .[18]

Aenesidemos, however, and especially Carneades, rejected the negative attitude of Pyrrho and Timon. Accepting the human burden of living despite the absence of a reliable theoretical guide, they transformed the same Sceptical epistemological assumptions into a positive guide to practice. Carneades maintained that even though all sense impressions are inherently unreliable, some are less unreliable than others, and a sufficient basis for practical choice and action can be found in the probable and the subjectively satisfying.[19] By introducing the concept of probability the Sceptics took a major step into an area which was alien to the speculation of the earlier period.

Carneades graded judgments according to their reliability and persuasiveness, classifying them as the apparently true and the apparently false. The class of the apparently true he

[e]There are many parallels between Hume's critique of metaphysics and the Sceptical critique of Peripatetic and Stoic thought. See Leon Robin, *La Pensee Grecque et les Origines de l'Esprit Scientifique,* p. 385.

subdivided into: (1) those which are probable in themselves, (2) those which are both probable and uncontradicted by any accompanying notions, and (3) those which are probable, uncontradicted by accompanying notions, and, moreover, "closely scrutinized," that is, tested by experience.[20f]

This method of analysis is designed to yield a reliable guide to action. Reliable action is based upon the analysis of action itself. Theory emerges from practice. Practice cannot emerge from theory, since reliability in practical applications is not a function of the logical consistency of abstract concepts.

Sceptical thought is thus the first glimmering of what we today call scientific method. These philosophers claimed that knowledge cannot be obtained directly but only indirectly—through a methodically controlled experience—and this is precisely what is done by any experimental scientist. By the same token, they maintained that no knowledge is absolutely reliable, since further experience may compel an alteration in one's views. This is also perfectly scientific.[g]

The idea that knowledge (theory) is the outcome of practice, rather than its cause, is the great discovery of the Sceptics. In seeking suitable rules of practical conduct in everyday life they discovered a method of investigation which is identical with the contemporary view of scientific method in taking into account the implications of the *negative instance*. This followed naturally from their desire to base knowledge on experience. Experience is manifold and contradictory, and if it is to be sorted out in some practical

[f]The words, *periodeumenai* or *dieksodeumenai*, are translated by Bury as "scrutinized" or "fully tested" (Sextus Empiricus, Loeb Edition, Vol. III, 529) and by Windelband as "verified in experience" (*History of Philosophy*, p. 207). The words appear in *Pyrrhonism* I, 227 and *Against the Logicians*, I, 181, 182, 187, 437.

[g]Bertrand Russell is mistaken in seeing a conflict between the Sceptical and the scientific mentalities because the Sceptics "assert the impossibility of knowledge Dogmatically" (*History of Western Philosophy* [New York, 1945], p. 234). In the first place, the Sceptics did not assert this dogmatically, but only withheld judgment (*Pyrrhonism*, I 237-238), but even if they had, this would not have been unscientific. Scientific knowledge is always only hypothetical—remaining valid until disproved by additional experience or experiments.

way, a procedure must be found which can incorporate negative cases. Hence the introduction of a doctrine of probability. Carneades' three classes of the "apparently true" represent three combinations of positive and negative instances—that is, three criteria of the reliability of experience, three probabilistic inferences.

The tables of instances compiled by Francis Bacon in the *Novum Organum* resemble the classes of Carneades and have the same function.[h]

All modern speculation about scientific method is only a continuation of the Sceptical effort to make methodical provision for the negative instance.

The fact that the Sceptics aimed to find a guide to practical behavior while "science" is concerned with the knowledge of nature does not affect this comparison. What is significant is that both the Sceptic and the scientist place practice (that is, experimental method) before theory and reject knowledge of causes in favor of the knowledge of sequences of events:

> In respect of things apparent [man] possesses a retentive sense of sequence, by which he remembers what things he has observed together with what, and what before what, and what after what, and from his experience of previous things revives the rest.[21]

Both thus recognize that knowledge of nature is tentative, remaining valid only until disproved by further experience.

The introduction of the negative instance into thought was a major advance of Scepticism over Aristotelianism, and it is this which ultimately places Aristotle outside the scientific tradition. Although he in many ways appreciated the significance of practice and experience, he cannot be said to have understood the importance of negative instances for the formulation of theory, since he tended to ascribe to the independent category of "chance" those events which did not accord with theory. The probabilistic approach of the Sceptics—which enabled them to extend their philosophic

[h]For further discussion of Francis Bacon see Volume II of this work.

vision to encompass *all* observed events and to subject them all to methodical analysis—is the opposite of Aristotelianism, which divides events into those which fall within the scope of philosophical analysis and those which fall outside it.

Both Scepticism and "science" posit utility as the criterion of knowledge.[i] The contemporary scientist means by utility the capacity of knowledge to produce some anticipated result in practice, and the Sceptic also proved the superiority of his doctrines by their practical consequences. This is seen from two anecdotes which the Sceptics told about themselves. In one the Sceptic propounds the *sorites* argument against a Stoic of the school of Chrysippos (*circa* 280-209 B.C.), and the Stoic declares that he "ought to halt while the argument is still proceeding and suspend judgment, to avoid falling into absurdity."[22j] Another is about Herophilos of Chalcedon:

> . . . he was a contemporary of Diodorus who, being given to juggling with dialectic, used to promulgate sophistical arguments against motion as well as many other things. So when Diodorus had dislocated his shoulder he came to Herophilos to get treated, and the latter jestingly said to him, "Your shoulder has been put out either in the place where it was or where it was not; but it was put out neither where it was nor where it was not; therefore, it has not been put out"; so that the Sophist begged him to leave such arguments alone and apply the treatment prescribed by medical *tekhne* as suitable to his case.[23]

The Stoic admits the superiority of the Sceptical argument by his *practical* behavior—he refuses to continue the argument. And Diodorus abandons his own doctrines when it becomes necessary to effect some practical result.

This latter example brings up another idea introduced into Greek thought by the Sceptics—that the relations obtaining in logic differ from the relations among the phenomena of nature. Sextus Empiricus writes:

[i]The Sophists had also maintained that utility is the criterion of truth, thus arousing the ire of Plato. Scepticism owes this idea to the Sophists.

[j]On the *sorites* see below, p. 275.

> . . . as regards all the sophisms which dialectic seems peculiarly able to expose, their exposure is useless; whereas in all cases where the exposure is useful, it is not the dialectician who will expose them but the experts in each particular *tekhne* who grasp the connections of the facts.[24]

making a distinction between logical relationships and the "connections of the facts." This distinction is, of course, parallel with the conflict in Greek medicine between *logos* and experience (since the "connections of the facts" are discovered through experience).[k]

Another sign of the awakening of the scientific mentality is the need for precision in particulars, as in the following passage:

> The exact blending of the simple drugs makes the product wholesome, but when the slightest oversight is made in measuring, as sometimes happens, the compound is not only unwholesome, but frequently even most harmful and deleterious.[25]

* * * * * * * * *

We have mentioned that the therapeutic doctrine of the Group I and IV Hippocratic writings stresses individualization of treatment. The doctrine itself is not an abstract body of knowledge but a set of rules. Medical practice is a skill learned by experience. Focus is on the individual practitioner.[l]

The themes of individualization, practical skill, and the reliability of knowledge link these medical writings with Scepticism—and later with the Empirical School. The Sceptics were concerned with the individual and problems of living. They sought reliable rules for skilful behavior by the individual in confronting practical problems of everyday life. Pyrrho deliberately left no writings but instructed by his own example and practical behavior. The Sceptics were not a

[k]Note also Paracelsus' distinction between "logic" and the "light of nature" (see below, pp. 372-374).

[l]See above, pp. 32-33.

group who subscribed to a single metaphysical doctrine but rather a group who confronted problems of life by following certain rules of behavior. "A Pyrrhonean is one who in manners and life resembles Pyrrho."[26]

In working out solutions to existential problems, however, these philosophers learned how to handle negative instances and degrees of probability. They hit on the idea of testing a doubtful judgment against practice or experience. These were later to prove invaluable to the Empirical physicians.

Herophilos of Chalcedon

Herophilos of Chalcedon, a contemporary of Arcesilaus, was the first physician consciously to apply the Sceptical philosophy to the practice of medicine.[27] For this reason he is rightly considered the spiritual father of the Empirical School founded by his pupil, Philinos of Cos.[28]

Herophilos studied medicine with Praxagoras of Cos toward the end of the fourth century and was brought to Alexandria by Ptolemy I in about the year 300.[29] He was a young man at the time, and his whole productive life was passed in Alexandria. His *floruit* is placed at between 270 and 260.[30]

Despite his training, Herophilos rejected the primary tenet of Rationalist medicine: the validity of causal knowledge of the organism. An aphorism attributed to him by many ancient writers is: "the phenomena must be considered as primary even though they are not."[31] Galen notes that he viewed proximate causes as "not discoverable,"[32] that "he dared not say anything about the nature of the first elements of the body," and that he even seemed to reject the procatarctic cause as an element of therapeutic doctrine.[33] Herophilos made experience "all-important."[34]

He criticized his contemporary, Erasistratos, for maintaining that the ultimate components of the organism, as well as some of its mechanisms, are cognizable by the *logos*. Herophilos accepted sense-perception as the sole criterion for distinguishing among the various components of the body—dividing them into the simple (meaning those parts made up of homogeneous substance, such as the brain, the sinews, and the arteries) and the compound (the hand, leg, head, liver, lung, etc.).[35]

Herophilos' view of logic has already been noted in Sextus Empiricus' tale of his dealings with Diodorus. He told his followers to avoid giving logical explanations of phenomena.[36] Instead, he emphasized their description. The fragments of Herophilos contain a number of his descriptions and definitions. They are based upon what is perceptible to the senses, and they seem to be as brief as possible.

In fact, many of these definitions are tautologies—a sign of Herophilos' refusal to speculate about causes. Thus, sudden death is due to paralysis of the heart.[37] Round wounds heal more slowly than long ones because the area of the wound is greater.[38] A strong pulse is due to the strength of the vital power (*zootikos dynamis*) in the arteries.[39] A good physician is the one who can distinguish between the possible and the impossible.[40] Medicine is the knowledge of healthy, morbid, and neutral conditions.[41] Disease is a disturbance of the humors. Or, a disease is something which is not always resolved in the same amount of time, but sometimes takes longer and sometimes a shorter time.[42] Drugs are classified as hot, cold, and in between.[43] The three types of physical constitution are the strong, the weak, and the neutral.[44] Tremor or shivering is an affliction of the nervous system.[45]

In his descriptions of diseases also, Herophilos stayed close to the sense-perceptible. Galen compliments him on his capacity for observation, stating that Herophilos proceeded with his analogy or induction as far as sense-perception permitted.[46] Caelius Aurelianus notes that Herophilos merely sets forth the symptoms (of paralysis) without going into its causes.[47]

He apparently wrote a work against accepted ideas or "common sense" in medicine (*pros tas koinas doksas*). All we know of it, however, is the title.[48][m]

[m]This may have been an attack on Rationalist etiological doctrines which appealed to common-sense arguments in favor of their validity. The Stoics were

Like the Empirics after him, Herophilos was an admirer of Hippocrates. He was the first to write commentaries on the Hippocratic works and compiled a collection of rare and unusual words encountered in them.[49] This concern with the meanings of words is natural to a man who considers the proper description of phenomena to be vitally important. Galen the Rationalist complains that "many have given concrete explanations of these expressions; Herophilos only gives verbal explanations."[50]

Herophilos made a major contribution to Empirical medicine with his doctrine of the pulse and its importance for prognosis.[n] He maintained that the pulse yields a direct reading of the movement of the *physis* and that rhythmic and other changes can be used to predict the course of disease.[51] He developed a body of pulse doctrine in which pulse rates were classified according to size, speed, strength, rhythm, order, disorder, and irregularity.[52] To make this knowledge graphic he based it on analogies with musical rhythms.[53] He also compared various pulses to the movements of the gazelle, the ant, and the worm.[54]

Of particular interest is his view that the "normal" pulse varies with age.[55] He measured disease by disturbance of the pattern normal to the particular age group.[56]

Herophilos' interest in prognosis is seen also in that he wrote a commentary on the Hippocratic work of that name.[57] He divided signs and symptoms into those which indicate the present, the past, and the future; it may be

teaching the doctrine of *communes notiones (koinai ennoai)*—that certain ideas are proven to be true by the fact that they are accepted by all. Such arguments were vulnerable to the Sceptical demonstration that experience provides many negative instances—that is, that many people do not share these common-sense notions (Windelband, *A History of Philosophy,* I, p. 204).

[n]C.R.S. Harris observes, "The real importance of his pulse-lore lies in the fact that Herophilos was, it would appear, the first to distinguish the pulse as a specific physiological reaction, and to recognize its importance as a clinical sign in diagnosis and prognosis . . . And though he is accused by Galen of a want of clarity in his exposition and of undue prolixity, there can be little doubt that his description of the different classes of pulse and their qualities and variations formed the basis of the teachings of the later physicians, notably Archigenes, Rufus, and Galen, who built upon the foundations which he had laid" (*The Heart and the Vascular System in Ancient Greek Medicine,* pp. 184-185).

assumed that pulse variations were among the most important of these signs.[58] He introduced a subtlety into the doctrine of prognosis—distinguishing between foreknowledge of an event and its prediction.[59] Although Galen calls this a false and sophistical distinction, Herophilos regarded it as genuine and not arbitrary.[60] The difference seems to have been between what will happen if external factors do not interfere and the actual prediction of events entirely under the physician's control.[61]

Herophilos is clearly an Empiric in his stress on sensory observation and description. Galen criticizes his pulse doctrine as a series of empirical facts and not a logical exposition.[62] A certain disregard for logic is also seen in his claim that a child's pulse is not necessarily small but can be large,[63] as also in his view that menstruation, instead of being beneficial to all women—as was claimed by the Rationalists on the grounds that it was a monthly cleaning process—is actually good for some women and bad for others.[64]

Herophilos is virtually unique among physicians in combining Empirical mistrust of the proximate cause with a tremendous interest in anatomy.[o] A modern writer calls him the "founder of systematic anatomy," and he was one of the foremost anatomists of antiquity.[65] Even Galen hardly ever contradicts Herophilos but merely elaborates on what he said.[66] He notes that Herophilos put the art of dissection on a firm basis and was outstanding in it.[67]

Herophilos was one of the first to dissect the human body. Aristotle had limited his investigations to the bodies of animals, but the transfer of the center of medical speculation to Egypt with its tradition of embalming the dead had given an important stimulus to the study of human anatomy.[68] Both Celsus and Tertullian, moreover, accuse Herophilos of

[o]Just as the followers of Aristotle could not handle the Empirical-Rationalist polarity of his thought but opted for the Rationalist side, so the followers of Herophilos went in two directions. Some became Empirics (see *infra*) while others, presumably inspired by his anatomical teachings, pursued an etiologically based medicine. See the description of the causes of difficult birth by the Herophilean Demetrios in Owsei Temkin, *Soranus' Gynecology* (Baltimore: Johns Hopkins University Press, 1956), pp. 177-182.

vivisection. Tertullian states: "Herophilos, that doctor, or rather butcher, has dissected countless persons, in that way investigating the *Natura*; he hated mankind in order to know him."[69] Celsus claims that he dissected condemned criminals.[70]

Herophilos opposed the Rationalists on several anatomical issues. He maintained that the arteries contain blood, not *pneuma.*[71] And he held that brain, not the heart, is the seat of the soul (the *anima,* the *psyche*).[72]

Only a tremendous intellect could withstand the temptation to use such extensive anatomical knowledge as the basis for etiological speculation about disease and health, and this is perhaps the clearest evidence of Herophilos' genius. He even admitted his inability to understand how the heart could be the principle (*arkhe*) of both the veins and the arteries.[73]

A very interesting problem is that of Herophilos' humoralism. Although Galen states that he accepted the humoral doctrine, the surviving fragments do not mention any humor other than the blood.[74][p] It may be surmised that he rejected the overelaborate humoralism of Praxagoras and the other early Rationalists and accepted the one humor whose presence could be detected unambiguously by sense-perception.[75]

In this he may have been following Erasistratos' doctrine which also centers on the blood (differing from the latter only in maintaining that the body is nourished by the blood through the arteries as well as the veins).[76] There was also precedent in Aristotle for assigning the blood a place superior to the other humors.[q]

In contrast to Erasistratos, Herophilos advocated bloodletting, as did his followers.[77] Why he did so, however, is a

[p]The view attributed to Herophilos by Celsus that "all the fault is in the wetnesses [*humidis*]" (*De Medicina, Prooemium,* 15) is not equivalent to support for Rationalist humoralism. The use of *humida* (plural of *humidum*), which means "wetnesses" or "wet parts", should rather be seen as an effort by Herophilos to evade the full force of Rationalist humoralism. Otherwise Celsus would have used *humor* (Greek: *chymos*).

[q]See above, p. 143.

mystery. It may have been for traditional reasons: blood-letting is mentioned in many of the Hippocratic writings.

In any case, Rationalist humoralism is rejected by both Herophilos and Erasistratos, although for different reasons. While the latter dissolves the humors into atoms, the former finds them not sense-perceptible.

Little is known of Herophilos' therapeutics. He treated diseases of the simple parts of the body empirically, those of the compound parts rationally.[78] He used gymnastics and dietary treatment, as well as phlebotomy.[79] And he was one of the great pharmacologists of antiquity, calling botanical drugs the "gifts of the Gods."[80] Pliny notes that he thought some so powerful as to be curative if only stepped upon.[81] Celsus states that the Herophileans treated no diseases without drugs and that of all the ancient schools they used drugs and herbs the most.[82]

Leaders of the Empirical School

The Empirical School arose during the lifetime of Herophilos or shortly after his death. In the year 250 it was headed by his pupil, Philinos of Cos.[83] The latter's younger contemporary, Serapion of Alexandria, was the other founder of this School and called himself the first "non-Dogmatist" physician (*primus medicorum indogmaticus*).[84]

None of the writings of these physicians have survived,[r] and we know their ideas only through references and comments in the works of others. The three topics which they treated were therapeutics, pharmacology, and Hippocratic exegesis—all of which had been stressed by Herophilos.[85]

Philinos wrote on pharmacology and Hippocratic exegesis.[86] He was also concerned with that fundamental problem of Empiricism—the meaning and value of sense perception.[87][s] Serapion wrote on therapeutics and on the critical side of Empiricism.[88]

[r]But see discussion of Celsus on following page.

[s]Erasistratos' polemical work against the opponents of causal analysis in medicine (*anaitiologetoi*) must have been directed against Philinos (Deichgraeber, *op. cit.*, p. 255).

Some thirty years later Apollonios the Empiric polemicized against the Epicureans over the interpretation of sensory data, maintaining that they did not yield ultimate knowledge. Apollonios also occupied himself with Hippocratic exegesis.[89]

His contemporary, Glaukias of Tarentum, wrote on the theoretical side of Empiricism as well as on therapy, pharmacy, and the Hippocratic Corpus.[90]

In the early part of the first century B.C. Empiricism recruited its ablest spokesman, Herakleides of Tarentum, from among the Herophileans. He was the first of the ancient physicians to write commentaries on all the Hippocratic works.[91] He pursued research in pharmacology as well, and all succeeding writers on pharmacology, including Galen, worked with the materials he left.[92]

One of his disciples, Lykos of Naples, also wrote commentaries on some of the Hippocratic writings.[93] Another famous Empiric of this time, a certain Zopyros, was the physician who supplied Mithradates with antidotes against poisons.[94]

In the first century A.D. an Empiric named Zeuxis wrote commentaries on the whole of the Hippocratic Corpus; these were later used by Galen.[95]

In Rome, at the court of Tiberias Caesar, there was an Empirical physician named Cassius who wrote on medicine and also composed a work against Zeno the Stoic.[96][t]

The Empiric who made the greatest impact on Galen's thought was Menodotos of Nicomedia, who lived at the beginning of the Christian era. Galen drew on him for some of his knowledge of Empiricism and wrote attacks on him as well.[u] Menodotos seems to have been the first to systematize

[t]We accept Max Wellmann's view that Celsus' *De Medicina* was patterned on one of the existing Empirical therapeutic compendia. Wellman suggests that Celsus rewrote in Latin a work by his friend, Cassius (Max Wellmann, *A. Cornelius Celsus: Eine Quellenuntersuchung*. Berlin: Weidmannsche Buchhandlung, 1913). See below, pp. 202-203.

[u]Galen's very important book on the Empirical School, *De Subfiguratione Empirica*, is thought by Deichgraeber to be based on the writings of Menodotos (Deichgraeber, *op. cit.*, p. 18). It was lost for centuries and is not included in the collected editions of Galen's works. The Greek original has not been found, and

the use of negative instances as the criterion of the reliability of medical experience and medical judgments.[97] He wrote works against both the Rationalist and the Methodist schools.[98]

The last of the Empirics is Sextus Empiricus, about 200 A.D., and shortly after his time the Empirical School as such disappears from history.[99v]

According to Diogenes Laertius there was a direct personal relationship between many of the Sceptical philosophers, starting with Timon of Phlius, and the Empirical physicians.[100] He states, in particular, that Aenesidemos was a pupil of Herakleides and a friend of Zeuxis.[101]

Whether or not this is an exaggeration, the overwhelming parallels between Sceptical thought and Empirical medicine make an association between these two groups of learned men highly likely.[w] Although we cannot know precisely at which date it began, the period of Philinos' study with Herophilos seems the most probable starting-point for the introduction of Sceptical ideas into medicine.[102]

Menodotos was an admirer or Pyrrho[103] and (if the *De Subfiguratione Empirica* really represents his views) has given the best statement of the relationship between the two groups: *qualis est secundum totam vitam scepticus, talis est circa medicativam empiricus.*[104]

The Empirics and the Hippocratic Corpus

The Empirics and Herophilos were antiquity's leading commentators on the Hippocratic Corpus. Herakleides and Zeuxis wrote on all of the Hippocratic writings, while others of the Empirics dealt with one or several of them.

we have only the Latin translation made by Niccolo à Reggio in the fourteenth century. This was first published in the sixteenth century and is included in Deichgraeber's *Griechische Empirikerschule,* pp. 42-90.

Albert Favier's *Menodote de Nicomedie: Precurseur de la Methode Experimentale Moderne* (Paris: Rousset, 1906) discusses Mendotos as an influence on the modern theory of scientific method.

[v]See below, p. 321, note.

[w]For discussion of these parallels see below, pp. 262-274.

We have been suggesting that the Empirical School drew inspiration from the works of Groups I and IV or, as is more probable, that the continuing medical tradition represented by these writings came to the surface in mid-fourth-century Alexandria and called itself the Empirical School.

The emergence and self-definition of the Empirical School was a response to the claims of the Rationalists to represent the true therapeutic method.[x] But the Empirical ideas must surely have remained in existence from the time of their formulation by Hippocratic writers in the fifth century.

The thesis of a connection between the Empirical doctrines and the therapeutic method of the Group I and IV Hippocratic works is substantiated not only by the congruence of these two bodies of ideas but also by the attitude of the Empirical physicians toward the Hippocratic Corpus: all available evidence suggests a preference on their part for the Group I works (and, to a lesser extent, those of Group IV) and a relative lack of interest in the Group II and III writings.

The one complete therapeutic handbook of the Empirical School which has survived from ancient times, Celsus' *De Medicina*, draws inspiration overwhelmingly from the Group I writings. W.G. Spencer finds that Celsus makes more than 200 references to the *Aphorisms*, 77 to *Prognosis*, 30 to *Prorrhetic I,* 4 to *Coan Prognosis,* and 2 to *The Art.*[105][y] Furthermore, Book VIII of *De Medicina* (volume two of the Loeb Edition), dealing with surgery, is "practically an epitome" of the Hippocratic surgical works (*On Fractures-On Joints, Mochlicon, Wounds of the Head,* and *In the Surgery*).[106] On the other hand, Celsus makes only three references to Group II works (1 to *Diseases I* and 2 to *Affections*) and ten references to Group III works (4 to *Regimen I* and *II,* 4 to *Breaths,* 1 to *Airs Waters Places*, and 1 to *Nature of Man*). Ten other Hippocratic references in *De*

[x]Deichgraeber suggests that the Empirics did not form a true school or a sociological unity characterized by a relationship to a particular body of doctrine and were perhaps held together primarily by their common rejection of Rationalism (*op. cit.*, pp. 253-254).

[y]See below, pp. 244-247.

Medicina are to works dated later than the ones analyzed by us above.

The evidence from Celsus indicates an overwhelming preference for the Group I writings, while little attention is paid to those of Groups II and III.

Additional information on this point is provided by the Empirical Hippocratic exegesis contained in the fragments preserved mainly by Galen. While their interpretation raises a number of problems, it is interesting to note that their distribution is similar to that found in *De Medicina*. These fragments make 4 references to the *Aphorisms*, 5 to *Prorrhetic I*, 7 to *Epidemics III*, 2 to *Epidemics I*, 2 to *Prognosis*, 9 to the surgical works, 1 to *Regimen in Acute Diseases I*, and 1 to *The Art*. There are no references to any writings of Groups II and III, but these fragments contain 37 references to other Hippocratic writings (*Epidemics II, IV, V, VI, Places in Man*, etc.).[z]

Thus the evidence of the Empirical fragments indicates a preference for Groups I and IV over Groups II and III.

But, leaving aside this somewhat circumstantial evidence, the texts themselves reveal a dichotomy in the Empirical attitude toward the Hippocratic Corpus. For, on one hand, the Empirics called Hippocrates an Empiric and the founder of their School, stating that "almost" everything he said was true, while, on the other, Galen alleges that Lykos "calumniated" and Serapion "impudently attacked" Hippocrates.[107] Bearing in mind that for Galen "Hippocrates" was the Rationalist author of *Nature of Man*, [108][a] one may reasonably assume that the Empirics disliked precisely those themes and currents in the Hippocratic Corpus which Galen accepted as the veriest proofs of the true Hippocratic doctrine.

In other words, the Empirics must have rejected the four humors and the search for proximate (humoral or pneumatic) causes. They must have preferred observation and description to logical analysis.

[z]See below, pp. 205 and note, 240-241.

[a]See below, pp. 305 note, 306.

And we find Galen accusing them of precisely these sins: "Hippocrates posited the hot, the cold, the wet, and the dry as causes, also the ambient air in the bodies of animals; thus he says that the four humors differing among themselves in *krasis* are the causes of diseases and of health. But the Empirics who have explained some book of Hippocrates according to these principles act as though playing a role in a comedy—acting the part of another person . . . they err with respect not only to the intent of Hippocrates but also to the truth of things, and are thus to be doubly reproached."[109]

Compelled by tradition and respect for the name of Hippocrates to write comments on all the works supposedly from his hand, the Empirics did so—but only paid lip-service to the Rationalist writings and refused to enter wholeheartedly into the argument. This is undoubtedly why they accepted "almost" all (and not "all") of Hippocrates as truth.

Thus they rejected the four-humor theory with its whole metaphysical structure of hypothesized proximate causes. Their commentaries on *Aphorisms* III: 11:

> As for the seasons, if the winter be dry and northerly and the spring wet and southerly, of necessity occur in the summer acute fevers, eye diseases, and dysentery . . .

were not based upon acceptance of the four humors and held that the relationship between season and illness was discovered only through observation. Thus Galen accuses them of disregarding the words of Hippocrates ("of necessity").[110] In a case with an unanticipated ending the Empirics observed that logic would have led the physician astray: "Hippocrates maintained that faith should never be placed in the plausible arguments of the Dogmatists but only in what was known and clear through experience."[111]

They urged the physician to trust the eye more than the word,[112] experience more than the *logos:* "judgment" (*Aphorisms* I:1)[b] to them meant that which can be determined from experience, while to the Rationalists it was equivalent to the *logos.*[113]

[b]"Life is short, the art long . . . judgment difficult."

They held that Hippocrates individualized treatment, separating the symptoms common to all from those of the particular patient, and treated by similars.[114]

They healed pleurisy by the method set forth in *Regimen in Acute Diseases.*[115]

They claimed that Hippocrates was more concerned with environmental factors and external causes than with the place affected, the internal cause, or the "disease" itself.[116]

They entirely accepted the Hippocratic surgical works, followed them, and wrote illustrated guides to them.[117] They urged that the best surgeon is made by practice.[118] Galen singles out Herakleides as the best witness on matters involving dislocations: "Not lying for the sake of his doctrine, as many of the Rationalists would do."[119]

Generally the Empirics viewed the Hippocratic Corpus as an internally consistent whole, designed to be used as a practical guide to treatment.[120] They held that Hippocrates taught by enumerating particular cases and not by pronouncing general principles.[121] Thus they regarded the books of the *Epidemics* as containing source material for the summaries set forth in the *Aphorisms.*[122]

Seeing the Hippocratic writings as detailed accounts of individual cases, they tried to limit the universality of the conclusions drawn from them.[123] For the same reason they were extremely interested in the precise meaning of obscure words and constructions.[124][c] They were the first, and the greatest, of the ancients to engage in philological research on the Hippocratic works.[d] Galen, who made extensive use of

[c]For instance, one of the Empirical fragments contains a discussion of the meaning of "hidden diseases" as set forth in *The Art* (cap. X: see above, pp. 80-82), showing the perennial concern of the Empirical School with the problem of the invisible (Deichgraeber, *op. cit.,* Fr. 312).

[d]Three of the Empirical philological fragments (Deichgraeber, Fr. 315-317) refer to *Places in Man* (VI, 276-349, L.), a Hippocratic work from 350 B.C. which develops most of the themes discussed in the Group I and IV writings.

The organism is a whole all of whose parts interact and intercommunicate: the smallest part contains everything which is in the largest part (cap. 1: cf. Paracelsus' "microcosm" and "macrocosm"). The *physis* is the starting point (*arkhe*) of all reasoning (*logos*) in medicine, and all cure must be directed at this *arkhe* (caps. 2, 31). Cure is through coction, with crisis and empyema (caps. 12,14,17,18,21). Hence medicines must be administered at the correct time, their compilations, compliments them on their philological and other criticism and compares it unfavorably with that of the Rationalists.[125]

Thus, although the fragmentary nature of the material makes the problem not completely soluble, we may accept Deichgraeber's conclusion that: "Two currents are to be distinguished [in the Empirical Hippocratic exegesis], one which sees in him the founder of Empiricism and another . . . which sees in him a Dogmatist and tries to interpret him as such."[126]

The close resemblance between the Empirical teachings and those of the Group I and IV writings will become even more apparent below, in the discussion of the Empirical doctrines themselves.

neither too soon nor too late (caps. 17,27).

Cure by similars, which had been suggested in the Group I and IV writings (see above, pp. 29, 85), is developed extensively. Not only are fevers treated with heating remedies (cap. 27), expectoration and coughs with medicines which provoke expectoration and coughing (caps. 17-19), and phlegmatic diseases with liquids (cap. 42), treatment by similars is proposed as a general principle: diseases are caused by similars, and by the similars which he takes the patient is saved; what causes strangury also cures it; coughs are caused and cured by the same things; fever is suppressed by what produces it and produced by what suppresses it (cap. 42). Strong remedies are suited to a strong *physis* and weak remedies to a weak *physis:* the treatment must be adjusted to the *physis* of the patient (cap. 45: see *Precepts,* cap. IX, p. 255 *infra*).

But "similarity" lies between the medicine and the *physis,* and this means "contrariety" between the medicine and the disease. Pain is caused by cold in those of warm constitution, by warmth in those of cold constitution, by wetness in those who are dry, and by dryness in those who are wet: "These changes occur whenever there is a change and corruption of the *physis*" (cap. 42). Hence such pains are cured by contraries: a warm constitution which has become painful through cold is cured by a warm medicine (cap. 42). If "similars" fail, "contraries" should be attempted (caps. 12,27,42: see below, p. 259).

This treatment of the relationship between organism and environment differs from that proposed by Diocles and the Rationalists (see below, pp. 225, 233) and resembles that of Group I (see above, p. 30).

Furthermore, medicines cannot be classified as exclusively "similar" or "contrary," since the same medicine can have opposite effects, even in the same person (cap. 41). This is why medicine is unstable and difficult to learn: it is a matter of degree or measure (cap. 44).

The author assimilates "similarity" and "contrariety" to the theory of coction. Purgatives are not the contrary of astringents, since an astringent can cause purgation. Thus they can have the same effect (cap. 41). Purgatives become non-purgatives (cap. 44). "Dry" medicines are actually attenuating; purgatives which attenuate are actually heating; whatever cools the stomach is a purgative (whether intrinsically "hot" or "cold"), and, if it does not purge, it is "heating." "Hot" things which cause evacuation are cooling, and, if not, they are "heating" (cap. 45), etc. (cf. *Ancient Medicine,* caps. XIII-XVI: above, pp. 85-88).

What is important is to drive the disease out by the most direct route (caps. 21, 45), and the author discusses disease suppression: "If a flux goes elsewhere, wherever that may be, it will cause a more serious illness" (cap. 11); a flux which is blocked, whether through the skin or through the stomach, will cause aches in the joints (cap. 22).

He holds that the curative method has been discovered, and that the one who knows it need not rely on chance (cap. 46). Good luck is the equivalent of skill, while bad luck indicates lack of skill (*loc. cit.*). Littre notes here the parallels with *Ancient Medicine*, cap. II, and *The Art,* cap. IV (see above, pp. 72, 92-93), as well as the numerous other parallels between *Places in Man* and *Aphorisms, Prognosis,* and *Coan Prognosis.*

At the same time, this work contains much physiological explanation of disease processes. Hence it is eclectic but relies ultimately on the Empirical postulates. Together with *Nutriment* and *Epidemics VI* (see below, pp. 240-241) it forms a connecting link between the Group I and IV writings and the Empirical doctrine which emerged a century later in Alexandria.

NOTES

[1]On the history and teachings of Scepticism see Eduard Zeller, *Stoics, Epicureans and Sceptics* (New York, 1962); R.D. Hicks, *Stoic and Epicurean* (New York, 1962); Edwyn Bevan, *Stoics and Sceptics* (Oxford, 1913); Windelband, *A History of Philosophy* and *A History of Ancient Philosophy.*

[2]Sextus Empiricus, *Pyrrhonism*, I, 19. This seems to be derived from Democritus' views on the subjectivity of sensation (Zeller, p. 515).

[3]Sextus Empiricus, *Pyrrhonism*, I, 36-125. Hicks, p. 376ff.

[4]Hicks, p. 390ff. Since Aenesidemos does not seem to have made this distinction, it probably arose only at the very end of the Sceptical tradition and may have been discovered by Sextus Empiricus himself.

[5]Sextus Empiricus, *Pyrrhonism*, II, 100-102. *Against the Astrologers*, 104.

[6]Sextus Empiricus, *Against the Logicians*, II, 156-158. Leon Robin, *La Pensee Grecque et les Origines de l'Esprit Scientifique* (Paris, 1963), p. 385.

[7]Sextus Empiricus, *Against the Logicians*, II, 188; *Pyrrhonism*, II, 97-100.

[8]Hicks, p. 387ff.

[9]Sextus Empiricus, *Pyrrhonism*, I, 180-186.

[10]*Ibid.*, III, 30-62.

[11]*Ibid.*, III, 17-30.

[12]*Ibid.*, II, 205-210.

[13]*Ibid.*, II, 211.

[14]*Ibid.*, II, 213-214.

[15]*Ibid.*, II, 204. Robin, *op. cit.*, p. 385.

[16]*Ibid.*, II, 116-117.

[17] *Ibid.*, II, 196, 198-199.

[18] *Lives of the Philosophers*, IX, 74.

[19] Sextus Empiricus, *Against the Logicians*, I, 158, 166. Zeller, p. 562; Windelband, *History of Philosophy*, p. 206.

[20] Sextus Empiricus, *Against the Logicians*, I, 166-189.

[21] *Ibid.*, II, 288. Bevan, p. 125. Robin, p. 385.

[22] *Pyrrhonism*, II 253.

[23] *Ibid.*, II, 245.

[24] *Ibid.*, II, 236.

[25] *Ibid.*, I, 133.

[26] Diogenes Laertius, *Lives of the Philosophers,* IX 70.

[27] K. Deichgraeber, *Der Listensinnende Trug des Gottes,* (Goettingen, 1952), p. 104; F. Kudlien, "Herophilos und der Beginn der Medizinischen Skepsis," *Gesnerus* (1964), XXI, 1-13, at p. 4.

[28] K XIV 683. The best work on Herophilos is K.F.H. Marx, *De Herophili celeberrimi medici, vita, scriptis, atque in medicina meritis.* Goettingen: Dieterien, 1840.

[29] Kudlien, p. 2. K VIII 723.

[30] Jaeger, "Vergessene Fragmente," p. 39.

[31] K X 107. See, also, K VIII 869. In *Anonymus Londinensis* it is given as: "Let those things be called primary that appear to be primary, even though they are not really so" (Jones, *Medical Writings of Anonymus Londinensis*, XXI: 26). Timon of Phlius had stated: the apparent is omnipotent, wherever it goes (Diogenes Laertius, IX 105). See also Sextus Empiricus, *Against the Logicians*, I, 30.

[32] *Galeni De Causis Procatarcticis Libellus a Nicolao Regino in sermonem Latinum translatus*, C.M.G. Supp. II (Berlin, 1937), p. 53.

[33] *Loc. cit.* K X 462. He did not even like to ask a patient if the fever might have been caused by exposure to heat or cold or by overeating. Pliny states that he investigated disease causes, but this must have been in order to criticize the concept (*Natural History*, XXVI: viii; Kudlien, *op. cit.*, p. 6).

[34] Richard Walzer, *Galen on Medical Experience* (Oxford University Press, 1947), p. 110.

[35] Jones, *Medical Writings of Anonymus Londinensis*, c.XXI-XXII. He thus accepts Aristotle's second and third levels of explanation of the organism.

[36] K X 110.

[37] Caelius Aurelianus, *m. chr.* II 15.

[38] Marx, p. 54. This seems to have been a traditional problem in ancient medical speculation. See Aristotle, *Posterior Analytics* 79a 13-15.

[39] K VIII 645.

[40] Kudlien, p. 5, note 9.

[41] X XIV 688. Sextus Empiricus gives the same definition (*Against the Ethicists*, c. 186).

[42] Marx, p. 38.

[43] K XI 421.

[44] K VI 388. Marx, *op. cit.*, p. 38.

[45] K VII 605, i.e., Herophilos refused to consider the shivering an impairment of some natural faculty. Galen accuses him of failing to distinguish between the faculty and the instrument.

[46] K IX 278.

[47] Caelius Aurelianus, *m. chr.* II 49.

[48] Kudlien, p. 3.

[49] K XIX 64-65; Marx, pp. 8-9. George Sarton, *A History of Science: Ancient Science Through the Golden Age of Greece* (Cambridge, 1952), p. 351.

[50] K XIX 64.

[51] K VIII 645, 723, 744, 911.

[52] K VIII 592.

[53] K IX 463ff.

[54] Harris, *The Heart and the Vascular System in Ancient Greek Medicine*, p. 191.

[55] *Ibid.*, p. 194.

[56] *Loc. cit.*

[57] Caelius Aurelianus, *m. chr.*, IV, 113.

[58] K VIII 911.

[59] K XVIIIB 12. K XVI 489.

[60] K XVIIIB 12.

[61] *Ibid.*, 13. Marx, p. 39.

[62] K IX 278.

[63] K VIII 871; K VIII 853.

[64] Kudlien, p. 7.

[65] J.F. Dobson, "Herophilos of Alexandria," *Proc. Royal Soc. of Medicine, Sect. Hist. Med.*, IV (March 18, 1925), 19-32, at p. 19.

[66] K II 901; K IV 597.

[67] K V 650; K II 895.

[68] K II 895.

[69] Tertullian, *De Anima*, ed. J.H. Waszink (Amsterdam, 1947), c. 10.

[70] Celsus, *Prooemium*, 23.

[71] K IV 731. Jones, *Medical Writings of Anonymus Londinensis,* cap. XXVIII.

[72] K XIX 315; Dobson, "Herophilos of Alexandria," p. 19.

[73] K V 543.

[74] K V 684. K IV 731. K XIX 391. K XIV 698.

[75] He did, in fact, reject a number of the doctrines of his teacher, Praxagoras (K VII 594; K VIII 723).

[76] Jones, *Medical Works of Anonymus Londinensis,* cap. XXVIII: 28.

[77] K XI 163. Caelius Aurelianus, *m.a.*, II, 218.

[78] K X 184.

[79] K V 879. K XI 163. K XIX 64-65.

[80] Marx, p. 47

[81] *Natural History*, XXV, v, 15.

[82] Celsus, *De Medicina*, Bk. V, cap. 1.

[83] K XIV 683.

[84] Deichgraeber, *Die Griechische Empirikerschule*, p. 86 (*De Subf. Emp.).*

[85] *Ibid.*, p. 255.

[86] *Loc. cit.*

[87] *Ibid.*, p. 255 and Fr. 164.

[88] *Ibid.*, p. 256 and Fr. 145 to 148.

[89] *Ibid.*, p. 257.

[90] *Ibid.*, p. 258.

[91] *Ibid.*, p. 260 and Fr. 319

[92] *Ibid.*, p. 261 and Fr. 193. Marx, p. 51.

[93] *Ibid.*, p. 261.

[94] *Ibid.*, p. 262.

[95] *Ibid.*, p. 263.

[96] *Ibid.*, p. 264.

[97] *Ibid.*, p. 265.

[98] *Ibid.*, p. 264 and Fr. 292.

[99] *Ibid.*, p. 268.

[100] Diogenes Laertius, IX, 116.

[101] *Ibid.*, IX, 106, 116.

[102] Bevan (*Stoics and Sceptics*, p. 136) suggests the first century B.C.

[103] Deichgraeber, *De Subf. Emp.*, p. 84.

[104] *Ibid.*, p. 82.

[105] Celsus, *De Medicina* (Loeb Edition), Vol. III, pp. 624-627.

[106] *Ibid.*, Vol. III, p. 624.

[107] Deichgraeber, *Die Griechische Empirikerschule*, p. 86 and Fr. 310. K XVIIB 415.

[108] K II 132. K XVIIB 347.

[109] Deichgraeber, *Die Griechische Empirikerschule,* Fr. 309 (K XVIIA 507).

[110] *Ibid.*, p. 28 and Fr. 363.

[111] *Ibid.*, Fr. 356 (K XVIIB 94).

[112] *Ibid.*, Fr. 164.

[113] *Ibid.*, Fr. 362.

[114] Celsus, *De Medicina, Prooemium,* 66. *Galeni in Hippocratis De Officina Medici Commentariorum* (C.M.G. *Supplementum Orientale* I), Translated from the Arabic by Malcolm Lyons, Berlin, 1963, pp. 73-74. Deichgraeber, *op. cit.*, Fr. 359c.

[115] Deichgraeber, *Die Griechische Empirikerschule*, Fr. 16.

[116] *Ibid.*, Fr. 314.

[117] *Ibid.*, Fr. 175, 266, 282, 322.

[118] *Ibid.*, Fr. 282.

[119] *Ibid.,* Fr. 175 (K XVIIIA 735).

[120] *Ibid.*, Fr. 329, 331, 353, and p. 319.

[121] *Ibid.*, Fr. 353, 363.

[122] *Ibid.*, Fr. 329, 331.

[123] *Ibid.*, Fr. 321 and 365.

[124] *Ibid.*, Fr. 311, 311a, 312, 313, 315, 316, 318, 320, 322-328, 330, 337, 344, 350, 352, 355, 358, 364.

[125] *Ibid.*, Fr. 350.

[126] *Ibid.*, p. 318.

PART THREE

GREEK MEDICINE IN ROME

PART THREE

GREEK MEDICINE IN ROME

Pliny the Elder testifies that "the Roman people for more than 600 years were not, indeed, without medical art, but they were without physicians." Until perhaps the second century B.C. medicine was a despised profession in Rome, and the city and republic made do with religious incantations and folk remedies.

A Greek surgeon named Archagathus received Roman citizenship in 219 B.C. but shortly afterwards was expelled from the city as a "butcher" for using the knife and cautery too liberally.

The infiltration of Greek medical practitioners into Rome had begun, however, and it accelerated as this city became an imperial center, while Athens and Alexandria were reduced to provincial capitals. By the first and second centuries of the Christian era Rome had well made up for its prior neglect of the medical arts—at least six different medical schools competed there for the patient's attention and patronage.

The Herophileans, Erasistrateans, and Pneumatists[a] need not concern us, as they were doctrinal sub-species of the three most prominent schools: the Empirics, Rationalists, and Methodists.[b]

[a]The Pneumatic School took its origin in Rationalist musings about the role of the *pneuma* in physiology. The fragments of this school have been collected in Max Wellmann, *Die Pneumatische Schule* (Berlin: Weidmann, 1895). Its history is set forth in Harris, *The Heart and the Vascular System in Ancient Greek Medicine*, pp. 235-251.

[b]Galen states that most physicians of his day were not Rationalists, but otherwise we have no information on the relative sizes of these schools (K X 32). My own suspicion is that by Galen's time the Methodists were in the majority, while the Empirics and Rationalists were smaller groupings.

And since the Methodist doctrine itself was philosophically insignificant, being nothing more than the *reductio ad absurdum* of Rationalism,[c] the major ideological conflict was between the Rationalists and the Empirics.

As we stated in the Introduction, the Rationalists accepted the proximate cause as an element of the medical *tekhne* while the Empirics rejected it. The pseudo-Galenic work, *Medical Definitions,* calls the Rationalist School "the sect which follows the science [*episteme*] of hidden things" and the Empirical School "the sect of those things which are seen frequently and in the same way."[1]

This conflict over the proximate cause, which is fundamental, has often been obscured in historical treatments of this issue by the other major dispute between the two schools: reliance on experience vs. reliance on logic or reason (*logos*). However, the Empirics sought to base medical knowledge and practice on experience *because* they held proximate causes to be unknowable. And *because* the Rationalists held the opposite, they claimed that medical knowledge could be built up through logical manipulation of these causes.

Both schools recognized the need to apply intellect to the solution of medical problems.[d] They differed with respect to the materials amenable to treatment by the intellect, the Empirics holding that such materials were limited to the data of sensory observation. Celsus epitomizes this position in stating: "I think that medicine ought to be rational, but to draw instruction from evident causes, all obscure ones being rejected from the art . . ."[e]

The Rationalists posited a direct analytical relationship between intellectual operations (using the categories of formal logic) and the processes of physical reality. The thinking physician could thus achieve true and reliable knowledge of matters which he could not perceive with his senses.

[c]In a precise parallel to Erasistrateanism, two centuries earlier.

[d]See *The Art,* cap. XI and discussion above, pages 81-83.

[e]"*rationalem quidem puto medicinam esse debere, instrui vero ab evidentibus causis, obscuris omnibus . . . ab ipsa arte reiectis*" (*Prooemium,* 57).

The Methodists accepted the Rationalist doctrine of proximate causes but simplified it so that only two classes of such causes were of significance to medicine: those indicating a slack condition of the body (*status laxus*) and those indicating a rigid or constricted state (*status strictus*). These were the "common elements" (*communia*) of all diseases, and the Methodists sought to base treatment on these "common elements."[f] According to the *Medical Definitions:* "The Methodist sect is the knowledge of apparent common elements: strict, lax, or mixed."[2]

Finally, Galen aimed to restore the true doctrine of Hippocrates–which he took to be identical with an enlightened Rationalism. To this end he trimmed off the rough edges of Rationalism and made it internally consistent.

[f]"They . . . maintain that medicine should examine those characteristics which diseases have in common" (Celsus, *De Medicina, Prooemium,* 57).

NOTES

[1] K XIX 353. See, also, Deichgraeber, *op. cit.*, p. 50 (*De Subf. Emp.*).
[2] K XIX 353.

CHAPTER VI

THE RATIONALIST SCHOOL

The Rationalist School in Galen's time professed adherence to certain of the Hippocratic works, the philosophy of Plato and Aristotle, and the medical doctrines of Diocles, Praxagoras, and Mnesitheos.[a]

Pathology

The hallmark of Rationalist medicine was the conviction that therapeutics is based upon pathology and that before proceeding to treatment the physician must ascertain the patient's pathological state..

Several centuries of philosophical development had resulted in the acceptance by this school of the four humors as the key to the organism's functioning in sickness and health.[1] These were blood, phlegm, yellow bile, and black bile. Blood was hot and wet, phlegm cold and wet, yellow bile hot and dry, and black bile cold and dry.

Some members of this school felt that blood was not a separate humor but rather a mixture of all the humors.[2] Blood is produced by the innate heat when the nutriment is in proportion, the other humors when it is not in proportion.[3] Similarly, the role and function of black bile were not always defined in the same way—suggestions being made that it was a toxic humor, not found in the healthy organism, etc.[4]

[a]In Greek the Rationalists are known as *dogmatikoi* (from *dogma:* opinion or tenet) or *logikoi* (from *logos:* reason, logic, *ratio*). In later tradition this school has been known as the Dogmatic or Dogmatist school. But in view of the competing meanings of "dogmatic" in the modern European languages (viz., "authoritarian," "imperious," "arrogant") "Rationalist" seems a preferable rendering. Celsus describes them as *"ii qui rationalem medicinam profitentur"* (*De Medicina, Prooemium,* 13).

On the whole, however, Rationalist theory held that health results from the correct mixture of these four humors (in the body as a whole and in each of its organs and parts)[b] and disease from their improper mixture (dyscrasia)–i.e., from the preponderance of one humor and its localization in some part of the body.[5]

The different dyscrasias were associated with different kinds of illness: phlegm with quotidian fever, yellow bile with erysipelas and tertian fever, black bile with quartan fever, etc.[6]

The presence of the dyscrasia was thought to inhibit or pervert one of the body's natural functions.[7] But the disordered function was not to be taken as the disease itself since, strictly speaking, it was merely the consequence of the "disease"–of the dyscrasia.[8] Hence the ordinary expression, "disease," could be subdivided into: (1) the dyscrasia (the proximate cause), (2) the damage to the function, and (3) the symptoms.[9]

Diagnosis, Symptoms, Diseases

When the physician sees his patient, it is the symptoms which first engage his attention. And the Rationalist saw his initial task as being to obtain an idea of the underlying dyscrasia from his observation of the symptoms of disordered function.

Thus the physician was not to attempt to note all the patient's symptoms, as this would only plunge him into a morass. Many of the symptoms are not even useful; the physician must separate the useful from the useless, and this he does by the *logos.*[10] Just as the sounds of the voice are infinite and only become useful for communication when organized by the grammarian, so must the symptoms of

[b]Galen's 16th-century translator, Nicholas Culpepper, writes: "Whereas Galen saith a good constitution consists of heat, cold, driness, and moisture, equally tempered, you must not imagine they are so all over the body, but according to place, for the Heart is and should be hotter than the Brain, etc., but each part exceeds not its due proportion in these, the brain is not hotter, colder, drier, or moister than it should be, judge so by the heart, liver, etc., and beleeve me such a man is a rare bird to find, almost as rare as a *Phoenix.*"

disease be organized by the physician in such a way as to be useful for therapy:

> So also with the kinds and varieties of musical sounds: they, too, are very numerous in loudness and softness, strength and lightness, and memory cannot hold them all and confine them without the *logos,* but rather the *logos* alone, which musicians make use of, encloses and confines them, bringing them within finite categories.[11]

The Rationalist physician also argued that, the functions of the body being finite in number, the useful symptoms—reflecting derangements of these natural functions, must themselves be finite in number.[12]

The physician knows that a given symptom is indissolubly tied to a particular internal pathological alteration because the doctrine of signs can be applied to medicine. The symptoms are indicative signs, revealing the presence of phenomena otherwise invisible.[13]

Thus, a hard pulse indicates a dry heart, a soft pulse a moist heart; a slow pulse indicates a cold heart and a fast pulse a hot heart. Signs of a hot liver are distended veins, hot blood, and much yellow and black bile. Those in whom the veins are narrow and thin, whose bodies are off-color, and who suffer a pain in the right side after eating, have too small a liver. Fickleness of opinion shows a hot brain and stability of opinion a cold brain. Other signs of a hot brain: the forehead is reddish and hot, the veins in the whites of the eyes are red, the hair is hard and curly, and the person becomes bald. Other signs of a cold brain: the hair is black, soft, and not curly; the person easily suffers from cold, has a pale face and a cold forehead, is dull-witted, and sleeps a lot.[14]

The symptom is to internal change as sign is to antecedent—the direct consequent of the disease and based on its very cause and nature.[15] At the same time it is an ephemeral phenomenon and does not in itself describe the internal pathological change. Just as one could see any number of fathers and sons together without being able to tell—with respect to two unknown men—whether or not they stood in this relationship to one another, so the physician needs additional knowledge to perceive the relationship between symptoms and diseases.[16] This additional knowledge is supplied by formal logic and the syllogism.[17] No role is played here by experience.[18]

Thus the useful symptoms contain something more than what is visible to the senses, and this "something" is revealed by the *logos*.[19] There can be no observation in and of itself, i.e., without participation by the *logos*.[20] Observation based on the *logos* is rational observation, and this is what the physician's training qualifies him to do.

The main symptom which the physician seeks (employing the *logos*) is the one indicating the disease cause, i.e., the humoral dyscrasia.[21] But if he cannot immediately find an indication of cause, he should try to obtain a harmonious picture of all the symptoms; this will reveal to him the nature and cause of the disease.[22]

Other important indications are the one revealing the disease *locus* (the place where the peccant humor has collected) and the one telling of the patient's vitality.[23] The latter is often found from the pulse.[24]

Symptoms falling outside these three classes do not indicate the main features of the disease and are less important for treatment.[25] Such other symptoms are the supervening symptoms appearing during the course of treatment as well as any symptoms which only point to a damaged function and are not associated with an underlying dyscrasia.[26] These and many others are neutral and do not yield an indication for treatment.[27]

The physician studies anatomy and physiology to recognize the normal organism and to become acquainted with the etiology of disease.[28] Vivisection is used to the same end.[29] Knowledge of the normal organism is especially needful when the physician sees his patient for the first time after he is sick and has no opportunity to observe him in health.[30] "When we lack knowledge of the patient's customary state of health, in order not to be totally at a loss, we resort in practice to an evaluation of aspects of the patient's case which he has in common with others. This is the advantage of the one who knows the *tekhne* over the one who does not."[31] The symptoms found in all cases of the given disease are of primary importance and others are of only secondary importance.[32] The greater the deviation from normality, the more severe the illness.[33]

Lacking knowledge of the patient's normal state of health the physician may also proceed by referring to the scientific classification of diseases.[34] This classification is based upon the logical differentiation of diseases, first according to genera and then according to species.[35] Fever may be considered a primary disease.[36] Some have said that there are four main diseases, others eight, and still others—seven.[37] There are eight kinds of weakness of the stomach and five principal diseases of the brain.[38] Further diseases are developed out of these major ones by adding *differentiae*—the symptoms differentiating one disease within the genus from another.[39] In this procedure, however, not every symptom is important—only the ones generated by the division of the genus itself.[40]

Mistakes in therapy are often due to an incorrect system of disease classification.[41]

Therapeutics

Therapeutics is based upon knowledge of the disease cause. And since this cause is defined logically as an intermingling of the four qualities or elements, with cure resulting from exhibition of the remedy of opposed quality or qualities, the remedies must also be analyzed in terms of their qualities.[42]

All medicines and foods have both primary and secondary qualities, the former being their shape, color, taste, smell, etc. and the latter being their effect upon the organism when ingested. The Rationalist physicians maintained that, in principle, secondary qualities could be determined analytically from an examination of primary qualities—just as the disease cause could be ascertained analytically from an examination of the symptoms.

Thus medicines which are hot or cold to the taste have the same effect on the disease cause.[43] Also the part of the plant from which the medicine is taken will yield a curative indication: Mnesitheos was correct in maintaining that the roots, containing the crudest juices, are harder to digest than the upper parts of the plant.[44] The color of a medicine will yield an indication: persons suffering from hemorrhage should avoid anything red, and those suffering from jaundice should avoid anything yellow.[45c] In all of these instances the *logos* indicates the remedy.[46] Furthermore, the compounding of remedies is a logical procedure.[47]

Armed with a variety of medicines, simple and compound, with whose qualities he is familiar, the physician proceeds to treatment.

The main curative indication is taken from the disease cause.[48] Once the cause has been elucidated, the correct treatment presents itself automatically.[49] The cause, so to speak, indicates its own treatment.[50] One automatically opposes the cause of the disease just as one instinctively pulls out a splinter embedded in the flesh, without reasoning about it beforehand.[51]

Treatment can be either qualitative (opposing or neutralizing the predominant humor inside the body) or quantitative (evacuating this peccant humor from the body).[52] Or the two types of treatment can be combined.

Qualitative treatment means opposing hot to cold, wet to dry, hot and wet to cold and dry, etc.[53] If the patient has a burning fever, the correct treatment is with cold water.[54] The patient, however, may have different disorders in different parts of his body: his stomach may be too cold, for example, and his head too hot.[55] If the disease consists of ten parts heat and seven parts dryness, the remedy should be ten parts cold and seven parts moist.[56] Remedies of opposite qualities (hot and cold, wet and dry) may be compounded together and administered when the state of the patient's health so requires—i.e., if his dyscrasia contains this mixture of opposed humors.[57]

[c]See discussion of similars below, p. 224.

While the powers of simple drugs are often revealed by experience, drugs are mixed together and compounded on logical grounds.[58]

Quantitative treatment involves removing the peccant humor from the body by administering vomitives, purgatives, sudorifics, or diuretics. It is especially useful to evacuate putrified humors in this way.[59] Bloodletting is another major technique of quantitative treatment, since blood is often in excess—whether absolutely or only in regard to the patient's strength.[60] A very common ailment is "plethora" (excess blood)—whose symptoms are gluttony, constipation, listlessness, redness of the skin, weakness, and swelling of the blood vessels.[61] Phlebotomy, however, can be used in any severe disease if the patient is too weak to support a large amount of blood in his system.[62]

Sometimes local and general quantitative treatment are combined. Thus, if much blood has flowed into one member, so that not only the large veins but the small ones also are distended, there is danger that what is spilled out of the veins will pass to the other parts of the body. But if the whole body is overfilled with humors, this member cannot be evacuated, since there is no place for the blood to flow. The cure is first to evacuate the body as a whole and then proceed to the affected part, dispersing its humors with cooling remedies and tight bindings.[63] Baths and gymnastics, as well as certain drugs, can also be used to drive humors from one part of the body to another.[64]

Erasistratean techniques are sometimes used: a man whose liver passages are too narrow is cured by an "extenuating" diet.[65]

When the disease is attended with complications, the most serious are to be cured first.[66]

As mentioned earlier, the indication of *locus* tells the physician where to apply the remedy, and the indication of the patient's strength tells him how powerful a remedy is needed:

> If he be strong and in the prime of life, and if the season be spring and the region temperate, you cannot go wrong

> in opening a vein and letting out as much blood as the condition demands; but if the patient be weak or quite a small child or a very old man . . . under these circumstances nobody would venture to carry out venesection.[67]

If the cause is the same, but the *locus* is different (the patient's strength being unchanged), the physician will apply the same treatment to a different part of the body; but if the cause is not the same (the *locus* and the patient's strength remaining unchanged), the physician will apply a different treatment to the same part of the body and to the same degree.[68]

Treatment is always based upon the principle of contraries.[69] Disease is an excess in one direction, and treatment must aim to oppose this excess.[70]

The principle of similars has no place in therapeutics, as like things only intensify likes. Similar medicines exacerbate the disease.[71] The principle of similars, however, has a place in hygiene. If a person's constitution is humid, a humid regimen will preserve him in health.[72] Healthy bodies are treated according to their nature and sick ones by contraries.[73]

Thus it is highly doubtful that the bite of a mad dog is cured when the patient eats a piece of its liver.[74] While the Empirics maintain that Hippocrates espoused the principle of similars, this would be impossible, since such a doctrine is illogical.[75] Hippocrates was always logical, and he said that contraries are the cure for contraries.[76] The Empirics also say that a chilled person can be heated up by immersion in cold water, quoting *Aphorisms* V: 21.[d] While this is partially true, it is not a case of cure through similars. The effect is observed only in a person with a large reserve of inner heat; immersion in cold water causes the skin to become tight, the heat which previously escaped from the body is blocked, and he appears to warm up. But if the body had no innate reserve

[d]"Sometimes in a case of tetanus without a wound, the patient being a muscular young man, and the time the middle of summer, a copious affusion of cold water brings a recovery of heat."

of heat, application of cold water would only cool it still more.[77] It is also true that nausea can sometimes be cured with an emetic, but this also is not a case of cure through similars; the emetic is administered to clear the stomach at a stroke of all the moisture which produces nausea and vomiting. Since this moisture clings to the lining of the stomach, sometimes it can be dislodged only by an emetic. In the same way, the moisture in the chest which causes coughing can be cleared out by medicines which provoke more violent coughing, but all these cures are still through contraries and not through similars.[78]

Seasons affect diseases in the same way—by contraries and not by similars. *Aphorisms* II: 34, alleging that diseases are *less* dangerous in their own seasons,[e] was rightly criticized by Diocles:

> What do you mean, Hippocrates? Can an ardent fever which gives rise to boiling inside because of the quality of the [morbific] matter, intolerable thirst, insomnia, and all the other symptoms observed in the summer, can it be more benign because of the affinity with the season, seeing that all of these troubles are even more acute in the summer than in the winter—when the force of the movement is diminished, its sharpness weakened, and the whole illness made milder?[79]

The *Problemata* also support the view that a disease is worse in its own season: "Why is it that a dry summer and autumn in which northerly winds prevail is unhealthy for those who are bilious? Is it because their bodily condition and the season have the same tendency, and it is like adding fire to fire?"[80]

In applying a treatment which opposes the cause one must avoid confusing proximate causes with external (exciting, procatarctic) causes.[81] Typical of the latter are wounds, bruises, hunger, surfeit, heat, cold, animal bites, etc.

[e] "In diseases there is less danger when the disease is more nearly related to the patient in respect of constitution, habit, age, and season, than when there is no such relationship." See, also, *Places in Man*, cap. 42 (*supra*, p. 205 note).

Knowledge of such causes can be useful to the physician—for instance, he can adjust his treatment of a dog bite if the dog was rabid,[82] but the exciting cause cannot be said to yield a curative indication in the same way as the proximate cause.[83] That is because the physician cannot give a remedy which opposes the exciting cause; he can only oppose the proximate cause which is the consequent of the exciting cause. Therapy is based on the proximate cause; the exciting cause falls in the realm of disease prevention, not therapeutics.[84]

The Rationalist physicians emphasized that their treatment was not symptomatic but was directed against the disease cause:

> [Diocles does] not infer the kind of treatment to be given from the symptoms which appear in the inflamed part, but from the nature of the disease itself. For [he does] not consider whether there is an unnatural or resistant swelling or a painful pulse, but whether there is an influx and obstruction in the ends of the arteries or a stoppage in the ends of the veins or a certain putrefaction of the humors . . . Thus [he] takes the indications for the medicaments from the status of the inflamed part and not at all from the symptoms which only accompany this status.[85]

The symptom is only the sign which the disease cause presents to the sense-perception of the physician; he does not treat this sign but rather the entity which he infers to be inside the body.[86] Nor does he treat the injured function; he treats the disease entity which is injuring the function.[87] The disease is an entity which has an existence of its own quite apart from the body in which it is lodged.[88] When this entity has been removed by appropriate treatment, all associated symptoms will disappear.[89]

Theory and Practice

To the Rationalists medical "science" (*tekhne* or *episteme*) was a body of logical knowledge about the functioning of the organism and its *physis* in sickness and health: "the knowledge of things healthful, unhealthful, and neutral."[90]

> They, then, who profess Rational medicine propound as prerequisites, first, a knowledge of the hidden causes of diseases, next, of evident causes, next, of the actions of the *Natura,* and, lastly, of the internal parts.[91]

> It is impossible, without having acquired a thorough knowledge of the *physis* of the body, to find out anything about the differences of diseases or to be well versed in remedies.[92]

> How will you be successful in treatment if you do not understand the real essence [*ousia*] of each disease?[93]

> The Dogmatists begin with an examination of the *physis.*[94]

Medical practice, therapeutics, is based upon this preexisting theory.[95] The connection between theory and practice is supplied by the doctrine of contraries.

The Theory

The Rationalist theory of the *physis,* their physiology, was a logical structure because these physicians identified the reality of the living organism with the categories of Aristotelian logic. Galen writes in his short work, *The Best Physician is Also a Philosopher,* that, while everyone admires Hippocrates, few follow his example of basing medical practice upon logical knowledge of the organism:

> Will you say that a person who is master of himself, temperate and disdainful of riches, is an honorable doctor but not a philosopher? . . . that knowledge of the body, functions of organs, differences between diseases, etc., is not acquired by the exercise of logic? . . . To know the *physis* of the body, the differences among diseases, the therapeutic indications, [the physician] should be well

> versed in the *episteme* of logic . . . it is true that philosophy is necessary for medicine.[96f]

For this reason Galen advises beginners in medicine to read first his works on logical demonstration.[97]

In addition to their assumption that the organism functions according to logical patterns the Rationalists brought other assumptions to their analysis of medicine: (1) that "diseases" are discrete entities, finite in number; (2) that these entities can be classified; and (3) that theorems can be deduced from observation of these entities, to guide the physician in diagnosis and therapeutics.

We have already seen above that the Rationalists assumed diseases to be discrete entities and finite in number. There are only four humors, and the functions of the organism are finite; hence, diseases also must be finite. "How, indeed, could anybody be a diagnostician and healer of diseases who does not know what diseases there are, how many, and of what kind? This truth was well known to Hippocrates, Praxagoras, Phylotimos, and Aristotle."[98] Praxagoras wrote a book on *The Kinds of Acute Diseases,* naming a number of them.[99]

The observed fact that diseases are infinite in number and overlap any nosological classification was explained by the hypothesis that several different diseases can coexist in the body at the same time,[100] or that diseases occasionally take on a form other than their "normal" or "natural" one. Galen speaks of "legitimate" and "illegitimate" fevers and of fevers with "extra" symptoms.[101]

The doctrine of "associated" or "supervening" signs and symptoms was another technique used by the Rationalists to

[f]The tone of this writing resembles that of the Hippocratic work, *Decorum:* "For a physician who is a lover of wisdom is the equal of a God. Between wisdom and medicine there is no gulf fixed; in fact, medicine possesses all the qualities that make for wisdom. It has disinterestedness, shamefastness, modesty, reserve, sound opinion, judgment, quiet, pugnacity, purity, sententious speech, knowledge of the things good and necessary for life, selling of that which cleanses, freedom from superstition, preexcellence divine" (Jones, II, 287). Edelstein dates *Decorum* from the Hellenistic, or even the early Christian, era ("The Professional Ethics of the Greek Physician," *Bulletin of the History of Medicine,* XXX (1956), pp. 391-419, at p. 400).

adjust the observed infinite variety of diseases to their logical nosology.[102]

Furthermore, these discrete entities can be organized into a logical structure: "the true physician . . . endeavors to follow the rational method in order to learn how to distinguish the genera and species into which diseases are divided and to grasp the therapeutic indications for each. This is the method revealed to us by the very *physis* of the body."[103] Mnesitheos, as has been noted, was the one who "proceeded from the first and highest genera to other genera, species, and *differentiae;* dividing these logically until he ultimately defined each individual disease."[104]

With this classification in mind the physician proceeds to develop the theorems which make up medical doctrine. He develops them by using the mode of reasoning called "analogy" (*analogismos*)—defined as reasoning from the evident to an understanding of the non-evident.[105]

Thus, matters which escape the senses are to be known by unnatural pains, functions, swellings, etc. Madness is the sign of an afflicted brain. The combination of difficult breathing, trembling, and fever indicates an afflicted heart. One determines the nature of an afflicted stomach by the quality of the humor vomited.[106] The existence of pores can be deduced from the appearance of sweat; or you see several persons dead of heart wounds and conclude that heart wounds are fatal.[107]

The above *analogismoi* are based directly on the visible. Others, however, can be abstracted from the phenomena: using his *logos* the physician can determine that such-and-such symptoms indicate liver trouble, such-and-such other symptoms kidney trouble, etc.[108] Still others are based upon proven premises: since it has been proven that coction occurs and that substances submitted to coction melt and liquefy and are distributed from the stomach through the body, and since it is also proven that sick people need food which is easy to assimilate, the theorem that "feverish persons need a liquid diet" (*Aphorisms* I: 16) is proven.[109] Others yet are obvious to common sense: all excess is contrary to the *physis,* and, thus, if the disease is caused by surfeit, it is cured by fasting (*Aphorisms* II: 22, 51).[110]

The truth of the *analogismos* is judged from its congruence with the principles of the *tekhne.* Sometimes this congruence is clear, and sometimes it must be demonstrated through the intermediary of a sign.[111] Visible things are judged by common sense, and those which are grasped through demonstration are judged by their conformity with other things generally recognized as true.[112]

The usefulness of an *analogismos* is judged by its relationship to the purpose of the *tekhne.*[113] Since the purpose of the *tekhne* is, of course, the production of health, any *analogismos* which leads to the patient's recovery may be considered useful.[114]

The *analogismoi* must be not only true and useful but also logically consistent with one another. Just as the subjects of the state are subordinate to the monarch, so are the *analogismoi* subordinate to the aim of the *tekhne.*[115]

The technique used by the Rationalists to expand knowledge, in other words, to apply the principles of the *tekhne* to new diseases, was the syllogism—defined as "the necessary derivation of something previously unknown from known postulates."[116] When encountering a new diseased state these physicians first attempted to deduce the cause from an examination of the symptoms; if unsuccessful, they reasoned from diseases with similar symptoms to the conclusion that the causes were also similar.[117] Then, using the syllogism, they transferred the previously known treatment to the new case.[118]

The body of knowledge contained in the theorems was organized in several ways. The most common division was: physiology, pathognomics, and therapeutics. Pathognomics was in turn divided into etiology and semeiotics (interpretation of symptoms), while therapeutics was divided into dietetics, *materia medica,* and surgery.[119] Another division was: physiology, etiology, pathology, diet of the healthy, semeiotics, and therapeutics.[120] Both divisions, however, emphasize the split between physiology ("the study of the *physis*") and pathology or pathognomics ("the study of those things which are unnatural" [i.e., contrary to the *physis: para physin*]), on one hand, and the practical parts (diet, surgery, therapeutics) on the other—with the latter subordinate to the former.

The Practice

The theoretical part of medicine is inherently precise and reliable because based upon inherently precise logic and philosophy. Thus, medicine cannot be called a conjectural science.[121] In practice, however, precision may be less, because of the improper education of many physicians and their inability to master the discipline; hence the practical side of medicine is often conjectural.[122]

In some writings Galen assimilates the distinction between theory and practice to the Aristotelian distinction between *episteme* (theoretical science) and *tekhne* (science in the field of production). Medicine is an *episteme,* but its correct application in the *tekhne* depends upon the physician's ability to penetrate to the underlying causes by correctly interpreting the signs.[123] Elsewhere he writes: "I discovered some [diseases] which presented a diagnosis according to *episteme* and others which fell under the sort of conjecture called *tekhne* and in which, consequently, the diagnosis had to be rectified frequently, since such is the strength of the conjecture according to *tekhne.*"[124]

The best physician, in any case, is the one who does everything on the basis of correct reasoning.[125]

* * * * * * * * *

While we have tried to do justice to the Rationalist physiological and therapeutic doctrine, the doctrine itself was inherently confused, being unable to distinguish clearly between (1) the *krasis* or proximate cause, (2) the disease entity, (3) the damaged function, and (4) the most prominent symptom or symptoms. The confusion is intrinsic to the method of analysis adopted, being inevitable when a vital entity such as the human organism is analyzed in the categories of Aristotelian logic.

In particular, the theory of the indicative sign was illogical and unclear. Symptoms can never be other than commemorative signs of some disease process, as was pointed out by Sextus Empiricus:

> And a similar criticism may be passed upon the rest of the "axiomatic" arguments, as they are called by the Peripatetics; and also upon arguments in the form, "If it is day, it is light." For the proposition, "if it is day, it is light," is capable, they say, of proving that "it is light," and the clause, "it is light," in conjunction with "it is day," serves to establish the proposition, "If it is day, it is light." For the hypothetical premise stated above would not have been considered valid unless the constant coexistence of "it is light" with "it is day" had already been observed.[126]

No symptom has an analytical relationship with liver disease or any other disease. The physician can never know anything more than the coexistence of certain symptoms with certain states of ill-health. Rationalist adherence to the indicative sign was due in part to the confusion between symptoms, entities, and causes, but mainly to the desire of these physicians to find an expanded role for logical analysis in medicine.

Thus the effect of Rationalism was to elevate the analytical and logical element in medicine above the observational and experiential component. When these physicians examined a patient, they could not see him in his uniqueness and difference from other patients. The symptoms and signs had no meaning except for what they told the physician about the hypothesized state of the humors. The physician's selection of "important" symptoms was itself a function of his *a priori* idea of the proximate cause. "Complications," "legitimate" and "illegitimate" fevers, etc. were all functions of some preexisting idea in the physician's mind of the "normal" in a fever or other disease. And even if the diagnosis itself was accurate, treatment by "contraries" had nothing to do with any real process of cure.

The Rationalist School continued the trend observed above (in the Group III Hippocratic writings) toward the transformation of a medicine based on observation and experience to one based on logical analysis. Observation itself was subordinated to *logos:* "Some phenomena are perceptible in themselves, others by a mediated observation."[127]

While the Rationalists professed adherence to many of the tenets of Hippocratic experiential medicine, their doctrine nullified these tenets or transvalued them. They sometimes urged attention to the individuality of the patient, for example, but individualized treatment was impossible in Rationalist medicine.[128] The theorems or analogies of which this doctrine was composed were deduced from classes of cases. They were thought to possess universal validity precisely for that reason.[129] But, being abstracted from a class of particular instances, they necessarily embodied the common or prominent symptoms of the class; there was no methodical provision in Rationalist doctrine for the idea of idiosyncrasy. The symptoms most important for treatment were those common to a class of patients.[130]

This meant disappearance of the *physis* from medical speculation, together with the associated concept of coction. As mentioned above,[g] these represent the experiential element in therapeutics; they must necessarily abandon the stage at the entry of an analytical doctrine. Coction was now identified with the digestion of food in the stomach,[131] and the operations of the *physis* were reduced to an arid clash among opposed qualities:

> Why is it that changes of the seasons and the winds intensify or stop diseases and bring them to a crisis and engender them? Is it because the seasons are hot and cold and moist and dry, while diseases are due to excess of these qualities and health to their equality? In that case, if the disease is due to moisture or cold, a season which has the opposite characteristics stops it . . .[132]

[g]See above, pp. 163-164.

Galen observes that in his studies he encountered many Stoic and Peripatetic philosophers who denied the existence of the *physis*,[133] and he notes that the physicians of his day understood it in a number of different ways.[134] He saw his own task as one of securing acceptance of the *physis* by his Rationalist colleagues, and to this end he evolved a new theory of the *physis* which is discussed below.

Prognosis was replaced by diagnosis. These physicians were not concerned with the course of disease; such an idea is alien to cure through contraries. The "associated" or "supervening" signs mentioned above are nothing other than the Hippocratic prognostic signs which have lost their integral connection with the disease process. And we have the testimony of Galen himself that prognosis was not practiced by the Rationalists at the time of his arrival in Rome:

> The misfortune of medicine has many aspects, but there is one point in it which I have resolved to deal with, since it belongs to what chiefly concerns myself. Should any one of the physicians who have learned medicine in the customary way forecast the occurrence in the patient of delirium, of a rigor, depression, hemorrhage, ear-abscess, or other kind of abscession in any part, an attack of vomiting, sweating, intestinal disturbance, syncope, or anything of the kind, he appears to the laity some strange monstrosity on account of the novelty of his behavior. So far, in fact, from earning their praise, the prognosticator may be glad if he is not taken for a sorceror. Some few there are, on the other hand, who, while they do not reject this point of view as impossible, yet straightway ask the forecaster himself, as well as other doctors, whether this sort of thing was known also to the older authorities or is simply a discovery of the forecaster himself. Thereupon those physicians who conceal their stupidity, as also perhaps some who are really ignorant, must needs say that none of the ancients ever wrote any such thing, and that he who brings forward such a forecast is a wizard. And the prognosticator himself does not dare to say that this subject was treated by many of

the ancients, and especially by Hippocrates, our leader in everything that is of good repute.[135]

* * * * *

Rationalist doctrine isolated the body from its environment. Exciting (procatarctic) causes were relegated to the realm of prevention and become important for treatment only if converted into proximate causes at work within the organism.[136h]

Rationalism isolated the physician from the patient and from society by founding medicine on the unseeable—by postulating the existence of a world of relationships cognizable only by those who had been initiated to their study and thereby admitted to the medical profession.[i]

Finally, this doctrine isolated medicine from history: the Rationalists held that all medical knowledge was discovered once and for all by Hippocrates.[137j] The refusal to see disease as a process, and lack of interest in its stages of development, was paralleled by indifference toward the historical development of medical knowledge.

[h]See above, p. 226.

[i]See below, pp. 322-333.

[j]Perhaps a misinterpretation of *Ancient Medicine,* cap. II, which only states that the correct *method of investigation* has been discovered (see above, pp. 92-93).

NOTES

[1]K II 139. K VII 334, 342, 345-346. K X 186. K XIX 363. Erich Schoener has discussed the four-humor doctrine extensively in "Das Viererschema in der Antiken Humoralpathologie," showing (p. 92) that the four qualities, humors, elements, seasons, principal organs, and most common fevers were associated as follows:

hot and wet	hot and dry	cold and wet	cold and dry
blood	yellow bile	phlegm	black bile
air	fire	water	earth
heart	liver	brain	spleen
spring	summer	winter	autumn
childhood	youth	old age	adulthood
continuous fever	tertian fever	quotidian fever	quartan fever

[2]Rudolph E. Siegel, *Galen's System of Physiology and Medicine* (Basel and New York: Karger, 1968), p. 217. See Aristotle, *Historia Animalium* 511b 1-10.

[3]K II 117, 122, 135-139.

[4]Siegel, *op. cit.*, p. 221. K II 131, 134. K V 144. K XVI 534.

[5]K II 121-122. K VI 2.

[6]Siegel, *op. cit.*, 196-332. K VII 334, 342, 345-346.

[7]K X 41.

[8]K II 126-128.

[9]K X 78, 86, 90, 92. See, also, Kurt Sprengel, *Histoire de la Medecine,* Vol. II (Paris, 1815), pp. 117ff.

[10]K I 110-11, 122-123, 139, 160.

[11]Walzer, *Galen on Medical Experience,* p. 89.

[12]*Ibid.*, p. 146. K X 93.

[13]K XIX 396.

[14]K I 322-337.

[15]K I 315. K X 101.

[16]K I 121.

[17]K I 54-55.

[18]K X 126.

[19]K I 121-122.

[20]K I 123-124, 134.

[21]K I 139, 157-159. K X 102, 157, 215. K XII 527.

[22]K I 126-128. K XI 9.

[23]K I 159-160.

[24]K XI 8, 10-11. K XVIIB 381-382.

[25]K I 139-140, 159-160. K X 65-70. K XI 8-9. K XVIIB 390. Sprengel, *op. cit.,* Vol. II, p. 123.

[26]K XVIIB 390, 399. K XVIIIA 56, 115.

[27]K I 359-365.

[28] K XIV 690.

[29] K XIX 357. Celsus, *De Medicina, Prooemium*, 26.

[30] *Galeni in Hippocratis De Officina Medici*, p. 103.

[31] K XI 3.

[32] *Galeni in Hippocratis De Officina*, p. 103.

[33] K XI 3.

[34] K XI 3. K X 22-26.

[35] K X 22, 26, 40. K XI 3.

[36] K II 121.

[37] K II 118. K X 22. Sprengel, *op. cit.*, Vol. II, p. 118.

[38] K I 319. K X 104.

[39] K X 128, 226. K XIV 690.

[40] K X 23.

[41] K XI 4.

[42] K I 381.

[43] Sprengel, *op. cit.*, Vol. II, pp. 122-123. K XI 813.

[44] K VI 455-457, 645-646.

[45] Walzer, *Galen on Medical Experience*, p. 151.

[46] K X 31, 209, 896.

[47] K XII 895. K XIV 222.

[48] K I 126-127. K X 157, 215. K XI 61.

[49] K I 131.

[50] K XIV 678.

[51] K I 127-128. K XI 32-35.

[52] K X 890-892, 895. K XVIIB 360,655, 660-661.

[53] K X 103. K XI 99-100.

[54] K XI 42.

[55] K I 375.

[56] K I 383.

[57] K I 374, 381, 382, 394, 398. K X 166-167, 215. See, also, *Problemata* 864a 19-22. K XIII 371, 374.

[58] K XVI 85.

[59] K I 382.

[60] K X 288. Sprengel, *op. cit.*, Vol. II, p. 119.

[61] K X 286. K XI 163.

[62] K X 288.

[63] K I 70, 394-395. K XI 62-63, 79-80.

[64] K XI 61-63.

[65] K I 379, 398-399.

[66] K X 219 .

[67] K I 71-72.

[68] K I 159-160.

[69] K I 381.

[70] *Problemata* 859a 1-9.

[71] Walzer, *Galen on Medical Experience*, p. 151.

[72] K I 381. K XVIIB 426.

[73] K XVIIB 427-428, 530-531.

[74] K XII 335.

[75] *Galeni in Hippocratis de Officina*, pp. 73-75. While Galen does not state that these are the Empirics talking, the context makes it evident.

[76] *Ibid.*, p. 79.

[77] *Ibid.*, pp. 75, 81.
[78] *Ibid.*, p. 79. See *Places in Man*, cap. 42 (VI, 337, L.).
[79] Diocles, Fr. 34 (K XVIIB 532).
[80] *Problemata* 860b 15-19. See, also, 859a 9-15 and 860b 8-13.
[81] K X 65. Celsus, *De Medicina, Prooemium*, 18.
[82] K I 73.
[83] K X 243.
[84] K X 876.
[85] K X 101.
[86] K X 100-102.
[87] K I 121. K X 92.
[88] K I 315. K X 152-156.
[89] K X 92.
[90] K I 307.
[91] Celsus, *De Medicina, Prooemium*, 13.
[92] K X 110-111.
[93] K II 127.
[94] K XIV 677.
[95] K XIX 351. K I 308.
[96] K I 59-62.
[97] K XIX 43, 53.
[98] K XVI 40.
[99] K XVIIA 889.
[100] K I 394-395. K X 219. K XVIIB 427-428.
[101] K XI 32-37, 42ff.
[102] K XVIIB 390, 399. K XVIIIA 7-8, 56, 115. K I 390.
[103] K I 59-60.
[104] K XI 3.
[105] K XIX 354.
[106] K I 352-356.
[107] K I 112-115.
[108] K I 112-115.
[109] K I 114.
[110] K I 114.
[111] K I 106-108.
[112] K I 110-111.
[113] K I 110-111.
[114] K I 115-117.
[115] K I 106-107.
[116] K XIX 354.
[117] K I 127-129. Celsus, *De Medicina, Prooemium*, 17.
[118] K I 127-129.
[119] Ludwig Englert, "Untersuchungen zu Galens Schrift Thrasybulos," *Studien zur Geschichte der Medizin*, XVIII (1929), pp. 1-104, at pp. 22, 23.
[120] *Ibid.*, p. 23. K XIX 351.
[121] K I 114.
[122] K I 114. K XIV 684.
[123] K I 308. See K XIX 350.
[124] K VIII 145.
[125] K XIX 355.
[126] *Outlines of Pyrrhonism*, II, 198-199.
[127] K I 126-127.

[128] K I 70.
[129] K I 114. K IX 841-842. K XIX 354.
[130] K X 128.
[131] Celsus, *Prooemium,* 20.
[132] *Problemata* 859a 9-13.
[133] K XIX 40.
[134] K XVIIB 529-532.
[135] K XIV 600-602 (translation by A. J. Brock).
[136] K I 368.
[137] Walzer, *Galen on Medical Experience,* p. 101.

CHAPTER VII

THE EMPIRICAL SCHOOL

The Empirical School was the conscious heritor of the tradition represented by the Group I Hippocratic writings. This is seen in their own view of "Hippocrates". But it is seen most strikingly in the identity of the Empirical therapeutic doctrine with that set forth in these Hippocratic works.

The physicians who accepted the Group I approach to healing were supplied with a philosophical instrument by Scepticism. By using it they were able to give verbal expression to the assumptions underlying their own therapeutic practice. By the second century A.D. the Empirical physicians had not only formulated a consistent philosophical justification for their method but had expanded the method itself to a high level of sophistication.

The method was predicated upon the same vitalistic interpretation of the organism seen in the Group I writings. The body's own reactive power was the chief weapon for combating disease. While the Empirical method was designed to afford the physician a variety of different ways of aiding the *physis*, the latter was still the key to healing.

The Physis and Coction

Max Neuburger has suggested that the *physis* was not an object of medical speculation in the early Hippocratic works but appeared later–specifically in *Nutriment* and *Epidemics VI:*[1]

> The *physis* is sufficient in all for all.
> (*Nutriment*, cap. XV: Jones, I, 347)
>
> The *physies* of all are untaught.
> (*Nutriment*, cap. XXXIX: Jones, I, 357)

> The *physies* are the physicians of diseases.
> (*Epidemics VI*, cap. V: V, 315, L.)
>
> The *physis* finds pathways by itself, not in consequence of deliberation . . . Though the *physis* is unschooled and uninstructed, she does what is proper.
> (*Epidemics VI*, cap. V: V, 315, L.)

But we have noted above that the *physis* is first defined in *Nature of Man* (as the product of the four humors) and that this definition is contested in *Ancient Medicine* which gives a vitalistic interpretation. Conscious awareness of the *physis* as agent of cure must therefore date from *Ancient Medicine. Nutriment* and *Epidemics VI* show that the vitalistic interpretation of the *physis* remained a force in Greek medical thought in the fourth century.[a]

In reaction to the Rationalist fixation on the four humors as the starting-point of medical speculation and practice, the proto-Empirics among the Hippocratic writers increasingly brought to the fore the holistic and vitalistic *physis*.

It can hardly be coincidence that 23 of the 68 surviving fragments of Empirical Hippocratic exegesis deal with *Epidemics VI.*[2]

In *Precepts*, an Empirical work dating from as late as the first or second century A.D.,[3] this interpretation of the *physis* is quite explicit:

> For the healthy condition of a human being is a *physis* that has naturally attained a movement, not alien but perfectly adapted, having produced it by means of *pneuma,* warmth, and coction [*katergasie,* literally: "overpowering"] of the humors, in every way, by complete regimen and by everything combined, unless there be some congenital or early deficiency.
> (*Precepts,* cap. IX: Jones, I, 327)[b]

And Celsus also sees the *physis* as the principal factor in cure: "Even where the resources of art are applied, the *Natura* can

[a]According to one ancient tradition the author of *Nutriment* was Herophilos (Jones, I, 340).

[b]Jones translates *katergasie* by "coction." See, below, p. 244.

do the most."[4] "With the *Natura* in opposition, the art of medicine avails nothing."[5]

Glaukias and Zeuxis wrote that the *physis* conquers the disease.[6] The Empiric, Apollonios Biblas, argued that the newborn baby should be nursed immediately, since to this end the *physis* has prepared the milk beforehand (in opposition to a Methodist who held that mother's milk is unwholesome for the first twenty days after birth).[7] Celsus held that the *Natura*, not number, must be the standard for frequency of sexual intercourse.[8]

As the passage from *Precepts* makes clear, cure is through "overpowering" the humors; in this the crisis is important.[9]

Here the author's failure to use the traditional *pepsis* may be significant, for the Empirical school was affected by the redefinition of "coction" by the Rationalist writers–its reduction to "digestion." And Erasistratos' introduction of the concepts of *anadosis* (distribution) and *diadosis* (assimilation) only compounded the confusion. The Empiric in Galen's *Medical Experience* cites this as a striking instance of the physiological incoherency of Rationalism:

> [They have very different opinions on] digestion and assimilation, and that to such an extent that one of them asserts that there is no such thing in this world as digestion, and another declares that digestion and assimilation exist indeed, but resemble the process of cooking, and another says that they do not resemble cooking at all, but rather decay–for this is what a man named Pleistonikos has said [Celsus, *Prooemium*, 20]–and another follows these two and imagines, just as men imagine things in dreams, that assimilation and digestion consist in the dissolving of food into a juice like the drink made from barley [*Regimen in Acute Diseases I*, caps. X-XII], and another is of the opinion that the food is ground and pounded, and another says that it is the work of the *pneuma* caused by a peculiarity contained therein. And you will find that Erasistratos has confused and mixed up many things, for he attributed a part of the process of assimilation and digestion to

warmth and the greater part to grinding and pounding, and has set forth in many passages his belief that this takes place only through the connexion of the food with the *pneuma*. And when one sees that the absurdity of these people goes so far in regard to one universally recognized fact of [the *physis*] . . ."

(Walzer, *Galen on Medical Experience*, p. 103)

Celsus writes that to the Rationalists *concoctio* is of the most importance, and the discussion indicates that *concoctio* means "digestion."[10] The Empirics, however, ask if "the process is *concoctio* or merely *digestio*."[11] The changing meaning of *pepsis*, Erasistratos' emendations of physiological doctrine, and (in the case of Celsus) the problem of translating these words into Latin, led to doctrinal difficulties even in Empiricism.

Digestio is from the verb, *digero, digerere,* meaning to "separate" or "distribute," and was the translation of *anadosis.* At some point, however, *digestio* became attached to the *transformation* of food in the stomach (as opposed to its subsequent distribution).[c] This is already seen in pseudo-Soranus' *Questiones Medicae* which state that, according to Hippocrates, the *digestio* is from the innate heat, according to Diocles it is putrefaction, and according to Erasistratos it is the breaking up of food in the stomach.[12]

A fragment of Dionysios Aigeus found in Photius' *Bibliotheke* also indicates the confusion in ancient thought with respect to these concepts. This work, which is a list of topics for debate, suggests that coction (*pepsis*) is due: to heat, to friction, to putrefaction, to the *pneumata*, or to the humors. Likewise, *anadosis* is referred to heat, to *pneumata,* or to *horror vacui.*[13]

Some have dated the latter work at the first century A.D., but Deichgraeber maintains that this is not certain and refuses to assign a date.[14] The Greek original of

[c]The confusion is seen in W.G. Spencer's translation of the above passage in Celsus: "nor does it matter how digestion takes place but what is best digested [*quid optime digeratur*] . . . and whether the process is concoction [*concoctio*] or merely distribution [*digestio*]." (Celsus, *Prooemium,* 38). In the same sentence *digerere* is translated as "digest" while *digestio* is translated as "distribution."

pseudo-Soranus has been lost, and thus we do not know the Greek word translated by *digestio*; nor do we know when the translation was made. Caelius Aurelianus, writing in the fifth century, contrasts *digestio*, in the sense of *pepsis*, with the "grinding up of food in the stomach and its penetration through all the narrow passages into the body."[15]

In any case, there was clearly confusion in the ancient mind over the meaning of digestion. Was it only applicable to food in the stomach or was it identified with the coction of morbific causes? It may have been this confusion which led the author of *Precepts* to abandon the word, *pepsis*, and maintain instead that the morbific humors are "overpowered."

In Celsus this ambiguity is important, since it is often unclear whether he is talking about concoction or digestion. His espousal of the theory of coction is seen from the following passages:

> The ancients tried to ensure *concoctio* by administering certain medicaments, because they dreaded crudeness [*cruditas*] most of all.
>
> (Celsus, III, 4: 2)
>
> Now thin and red urine is usual in severe *cruditas*, and often, before there is time for it to mature, it carries the man off.
>
> (Celsus, II, 6: 11)[d]
>
> Whitish urine indicates that *concoctio* is still going on, reddish that *concoctio* is complete.
>
> (Celsus, I, 2: 4)
>
> At times too the urine remains thin and crude [*cruda*] for so long that other signs are salutary, and from this condition an abscess often occurs below the transverse membrane which the Greeks call *diaphragma.*
>
> (Celsus, II, 7: 32)

[d]This is a clear reference to *Prognosis*, cap. XII (Jones, II, 27): "So long as the urine is thin and of a yellowish-red color, it is a sign that the disease is unconcocted." Spencer observes: "According to Hippocrates it is the disease, not the urine, which is 'undigested.' Here *cruditas* may be the subject of *maturescat.*" I.e., the above passage should perhaps read: "before there is time for the *cruditas* to mature, it carries the man off."

> When sinews tend to become painful, as is common in foot or hand ache . . . *concoctio* is a necessity, for *cruditas* is most harmful, and whenever the body is attacked, the faulty part feels it most.
>
> (Celsus, I, 9: 2)
>
> But just as *concoctio* has to do with all sorts of troubles, so has cold with some, heat with others; each person should be guided by his own bodily habit [*habitus corporis*].
>
> (Celsus, I, 9: 3)

But elsewhere *concoctio* clearly means the digestion of food in the stomach:

> *Concoctio* depends upon what the food is, and how much.
>
> (Celsus, III, 6: 12)
>
> Take food twice rather than once a day, and always as much as one wants, provided one digest it [*concoquat*]
>
> (Celsus, I, 1: 3)
>
> It is generally the case too that the more substantial the material, the less readily it is digested [*concoquatur*], but once digested [*concocta*] it nourishes the more.
>
> (Celsus, II, 18: 13)

Digestio and *digerere* in Celsus are usually to be understood in the Erasistratean sense of "dispersal" or "distribution"—although now it is mainly the humors, suppurations, morbific matter, etc. (not food) which are "dispersed" or "distributed":

> [Sweating treatments] are useful whenever humor is doing harm inside and has to be dispersed [*digerendus est*].
>
> (Celsus, II, 17: 1)
>
> The common effect of [sweating] is to disperse [*digerere*] whatever is oppressing the parts over the heart, or strangling the throat, or harming some limb.
>
> (Celsus, II, 17: 10)

> Suppurations may be dissipated by dispersive poultices [*quae digerunt*].
>
> (Celsus, III, 27: 4A)
>
> Rubbing is also to be employed . . . in order that the materials of the disease, which have been doing harm by collecting, may be dispersed [*digerantur*].
>
> (Celsus, IV, 29: 3)

However, he calls this class of remedies by a different generic name–*ad discutienda* (from *discutere*, to scatter, disperse).[16] And while *digerere* is also used to denote the distribution of food through the body,[17] in one passage Celsus uses *diducere* (to divide, distribute): "in order that the food might be distributed when the body was as far as possible fever-free."[18]

The point is that many diseases involve digestive disturbance. Furthermore, dietary treatment of disease was an integral component of Empirical doctrine.[19] Hence there were solid medical grounds for assimilating coction to digestion, for considering *cruditas* the equivalent of indigestion, and for focussing on the stomach in the treatment of most diseases. When Celsus observes that sweating, clysters, and bloodletting should not be employed in *cruditas*,[20] or that *cruditas* can convert a quartan fever into a quotidian,[21] *cruditas* can be interpreted equally well in both senses.

The Empirics prior to Celsus seem to have attached the pristine Hippocratic meaning to "coction" and "crudeness." Lykos of Naples, for instance, held that incipient furuncles and indurations, whether crude or concocted (*vel cocto vel crudo*), should be treated with a salve.[22] Zopyros held that sudorific medicines mature the humors.[23] In one of the fragments of Herakleides the contrasting meanings of *cruditas* come out in the comments of Caelius Aurelianus. When Herakleides suggests purging with scammony in a case of phrenitis from *cruditas*, the Methodist observes with indignation:

> We might have thought that Herakleides has in mind *cruditas* of the humors for the sake of recognizing the

disease if he had not prescribed *scammonium*. For where does he think this *cruditas* is? in the bowels, the head, or the whole body? He seems to have left this decision up to the drug itself, hoping it would act like a conscious being, separating out from the normal parts of the body the alien substances, i.e., those which have been corrupted by *cruditas*, and removing these alone.[24]

Thus the Empirics, down through Cassius and Celsus, endeavored to abide by the theory of coction but were led into confusion by the ambiguity of this concept in the later medical tradition.

Semeiosis and Prognosis

Acceptance of the self-acting *physis* as the foundation of therapeutics implies renunciation of the search for proximate causes and reliance on purely sensory knowledge. If the *physis* is autonomous in the struggle against disease, by definition there can be no *a priori* knowledge of the pattern of its action in any individual case.

Hence the Empirics "refuse to investigate the *physis*,"[25] "reject contemplation of the *physis*."[26] "Those who are called Empirics . . . contend that inquiry about obscure causes and actions of the *Natura* is superfluous, because the *Natura* is not to be comprehended."[27]

They accepted the Sceptical critique of Aristotle's theory of causes. Even on such a simple matter as coction/digestion, they said, the Rationalists could not reach agreement.[28] And, since methods of treatment vary from one country to the next, the proximate causes must also vary.[29] When the exciting causes themselves do not disclose the appropriate treatment (as in wounds), how can treatment be revealed by the proximate cause?[30] Hence it was better to rely on that which is apparent to the senses—upon which all men can agree. "Since the [proximate] cause is as uncertain as it is incomprehensible, protection is to be sought rather from the ascertained and explored, as in all the rest of the arts, that is, from what experience has taught in the actual course of treatment."[31]

Hence, "experience" to them meant sensory perception of the patient's changing symptom-patterns: "the observation and memory of those things which are seen to occur frequently and in the same way."[32] While the Rationalists make a conjecture about the patient on the basis of the humoral elements, the Empirics do so on the basis of the visible phenomena.[33] While the Rationalists diagnose on the basis of indications about the state of the humors, the Empirics learn about the *physis* by examining and interrogating the patient.[34] Zeuxis and the other Empirics "all hold to visible phenomena alone."[35] They do not "differentiate the *physies* according to *logos*."[36]

Hence, the Empirics spoke of "semeiosis" (symptom analysis) rather than "diagnosis."[37]

Even when they determined that such-and-such patient had a "dry" *krasis*, it was on the basis of sensory data: a red complexion, pointed nose, small eyes, a crafty disposition.[38] Usually they preferred to say that the constitution of the patient was like that of a child or a women (not that it was moist), or a farmer or sailor (not that it was hard and dry).[39]

They denied that any sign could supply knowledge of internal physiological processes.[40] Only sensory observation is reliable, since things perceived by the senses are understood in the same way by everyone. Indicative signs are not instinctive but taught; although the sign itself is visible, men differ as to what it indicates, and it is thus unreliable.[41]

Rejecting the indicative sign, the Empirics rejected the disease entity which this sign was supposed to indicate. It was pointless to try and isolate the proximate cause, since any disease was the result of a number of such causes acting together.[42] The essence of the "disease" or disease cause was unknowable.[43]

They thus denied the Rationalist claim that "important" symptoms could be distinguished from "unimportant" ones by logical analysis:

> The assertion of the [Rationalists] that by means of the *logos* they can bring into unity things which are utterly opposed to each other gives one cause for the greatest

> astonishment at the excellence of their intelligence. If I but knew whether they are after things which we believe to be many and are not in reality a single thing, and which they then invert and revise and recreate in a new form, and change until they become something which they are not, or whether it concerns things which are one in themselves but which many people do not consider one . . . "Naturally," [the Rationalist] answers, "We make them one, although they are not uniform." If he says this, his words do not fall short of absolute ignorance and illiteracy in our view. If he says: "This is according to the second way," we would answer, "I should like very much to know if you are empowered to see the one thing which in itself is one, although it exists as a multiplicity, and we are unable to do so."[44]
>
> How is it that you have been granted the sovereign power to establish in your book all the symptoms which adhere to and affect conjointly one who suffers from phrenitis, as being symptoms belonging to a single person, while I have not this power, but because of me the phrenitic becomes not one but many, for they differ in respect of ages, lands, seasons, and physical conditions, activities, and temperaments.[45]

The thrust of Rationalist analysis was to group diseased persons on the basis of the common symptoms (*communia*). These common, general, and most frequently encountered symptoms designated the "entity" and were therefore the leading therapeutic indications.[46]

The thrust of Empirical analysis was precisely the opposite. As the above passages indicate, they denied the possibility of grouping patients into categories through logical determination of the proximate cause. Hence they distinguished patients on the basis of their symptoms.[47] They rejected the concept of the "disease", saying they had never seen a "disease" apart from the person who was suffering with it.[48] Hence they employed the expression, "symptom syndrome."[49] Each such syndrome they considered unique and irreproducible.[50] While they sometimes gave names to the syndromes, this was only for convenience and did not imply knowledge of the disease essence.[51]

The symptoms were defined as "commemorative signs"—meaning those things which are visible and recognizable from prior observation and thus remind the observer of what he has seen in the past.[52] Making the same impression on the mind of each observer, they are more reliable criteria (than the proximate cause) for distinguishing one patient from another.

The symptoms in the syndrome were divided into those common to many (*communia*) and those peculiar to the individual (*propria*).[53] The Empirics maintained that Hippocrates did the same.[54] The patient's habits and mode of life were among the most important of the *propria.*[55]

In direct contrast to the Rationalists, the Empirics held that the *propria* were *more* valuable for treatment than the *communia*:

> For the Empiric, examining what he calls the syndromes, which are the observation of symptoms which he has seen occurring many times in the same way, remembers them all equally. And when, from this observation, he has experience of many syndromes, he makes his judgment. Having seen some symptoms in many syndromes and others in one single syndrome, he comes to speculate about the *communia* and the *propria* . . . What is seen in many or all syndromes yields in importance to what is seen in a single syndrome; what is seen in several syndromes yields less, and what has been seen in two syndromes yields least in importance [to what is seen in a single syndrome].[56]

Thus they separated *propria* from *communia* with the aim of coming as close as possible to the idiosyncrasy of the patient.[57][e] While the Rationalist method effaced the differences among patients and aimed to treat classes of "diseases," the Empirics denied that there is any cure for a

[e] *Idiosynkrasia:* the patient's own peculiar temperament (*krasis*).

disease class.[58] The idiosyncrasy of the patient—that which distinguishes him from all similar patients—while unknowable in itself, was yet the basis of therapy.

> Even Erasistratos himself, who says that fever is produced by blood transfused into the arteries, and that this happens in an over-replete body, failed to discover why, of two equally replete persons, one should lapse into disease and the other remain free from anything dangerous; and that clearly happens every day. Hence, however true this transfusion, one can learn that it does not occur of itself when there is bodily fullness, but *when there is added something else.*
>
> (Celsus, *Prooemium*, 60-61)

The Empirical method was designed to single out this "something else" which distinguished the patient from all others of his class. Each sick person is unique in his sickness, and the sickness is unknowable in its essence.[f]

Thus there are general patterns of response by the *physis* to external morbific influences. At the same time each individual's response is different. The author of *Precepts* expressed this duality in stating: "it is through many turns and changes that all diseases settle into some sort of permanence" (cap. III: Jones, I, 317). The author of *Epidemics I* had urged the physician to form his judgment "from the common *physis* of all and the particular *physis* of the individual" (cap. XXIII: Jones, I, 181).[g] The *communia*

[f]Tolstoy expresses an identical view of disease in *War and Peace:* "The doctors visited Natasha individually and in consultation, talked a great deal in French, German, and Latin, attacked one another, prescribed the most variegated medicines possible for all the diseases they knew; but not one of them chanced upon the simple idea that they could not know the disease from which Natasha was suffering, just as none of the diseases to which the living body is subject can be known: for every living person has his own characteristics and always suffers from his own peculiar disease, one unknown to medicine; not the disease of the lungs, liver, skin, heart, nerves, etc. described in the medical books, but a disease consisting of one of the uncountable combinations of ailments of these organs . . ." (Part IX, Chapter 16).

[g]Celsus was undoubtedly referring to this passage when he wrote that Hippocrates distinguished *propria* from *communia* (*Prooemium,* 66).

reflect the "common *physis* of all," while the *propria* reflect "the particular *physis* of the individual."

The process of cure by the *physis* was divided by the Empirics into a variety of sub-processes, each constituting a particular symptom-syndrome. These sub-processes, which they called "divisions" or "determinations" (*diairoumenoi*) of the *physis*, were their answer to the Rationalist proximate cause.[59]

While they rejected the proximate cause, the Empirics accepted the exciting (procatarctic) cause—because it is visible to the senses and thus has the same meaning to every observer.[60] "Medicine ought to draw instruction from evident causes, all obscure ones being rejected from the art."[61] They attributed some causality to these causes[62] and included them in the patient's syndrome as additional indications for treatment[63]—in contrast to the Rationalists for whom such causes fell outside the structure of the *tekhne*. "An evaluation [*aestimatio*] of the [exciting] cause often solves the malady."[64g]

Rejection of the proximate cause led to rejection of vivisection as a technique for ascertaining these causes. Being vitalists, they held that function was more important than anatomical configuration.[65] Cutting open a live person alters the very function which the anatomist is trying to elucidate.[66]

> Nor is anything more foolish, they say, than to suppose that whatever the condition of the part of a man's body in life, it will also be the same when he is dying, nay, when he is already dead . . . it is only when the man is dead that the chest and any of the viscera come into the view of the medical murderer, and they are necessarily those of a dead, not of a living man. It follows, therefore, that the medical man just plays the cut-throat, not that he learns what our viscera are like when we are alive.
>
> (Celsus, *Prooemium*, 42-43)

They wrote whole books against the Rationalist anatomical doctrines.[67]

[g]See discussion of *epilogismos* below, pp. 271 ff.

The Empirics have come down through history as a group which knew nothing of human anatomy, but this misrepresents their position. They urged the study of anatomy on corpses, to learn "positions and relations, which the dead body exhibits better than does a living and wounded man."[68] They held only that such knowledge does not yield a therapeutic indication: "[in pleurisy] it is not important to know whether the inflammation attacks the so-called membrane or enveloping tunic or some other part of the side; or even whether or not the lung itself is necessarily affected in its lobes, or completely exempt. They have already seen a number of pleuritics cured according to the method described by Hippocrates in the *Regimen in Acute Diseases*, and they know perfectly well which medicines will relieve him or harm him. They remember the distinctions based on apparent signs which indicate to them in which cases bloodletting is indicated or not. They also know of fomentations, cataplasms, diet, laxatives . . . "[69] Thus, while some general background knowledge in anatomy is useful, the physician has to guard against using it to formulate theories of disease causation. Celsus reflects their view in observing, after presenting a four-page description of the human anatomy: "Having made a sort of survey, as it were, of these organs, so far as it is necessary for a practitioner to know them . . ."[70]

They also held that the necessary anatomical knowledge could be acquired while treating the wounded or during surgical operations.[71] And the Empirics were among the most renowned surgeons of antiquity.[72] As noted above, they entirely accepted the Hippocratic surgical works, wrote comments on them, and urged that surgeons be formed through practice rather than through books.[73] Polybius divides the Empirical School into those who treated with drugs and those who treated by surgery.[74]

It is, in fact, to be presumed that the Empirics knew *more* anatomy than the Rationalists, rather than less. At the same time they refused to base theories of disease on anatomical speculation.

Their prejudice against Rationalist anatomical and other diagnostic techniques required—just as in the Group I Hippocratic works—a development of prognosis,[h] the technique for determining in advance the various stages of the disease in order to assist the *physis* in its passage through each stage. "Early determination of the patient's treatment—since only what has actually been administered will benefit; emphatic assertion is of no use—is beneficial but complicated."[75]

Celsus has a whole book on prognostic signs, stating in the introduction:

> Of impending disorders there are many signs, in explaining which I shall not hesitate to make use of the authority of ancient men, and especially of Hippocrates; for although more recent practitioners have made some changes in methods of treatment, they allow none the less that the ancients prognosticated best.
>
> (Celsus, II, *Prooemium*)

The Empirics divided symptoms into "diagnostic, therapeutic, and prognostic," or, according to another source, those which indicate the past, the present, and the future.[76] The "diagnostic" symptoms were purely descriptive, offering a convenient name for the sickness and implying no knowledge of arcane physiological processes.[77] The therapeutic signs—commemorative signs reminding the physician of past illnesses and their cures—were more valuable, while the prognostic signs were based on these therapeutic ones.[78]

Thus the Empiric's elucidation of the patient's illness proceeded along totally different lines from that of the Rationalist. The latter employed the *logos* to sort out the common elements in a series of cases, thus to define a recognizable disease entity; for purposes of treatment the common or striking features of the patient's illness were the most important. The Empiric used sensory observation to single out precisely the features in the given patient which

[h]The *De Subf. Emp.* gives a prognostic example from *Prognosis*, (Deichgraeber, *op. cit.*, p. 60).

distinguished him from others, which defined his unique way of being ill. Treatment was based upon these unique aspects of the patient's illness.

Therapeutics

Empirical therapeutics was predicated upon acceptance of the theory of coction. The primary curative process was the maturation, coction, and expulsion of the morbific cause or humor, and Empirical therapeutic doctrine is to be understood in this light. The contrast with Rationalism is striking, as the latter approached therapeutics from the point of view of contraries, even interpreting the process of coction in terms of the clash among contrary qualities.

As has been discussed above, cure by the promotion of coction means nothing more than seconding the efforts of the organism itself. "He who has taken the sick man in hand [should] display the discoveries of the *tekhne*, preserving the *physis*, not trying to alter it . . . Should there be [a congenital defect] in a patient who is wasting away, try to assimilate it to the fundamental *physis*." (*Precepts*, cap. IX: Jones, I, 325).

This approach to therapy has two salient characteristics: (1) the organism is viewed as a whole entity, and (2) symptoms are seen as positive phenomena–signs of the struggle of the *physis*.

Coction being a process in which the whole body participates, all cure must necessarily be directed at the body as a whole:

> Most emphatically, it is not enough for the practitioner to pay attention merely to the actual fevers, but also he must look to the habit of the body as a whole, and direct treatment to that.
>
> (Celsus, III, 5: 11)
>
> If sometimes not the whole body, but a part only, is affected, still the support of the strength of the whole body rather than the curing by itself of the part diseased is of more importance.
>
> (Celsus, III, 2: 4)

> [in painful sinews] as in all other bodily affections *concoctio* is a necessity, for *cruditas* is most harmful, and whenever the body is attacked, the faulty part feels it most.
>
> (Celsus, I, 9: 2)

Typical was the observation of Herakleides that his treatment of phrenitis was not designed to break down the disease, but to save the patient.[i]

The body's symptoms and signs were not viewed as harmful, but as beneficial—being signs of the struggle of the *physis* against disease. Madness is relieved by the formation of varicose veins, by dysentery, or by bleeding hemorrhoids.[79] The cause of epileptic fits can be discharged through the stools.[80] Watering of the eyes is benefited by diarrhoea.[81] Shoulder pains spreading to the shoulder-blades or hands are relieved by a vomit of black bile.[82] Prolonged diarrhoeas are suppressed by vomiting.[83] The vomiting of blood in women is relieved by epistaxis or the onset of menstruation.[84] Dysentery benefits enlarged spleen.[85] If epistaxis in children ceases, there is danger of headache, ulceration of the joints, or some debilitating disease.[86] Severe pains after childbirth are removed by epistaxis after twenty days.[87] Round worms in the stool at the disease crisis are a good sign.[88] If bleeding hemorrhoids are suppressed, a sudden and serious disease is liable to supervene.[89]

The Empirics realized that chronic diarrhoea should often be left alone, since its suppression could lead to swelling of the liver or some other organ.[90]

> Fever itself is in the end often a protection, which may appear very strange. For it brings to an end pains over the heart if there is no inflammation; and it also relieves a painful liver; and if it begins after spasm and rigor, it gives entire relief; and it removes the disease of the small

[i]Caelius Aurelianus, *m.a.*, I 17 173. Typical also was the response of the Methodist writer who calls this "utter foolishness. For . . . the patient is saved by the very means by which the disease is relieved . . ."

> intestine arising from urinary difficulty if by its heat it promotes urination.
>
> (Celsus, II, 8: 17-18)
>
> It is the part also of a circumspect man at times to renew and increase a disease and to inflame fevers, for when the existing condition does not answer to a treatment, that which is to come may do so.
>
> (Celsus, III, 9: 4)

These signs all indicate progress in the body's overcoming of morbific causes. Diseases pass through cycles with periodic crises (*accessiones*).[91] If the crisis is unsuccessful, the disease may pass into the stage of abscess-formation.[92] Sometimes a disease is resolved by a skin eruption[93] or by an eruption with fever.[94]

Diseases move downward in the body in the process of cure; if a disease moves upward, it is a very dangerous sign.[95]

Since the aim of therapy was to further the natural course of the disease, the symptoms—representing the organism's struggle against disease—were to be intensified. This meant treatment with similars, in contrast to the Rationalist contraries. Galen comments that, while bodies in an unnatural state are healed only by contraries, the Empirics and Herophileans do not realize this.[96] Celsus divides medicines into *secunda*, which second or promote the body's own healing effort, and *contraria.*[97] In another writing Galen mentions a group whose views resemble "the doctrines of the rhetoricians" and who treat by similars; the context indicates that he has in mind the Empirics.[j]

While the Empirics used dietary treatment primarily when treating internal diseases,[98] they also employed vomitives, purgatives, medicines "to mature abscessions and

[j]*Galeni in Hippocratis De Officina,* p. 83. The reference to "rhetoricians" reflects the Empirics' concern with the correct meaning of words, natural in a school which strove for accurate descriptions of phenomena. Their Hippocratic exegesis was largely devoted to grammatical analysis and elucidation of the meanings of obscure words. Galen frequently calls the Empirics "hair-splitters" and Sophists for the same reason (Deichgraeber, *op. cit.,* Fr. 165,358 and p. 87). The Herophileans resembled the Empirics in this respect: Pliny calls Herophilos the founder of an "over-subtle sect," and Galen calls him a "dialectician" (Pliny, *Natural History,* XXVI, vi; K X 28).

promote suppuration," medicines to "open mouths in the body," medicines to "draw out humors," etc.[99] These were all *secunda* which aided the coction of the morbific cause and its discharge from the body.

Coughs were treated with medicines which provoke coughing, nausea with emetics, and diarrhoea with laxatives.[100] Pleuritic patients who were coughing up sputa were given expectorants.[101] A fever patient was to refrain from drinking or was given hot water, wine, or some other substance to raise his temperature.[102] The patient with an inflamed stomach was to take lukewarm water.[103] If the stomach was bilious, the patient was to take dry wine and wormwood.[104] A man with a chill was warmed by being sprinkled with cold water.[105] An emaciated limb would fill out if tightly bandaged.[106]

Several of Celsus' remedies are so pronouncedly "similar" as to be described by Spencer as "homoeopathic."[107] He calls for black hellebore in diseases where black bile is present,[108] white hellebore in diseases with white phlegm,[109] and ox spleen as a remedy for enlarged spleen.[110] Embedded splinters are drawn to the surface by a poultice made of pole-reed because "of splinters the pole-reed is the worst because it is rough. There is the same harmfulness in fern. But by experience it has been learned that either, when pounded up and applied, serves as a medicament against the other."[111] Likewise, "the scorpion is itself the best remedy against itself. Some pound up the scorpion and swallow it in wine; some pound it up in the same way and put it upon the wound; some put it upon a brazier and fumigate the wound with it . . ."[112] The remedy for an earache with maggots is oil in which the maggots have been boiled.[113] Hydrophobia was treated by throwing the patient into a pond.[114]

Caelius Aurelianus, who was oriented toward contraries, often complains that the Empirical remedies and procedures will only exacerbate the disease. When the Empiric, Serapion, calls for sharp, stimulating, and dilating ointments in synanche, Caelius Aurelianus complains that these will only intensify the inflammation.[115] He states that Serapion's astringents in epilepsy actually constrict the parts that require relaxing and disturb the body at the very time it should be kept in a state of repose.[116] Herakleides' exhibition of clysters in pleurisy only adds to the existing diarrhoea and aggravates the concomitant inflammation.[117]

The Empirics had a second therapeutic principle: when the *secunda* fail, the physician should try the *contraria.*[118] Hence they sometimes used cold applications in fevers and inflammations,[119] checked the flow in diarrhoea, etc.[120] "Contrariety," however, had a different meaning to the Empirics than to the Rationalists. They did not recognize the existence of "secondary" qualities in drugs which could be deduced from their "primary" qualities by tasting, smelling, or observation of the medicine's shape or color. They classified medicines only in function of their effect on the body: emollients, laxatives, epispastics, caustics, dispersants, erodents, etc.[121] The "contrary" of a laxative drug was one which constipated; of one which healed over ulcers was one which kept ulcers open; of one which stopped bleeding was one which promoted hemorrhage, etc.

Jones observes that "in the treatment of fevers the *De Medicina* is more empirical than usual. It 'regards exclusively the clinical picture and the empirical remedy.'"[122] The physician could not know the essential nature of the remedy any more than he could know the *physis* of the patient.[123] All he could ascertain was the remedy's effect on the body. Each medicine was considered to possess its own specific property or power to affect the body in a particular way.[124] Sextus Empiricus calls this the medicine's "relative quality."[125] This power could not be isolated from the substance, and the remedy had to be considered as a whole.[126] The remedy's "relative quality" could be determined in only one way: through trial and error on the sick, that is, through experience.[127] This is how the ancients themselves discovered the uses of medicines.[128]

The Empirics were famous for their pharmacological knowledge and research. While it is not recorded, they surely agreed with Herophilos that medicinal herbs are the "gifts of the Gods." Celsus observes that pharmacology was held in high esteem by both Herophilos and the Empirical school, "inasmuch as they treated no kind of disease without them."[129] In the *De Medicina,* according to Jones, "drugs are recommended more than they are by Greek writers on medicine."[130k]

The surviving Empirical fragments contain many of their prescriptions—which were used by physicians of other schools as well.

They differentiated among foods but in a less far-reaching way than among drugs—classifying them as "more" or "less" digestible or as "strong," "weak," and "middling."[131]

They practised bloodletting, especially in plethora.[132] The pain of a headache was relieved by opening a vein in the forehead.[133] But they disagreed with Galen's contention that bloodletting should be employed in traumatic injuries and wounds.[134] Celsus and Menodotos warn against bloodletting in those who are too weak to bear it.[135]

The use of all of these medicines, diets, and other procedures was subordinated to the overall Empirical procedure of distinguishing the patient from all others of his class, and the remedy from all similar ones, in order to match the specific power of the remedy to the *proprium* (*idios*) of the patient.[136] This process of discrimination (*diastole*) was based upon symptoms because the *physis* of both the patient and the remedy were in themselves not directly knowable.[137] And they contrasted their *diastole* with the *diorismos* (discrimination) of the Rationalists which was based upon logic.[138]

They took therapeutic indications from the season, the climate, the exciting cause of the illness, and the patient's age and habits.[139] They held that treatment of similar conditions varied from one country to another.[140]

Their rationale of compounding remedies was different from that of the Rationalists. The latter mixed medicines of "opposite" qualities in order to have a substance with a quality against each proximate cause inside the body. The Empirics, however, mixed together substances whose "whole

[k]Books V and VI of *De Medicina* are on pharmacology.

natures" were *similar*—to have a compound with a composite quality covering variations in the disease due to variations in the patient's temperament.[141]

The disease categories of the Rationalists were fragmented by the Empirics. Galen complains that they insist on discussing putrefying ulcers, corroding ulcers, ulcers with gangrene, ulcers with erysipelas, painful ulcers, etc., thinking in this way to find essential differences among the ulcers. Actually (says Galen) these are only *differentiae* of the class, "simple ulcer."[142] The Rationalist confronted with a case of diarrhoea called for "constipating remedies," while the Empiric enumerated fifteen different ones with the appropriate indications.[143][1] Celsus argued against the Methodists:

> There are different kinds of constricting and of relaxing diseases, those in which there is a flux being the more easy to observe. For it is one thing to vomit blood, another bile, another food; it is one thing to suffer from diarrhoea, another from dysentery; one thing to be relaxed through sweating, another to be wasted by consumption. Humor may break out into particular parts, such as the eyes or the ears; from a risk of this kind there is no human member free. No one of these occurrences is treated in the same way as another.
>
> Hence the art descends down from a consideration of the common characteristics [*a communi*] of a flux to the particular case [*ad propriam*]. Moreover, because the same remedies do not meet with success in all, even of similar cases, additional knowledge of peculiarities in such a case is often necessary. Although certain things act upon the bowels in most cases, whether as astringents or as laxatives, yet there are to be found some in whom the same thing acts differently than it does in others. In such instances, therefore, investigation of *propria* is salutary, that of *communia* the reverse.
>
> (Celsus, *Prooemium*, 67-68)

[1]See, also, Lykos of Naples' extremely far-reaching discrimination among cases of *ileus* and dysentery, with the indications for dozens of different treatments (Deichgraeber, *op. cit.*, Fr. 262).

Theory and Practice: The Empirical Definition of "Scientific Medicine"

One of the major problems confronting any therapeutic doctrine is the tremendous diversity of diseased states. Aristotle observed that "individual cases are infinitely varied,"[144] and this fact was well recognized by the Empirical School:

> The number of diseases and their accompanying symptoms are endless owing to the isolation of each case . . . we understand by endlessness the variations in their degrees and arrangement which complicate the diseases and their symptoms through some of them preceding and some following others.
>
> In the almost endless variety of their diseases and the symptoms of them, the sick themselves differ from one another . . . What is more manifold, more complicated, and more varied than disease? . . . How does one discover that a disease is the same as another disease in all its characteristics? Is it by the number of symptoms or by their strength and power? For if a thing be itself, then in my opinion, it must be itself in all these characteristics, for if even one of them is lacking, it is perverted, and ceases to be itself.[145]

When the Empirics emerged on the historical scene, they found that the Rationalists had already developed a therapeutic doctrine for coping with this diversity of diseases, based upon experience and the (logical) indication.[146] However, the Empirics did not accept this line of argument. They pointed out that, while the Rationalists claimed to act on logical grounds, whatever correct techniques they possessed had all been developed by experience.[147] "It was afterwards, when the remedies had already been discovered, that men began to discuss the reasons for them: medicine was not a discovery following upon reasoning, but after the discovery of the remedy, the reason for it was sought out. They ask, too, does reasoning teach the same as experience? If the same, it was needless; if something else, then it was even opposed to it . . ."[148]

If reasoning was so valuable to medicine, the Empirics said, philosophers would make the best physicians, but this is obviously not the case: "they have words in plenty, and no knowledge of healing at all."[149]

The Empirics concluded that the logical determination of proximate causes was a delusion and a waste of effort.[150]

Hence they sought a different approach, a different instrument to make the heterogeneity of diseases manageable, a different definition of "scientific medicine." This approach was based on the writings of the Hippocratic Corpus which abjured the use of logic in medicine, relied wholly on sense-perception, and founded therapeutics on the theory of coction.[m]

Reliance on sensory evidence is the necessary corollary of a vitalistic physiology, for, if the *physis* is spontaneous and self-determined, no *a priori* knowledge of its actions is possible.[n]

We cannot say why the Empirics accepted this set of assumptions about the organism and the nature of medical knowledge any more than we can tell why the Rationalists assumed that the organism is *not* a reactive entity and that *a priori* knowledge of its mechanisms *is* possible. Answers to these questions can be found only outside the theory of medicine and require an examination of the social context in which medicine is practised.[o]

In any case, the Empirics accepted these assumptions and based medical practice on the Hippocratic works which followed the same assumptions.

But medical thinking had not come to an end in the fifth century B.C. The Alexandrian era was distinguished, in particular, by an extensive development of pharmacological knowledge. The Hippocratic writings contained relatively

[m]As noted above (p. 202), the Empirical school almost certainly represents a continuing tradition which emerged to self-consciousness in the third century B.C. under the impact of Scepticism.

[o]See below, pp. 279-284.

[n]Apollonios the Empiric polemicized over the value of sense-perception *circa* 175 B.C., denying that it yielded knowledge of any underlying reality. He was arguing against the Epicureans who held that sense-perception *did* yield such knowledge (Deichgraeber, *op. cit.*, p. 257 and Fr. 164).

little pharmacology, and the Empirics were faced with the necessity of engrafting onto the theory of coction this volume of new information about medicinal drugs, of determining how the process of coction was affected in each case by drugs which were not known to the Hippocratic authors.

They had to devise a method for analyzing and subdividing the process of coction in function of these new medicines. Fortunately, the materials for such a method were available in the Sceptical philosophy which appeared in history at the same time as Empiricism and remained allied with it for centuries.

Scepticism and Empiricism have in common the conviction that day-to-day experience is the proper concern of the thinker. The Sceptics analyzed this experience and from it developed a method for surmounting the difficulties encountered in everyday life. The Empirics analyzed medical experience to discover a method of coping with problems of medical practice.

Under Sceptical influence the Empirics shifted the emphasis of medical thought from the physiological category, "coction," to the epistemological category, "experience." The Hippocratic writers had accepted a set of assumptions about the nature of medical theory and practice; of these the theory of coction was the most fundamental. The Empirics altered the terms of the argument somewhat by focussing on "experience" and interpreting coction in the light of an all-encompassing theory of medical experience.

They distinguished between "experience" (*empeiria, experientia*) and the single "experiment" (*peira, experimentum*). Both were defined as the reception of information by the senses and its storage in the memory, and medical *experientia* was the sum total of all the *experimenta* of medical practitioners. Sometimes the Empirics claimed that their whole *tekhne* was identical with experience, i.e., with observation and memory; sometimes they only claimed that experience was the principal component of the *tekhne*.[151] In any case, "experience" is fundamental.

But the experience of mankind is its history, and the Empirical stress on experience signified a deep interest in medical history. They held that medical theory is identical with the medical history of mankind (just as one might say today that the embryo in the womb passes through, and incorporates in itself, all stages of biological development of the race). Just as disease itself is a process, so the Empirical doctrine arose in a gradual process out of the accumulated *experimenta* of thousands of physicians and their patients:

> Even in its beginnings, [the Empirics] add, medicine was not deduced from such questionings, but from experience; for of the sick who were without doctors, some in the first days of illness, longing for food, took it forthwith; others owing to distaste, abstained; and the sickness was more alleviated in those who abstained. Again, some partook of food while actually under the fever, some a little before, others after its remission, and it went best with those who did so after the fever had ended; and similarly, some at the beginning adopted at once a rather full diet, others a scanty one, and those were made worse who had eaten plentifully. When this and the like happened day after day, careful men noted what generally answered the better, and then began to prescribe the same for their patients. Thus sprang up medicine, which, from the frequent recovery of some and the death of others, distinguished between the pernicious and the salutary.
>
> (Celsus, *Prooemium*, 33-35).

Celsus' account is taken from *Ancient Medicine* (cap. III), and it is no accident that this outstanding work of the Hippocratic Corpus is itself a history.

The crystallization of *experientia* from the medical *experimenta* of mankind was converted by the Empirics into a precise method whose three components were: 1) the perception of events (*autopsia, per se inspectio*), 2) accounts of events which had occurred in the past (*istoria, historia*), and 3) the passage-from-like-to-like (*omoiou metabasis, tran-*

sitio similis). These they called the "constitutive parts" of medicine.[152]

The first of these, the *per se inspectio*, was the observation of an event and its storage in the memory.[153] The event itself, or its observation (this was a matter of dispute), was the *experimentum*, and the sub-categories of the *per se inspectio* were: 1) observation of events occurring spontaneously, and 2) observation of events produced through human intervention.[154]

Spontaneous events, in turn, were subdivided into: a) events produced by the *physis* and b) events due to chance. For this reason the Empirics said that the *physis* and chance were their guides to discovery.[155]

Typical of the first would be a patient whose fever was alleviated or cured by a spontaneous nosebleed.[156] By observing this the physician learned one technique of the *physis* for curing fever and could subsequently employ it himself. "So we must conceive of our *physis* as being stirred and instructed under compulsion by the great variety of things; and the intellect, taking over from the *physis* the impressions, leads us afterwards into truth" (*Precepts*, cap. I: Jones, I, 313).

Typical of the second was the patient with headache who tripped and fell to the ground, cutting a vein in his forehead, and found that the ensuing loss of blood put an end to his pain.[157]

The category of events produced by human intervention also had two sub-categories: a) *experimenta* done in imitation of events seen in the past and b) *experimenta* which were not done in imitation of some other event, but at random.

The first of these, the imitative experiment, would be, for instance, using a plant or herb as a remedy because it was so used by a wild animal, or administering an enema after observing the ibis cleaning out its own colon in this way.[158][p] This category was greatly extended by the passage-from-like-

[p]On the discovery of the enema by the ibis, see above, 110, note.

to-like and is discussed below.[q] It was used mainly to expand pharmacological knowledge.

The second of these, the random experiment, seems also to have been the Empirical response to the profusion of new medicines in the Alexandrian period. A fever patient of his own volition drinks cold water or eats some fruit and is relieved. Or a person bitten by a wild animal feels a desire for some specific herb or plant and is cured.[159] Or a man suffering from a loathsome skin disease attempts suicide by imbibing a drink in which vipers have been soaked: instead of killing him, however, it acts as a cure.[160] Or a female slave brings her master wine from a bottle into which a snake had crawled and died: the drink acts therapeutically.[161] Celsus describes how the discovery was made that a person bitten by an asp should drink vinegar:

> The case of a certain boy is said to demonstrate this, for having been thus bitten, partly on account of the bite, and partly owing to excessively hot weather, he was tormented by thirst, and being in a dry place found no other fluid, so he drank the vinegar he chanced to have with him and was saved.
>
> (Celsus, V, 27: 4)

The Empirics professed to be uninterested in the origin of suggestions for the trials of remedies, claiming that knowing how to employ them correctly was more important.[162] When pressed, however, they mentioned dreams, chance, and accidents. Compound remedies were discovered in the same way—from dreams or because someone swallowed a mixture by accident and was thereby benefited.[163]

The second constitutive part of medicine, the *historia*, symbolizes the intimate concern of the Empirics with medical history. The *historia* was a verbal or written account of some *per se inspectio* which had occurred in the past.[164][r] They justified its use as follows (Galen speaking):

[q]See below, pp. 268-270.

[r]Deichgraeber observes (*op. cit.*, pp. 300-301) that the principle of the *historia* is found in *Ancient Medicine*, cap. II: "But medicine has long had all its means to hand, and has discovered both a principle and a method, through which

> Often there occur diseases for which the treatment has not yet been discovered from the *per se inspectio*. Consequently, in order to have some aid at hand, and not to have to await the natural outcome of the disease, [the Empirics] use the *historia.* Also to make instruction less lengthy, because they say it is impossible that the learner should encounter all the possible symptoms and make his observation on all. Hence they say that the *historia* is useful to the exercise of medicine, so that one should not remain a student all one's life but be able to apply the art at some point.[165]

Because "life is short, the art long" (*Aphorisms* I:1), the physician needs access to the experience of his forebears. Analytical knowledge of disease is foreclosed to him, and he must make use of others' experience. The Empirics said that in their day, because the *tekhne* was old, the *historia* was more important than the *per se inspectio.*[166]

However, the *historia* was not accepted uncritically. It was evaluated according to the author's reputation, the verisimilitude of the account (meaning its agreement or lack of agreement with other accounts or observations), and the techniques devised by the Empirics for testing the truth of experiential knowledge.[167s]

The third constitutive part of the Empirical *tekhne* was the passage-from-like-to-like—an expansion and development of the imitative experiment. It was a heuristic principle, providing a methodical basis for expansion of medical knowledge, and thus the Empirical equivalent of the Rationalist syllogism.

The passage-from-like-to-like was used in three ways: remedies found to be effective in illnesses of one part of the body could be applied to some other part, those effective in one disease could be transferred to a similar disease, and a

the discoveries made during a long period are many and excellent, while full discovery will be made, if the inquirer be competent, conduct his discoveries with knowledge of discoveries already made, and make them his starting-point." Also *Epidemics III,* cap. XVI: "The power, too, to study correctly what has been written I consider to be an important part of the art of medicine."

[s]See below, pp. 270-271.

medicine could be substituted for another of similar effect.[168] The transition had to be based upon sense-perceptible data.[169] It was a passage from the discovered to the not-yet-discovered.[170]

This technique had its antecedents in *The Art*:

> The physician sets about his task with healthy mind and healthy body, having considered the case and past cases of like characteristics to the present, so as to say how they were treated and cured.
>
> (*The Art*, cap. VII: Jones, II, 201)

Celsus describes it as follows:

> For even if there happened nowadays some unknown form of malady, nevertheless the practitioner had not to theorize over obscure matters, but straightway would see to which disease it came nearest, then would make trial of remedies similar to those which have succeeded often in a kindred affection, and so through its similarities [*similitudines*] find help.
>
> (Celsus, *Prooemium*, 37-38)

He recounts the case of "a lady from whose genitals flesh had prolapsed and become gangrenous [and who] died in the course of a few hours, whilst practitioners of the highest standing found out neither the class of malady nor a remedy" out of fear that "he might seem to have killed, if he did not save her . . ."

> In this sort of practice similarity [*similitudo*] is not always of service, and when it does prove serviceable, nonetheless, there has been a process of reasoning in the theorizing over similar classes of diseases and of remedies, as to which is the best remedy to use. When, therefore, such an incident occurs, the practitioner ought to arrive at something which may answer, even if perhaps not always, yet nevertheless more often than not. He will seek, however, every novel plan, not from hidden things, for these are dubious and unascertainable, but from those which can be explored, that is, from evident causes.
>
> (Celsus, *Prooemium*, 49-53)

In contrast to the Rationalist syllogism, the passage-from-like-to-like did not in itself yield reliable knowledge. It was only a procedural principle yielding a "possible judgment"[171] and had to be tested before the knowledge which it provided was considered reliable: "every transition of this kind is a road to discovery, but experiment is needed before it actually becomes a discovery."[172]

For the passage-from-like-to-like, the *historia*, and, indeed, the *per se inspectio* were subject to tests to determine their reliability.[173] And in developing these test procedures the Empirics came upon the principles of scientific method. Their research led them to (1) a technique for dealing with negative instances and (2) the scientific experiment.

In a manner similar to that later discovered by Francis Bacon the Empirics developed a method enabling them to distinguish knowledge into four grades of reliability. The highest grade consisted of those events which occurred invariably and without any contradictory instances. The second grade consisted of those which occurred with a few negative instances. The third grade consisted of events with a fifty percent probability of occurrence, and the fourth grade included events which happened only rarely, with negative instances predominating. They had a fifth category also: those events which occurred without any apparent order or pattern.[174]

But the major device developed by the Empirics to certify the reliability of their knowledge was the "expert experiment" (*tribike peira, trivica experientia*).[175] Since the only reliable knowledge was that of events which repeated themselves, the Empirics sought in the "expert experiment" a technique for duplicating events at will. The experiment could only be done by the physician who was skilled in the *tekhne*.[176] Knowledge obtained in this way was as reliable as if it had been obtained from events occurring many times.[177]

The analysis of negative instances originated in Carneades' classification of judgments, and the "expert experiment" is derived from his "closely scrutinized judgment."[t] Both were

[t]See above, pp. 189-190. This treatment of negative instances was known to Herakleides (Deichgraeber, *op. cit.*, Fr. 342 and p. 296).

put in their final form by Menodotos. This was how he applied *logos* to medicine.[178]

Favier has noted correctly that a technique for handling negative instances and the "expert experiment" are fundamental components of scientific method and that the Empirics were thus essentially scientific in their approach to therapeutics.[179]

Hence the Empirics and Rationalists do not represent a conflict between *logos* and experience. The Rationalists claimed to derive much of their knowledge from experience, and the Empirics made a large place for *logos*. The problem was rather one of how *logos* and experience were combined in the two doctrines.

The contrast is rooted in the opposed assumptions of the two schools about the reliability of sensory knowledge. The Rationalists held that it was ultimately unreliable, and the Empirics held the contrary. They rejected "the naming which is by man and demand[ed] that things be known according to the soul."[180] They rejected the Rationalist view that the *logos* yields direct knowledge of the essence of objects, as represented by the Rationalist identification of objects with their names.[181] But it would be ridiculous to think that they wanted the physician to dispense with thought, or even belittled the importance of thought. They merely viewed the soul (*anima, psyche*) as capable of a different function: "a capacity of weighing and considering what is acceptable and what is not."[182] This function they called *epilogismos*—a weighing of evident things, a mode of thought rooted in sense-perceptible phenomena and yielding results acceptable to all.[183] They contrasted their *epilogismos* with the Rationalist *analogismos*—defined as cogitation about non-evident things.[184]

When the physician had seen certain symptoms repeat themselves time after time, or had seen that a certain group of symptoms was always followed by death,[185] or had seen that certain medicines acted curatively in certain syndromes, he marked this down for future use. The proposition was inherent in the phenomena, not abstracted from them. The Empirics accepted *epilogismos* because it is "an inference commonly and universally used by the whole of mankind, and wherein men are unanimous, and where there is no such thing as schism and diversity of opinion."[186] It "prescribes the doing of what should be done on the basis of the good or evil which is inherent in the thing and accompanies it, whereas the conclusion known as *analogismos* prescribes action on the basis of the natures of things."[187]

> For a *logismos* is a composite memory of things apprehended with sense-perception. For the sense-perception, coming first in experience and conveying to the intellect the things subjected to it, is clearly imaged, and the intellect, receiving these things many times, noting the occasion, the time, and the manner, stores them up in itself and remembers. Now I approve of *logismos* also if it lays its foundations in incident and deduces its conclusions in accordance with phenomena. For if *logismos* lays its foundations in clear fact, it is found to exist in the domain of intellect which itself receives from other sources each of its impressions.
> (*Precepts,* cap. I: Jones, I, 313)

The Empirical *epilogismos* and the *logismos* of *Precepts* are identical with the *logismos* discussed in cap.XI of *The Art.*[u] All three are based on sensory data.

Herakleides and Menodotos recognized this function of the soul, adding it to sensory observation and memory.[188] The latter held that the application of *epilogismos* to the materials of the *per se inspectio,* the *historia,* and the passage-from-like-to-like, the weighing of positive and negative instances and the conduct of "expert experiments" distinguished the developed form of Empiricism from its more primitive beginnings.[189] He called "irrational" those physicians who did not apply the theory of negative instances.[190] Theodas, an Empirical physician living in the second century A.D., held that experience processed through the passage-from-like-to-like became "rational" (*rationabilis*).[191] Galen notes that the Empirics condemn an

[u]See above, pp. 81-83.

Empiricism which is "without a certain limitation" and contrasts the Empirics, who have a method, with the Methodists, who have none at all.[192] The author of *Precepts* advises the physician to "attend in medical practice not primarily to plausible *logismos* but to experience combined with *logos* [*tribe meta logou*]."[193]

Thus the medical tradition that the Empirics disregarded *logos* is incorrect. Specifically, Celsus' observation that "reasoning is necessary in medicine" and that "medicine ought to be rational" in no way precludes him from consideration as a representative of Empiricism.[194][v]

The weighing of the *per se inspectio* and the *historia* by employing *epilogismos* led to the crystallization of theorems (*theoremata*). When an event had been seen to occur many times in the same way (with all necessary qualifications), it became a theorem.[195]

The Hippocratic aphorisms are identical with the Empirical theorems and were by them accepted as such. This is seen from the more than two hundred references to *Aphorisms* in Celsus' *De Medicina.*

The Empirical *tekhne* consisted of all these theorems grouped together.[196] They defined the *tekhne* as the "conservation" or "guarding" in the memory of all that is seen to occur in medicine.[197] The theorems were divided into those dealing with: (1) the recognition of commemorative and prognostic signs, (2) therapeutics–subdivided into surgery, pharmacy, and diet, and (3) hygiene.[198] These were the "final" parts of medicine, as distinguished from the "constitutive" parts: the *per se inspectio,* the *historia,* and the passage-from-like-to-like.[w] While the latter served to build up the *tekhne,* the former indicated its various applications. Both "constitutive" and "final" parts, however, arose from

[v]Celsus observes that the passage-from-like-to-like involves a process of reasoning: *"id ipsum rationale est"* (*Prooemium,* 51).

[w]The Empirics disputed among themselves over the precise division of the "final" parts of medicine but recognized that this was of no significance and was, in fact, a mere quibbling over words (Deichgraeber, *op. cit.,* p. 53 [*De Subf. Emp.*]).

and were related to practice, and there is no division between "theory" and "practice" in Empiricism.

Rationalist Criticism of the Empirical Tekhne

Rationalist criticism of the Empirical *tekhne* reveals the different attitudes of the two schools to the problem of correct method in medicine. The Empirical method was based on an enumeration of particulars: "the whole *tekhne* has been set forth by observing some part of the final end in each of many particulars, and then combining all into a single whole" (*Precepts,* cap. II: Jones, I, 315). From the particulars they induced their theorems. In a more general sense, however, their method should be described as a testing of the data of sensory observation against the hypothesis that the organism cures through coction. The Empirical doctrine was a body of rules of practice based upon the hypothesis of coction. If the practice was done correctly, the hypothesis would be proved correct; knowledge was developed in the course of practice.

Hence the Empirics espoused a theory of knowledge identical with that which underlies scientific method. Theory (knowledge) arises out of practice and is identical with crystallized practice. The theory of medicine is only a reflection of the theory of the *physis*. The physician's practice can be nothing more than a copy of the practice of the *physis*.

Just as the author of *Ancient Medicine* had asserted that a knowledge of the *physis* can be obtained only through the practice of medicine, so Celsus writes: "all that is possible to come to know in the living, the actual treatment exhibits."[199] And Paracelsus said, fifteen centuries later, "the cure points to the cause."

This was the opposite of the Rationalist doctrine which held that theory is derived *a priori*, from analysis of the data of experience by the *logos* and the deduction of theorems. Practice was then based upon this preexisting theory. Hence the Rationalists asserted that a doctrine relying on *epilogismos* and the passage-from-like-to-like was not a *tekhne*.[200]

Their primary criticism was directed against the elucidation of truth through an enumeration of particulars. The Empirics recognized that a single *per se inspectio*—one occurrence of an event—had no probative value.[201] The Rationalists asked: How many times must an event be repeated before it can be accepted as "scientific" (i.e., belonging to the *tekhne*)?[202] How many times must a medicine purge before it can be accepted as a purgative?[203] If the individual case itself is not "scientific," the sum of these cases cannot have "scientific" value either. The Empirics have no standard for the number of times an event must be observed before it becomes "scientific."[204]

Here they raised the *sorites* (pile of sand) argument: how many grains of sand must be amassed together before they form a pile?[205][x]

Furthermore, the Rationalists held, when the medicine fails to work in a particular case, the Empirics cannot give the reason why.[206] Unless they make a distinction between important and unimportant symptoms, they will be reduced to treating only common cases, not rare ones.[207]

To avoid reliance on the enumeration of particulars, the Rationalists referred the phenomena to *logos* and distinguished among sense-perceptibles on that basis. Do the Empirics "desire to comprehend that which is infinite by bringing it into the category of temporal experience without making use of the *logos*?"[208] Logical consistency is a better criterion of reliability than the Empirical experiment. Information cannot be stored up *ad infinitum* in the memory: systematic recollection and recall require reduction to logical principles.[209] The sounds of speech and the words of language could not be remembered unless they had been reduced to order by the grammarians.[210] If the Empirics reject logic as the criterion, they must admit that their therapy is based upon random symptoms.[211]

The application of *logos* to medicine, they insisted, compels departure from the realm of the visible:

[x]No answer is possible, since the rejoinder is always: Does the pile cease being a pile if one grain of sand is taken away?

> One may legitimately call the phenomena the principle of the discovery of theorems; but the phenomena are not the principle of the *tekhne*. Thus one would say that the tracks are the principle of the discovery of the hare, but no one with common sense would call them the principle of the hare, since the hare is not made up of tracks. One would be right in saying that the phenomena are the principle of the discovery of theorems, considering that the founders of the *tekhne* constructed it by basing themselves on the phenomena; but the phenomena are not the principles of the *tekhne, since the principles have to be referred to the quality* [poiotes] *of the thing of which they are the principles.*[212]

They argued that no one could live long enough to try out all possible remedies in all possible diseases, thus to establish a *tekhne* on that basis.[213] Written records are unreliable and can be judged only by the credibility of the causal relations described.[214] They noted difficulties with the Empirical acceptance of the exciting (procatarctic) cause as one of the indications: how did the Empirics know where to draw the line, since the number of such causes is infinite?

> Tell me, why is it that lassitude, burning caused by the sun, drunkenness, overeating, exposure to a cold atmosphere, overstepping the limits with regard to coition, and indigestion are things which must be remembered and inquired into, and to which *logos* must be applied, but other things analogous to these need not be made the subject of investigation? I mean by analogous things inquiring into whether the sick man took a bath before the onset of his illness or not; whether he had stayed in the town or the village; whether he had stayed in a room or on the terrace, and if he had slept or lain awake, or if he had been depressed or had had worries, or if he had read some books. More remote from this would be the query as to whether he had worn a white garment before that time, or a red, or a black, or a crimson one. Furthermore, one might ask whether he had wrestled or

> had bathed with anyone, dined or slept with anyone. For all these and similar things, although there are others more remote than these, they must retain in their memories and investigate when they have even once refused to disown the memorizing of what they see of the salient causes.[215]

The Empirics recognized that Aristotelian logic did not yield a technique for transforming particular instances into general rules, but the ocean exists even though one could not state precisely how many cups of water would have to be put together to form this body.[216]

> I for my part adhere to and follow that which is known to men, and accept what is obvious without inquiring into the cause of each individual thing. Therefore, I say of what has been seen but once that it is not technical [possessing *tekhne*] just as the single grain of wheat is not a perfect heap: if, however, it is a thing that is seen many times in the same way, then I call it technical. For I observe that children, too, do not learn to write on seeing the letters of the alphabet only once, but they must hear and see them many times. How many times they must do so I shall not ask, since I gain no advantage thereby . . . You, however, prompted by your dilettantism in seeking to investigate what is neither useful nor necessary, trouble yourself with this and all other like matters.[217]

Thus they denied the relevance of formal logic to medicine altogether. Reliable knowledge is not that which is logically consistent but that which is seen to occur many times.[218] They held their method adequate to discover not only simple concepts and elementary knowledge, but complicated concepts as well and, in fact, the whole *tekhne* of medicine.[219] They transvalued the Rationalist categories, defining *logos* as the "selection of those aids which have been discovered by experience."[220] Instead of "definitions" they employed "descriptions."[221] Hence, *logos* was knowledge of appearances, not of the underlying reality.[222]

The general Empirical response to Rationalist criticism was that it had a political or economic aim: "to disparage and deprecate Empiricism and to prove that it does not advance along the lines of a *tekhne* and that it is neither credible nor reliable."[223] How could Empiricism not be a *tekhne*, they added, when its results demonstrate its existence?[224] Empiricism, in fact, "suffices to discover everything used in healing," and the Empirics, who do not rely on the Rationalist *logos*, heal just as well as, or better than, the latter.[225]

Where the author of *The Art* had argued:

> How is it possible for patients to attribute their recoveries to anything else except the *tekhne*, seeing that it was by using it and serving it that they recovered?
>
> (*The Art*, cap. IV: Jones, II, 195)
>
> Medicine . . . because it acts "through something" and because its results may be forecasted, has reality, as is manifest now and will be manifest forever.
>
> (*The Art*, cap. VI: Jones, II, 201)

the Empiric in Galen's *Medical Experience* states:

> With regard to the cause . . . which makes it completely technical and when it begins to be completely technical, I am of the opinion that it is useless to demand this. For I find that not a particle of harm befalls *tekhnes* and men in their modes of life and activities for being ignorant of such things . . . If you should get no answer to your questions, you have no right to reproach us or to make a charge against us that the fact does not exist, for it is assuredly clear that it does exist . . . And yet do you command me not to believe that which is evident to the senses, since I cannot explain how a thing is truly technical that has been observed very many times? I am no Sophist whose business it is to refute errors or to compound them and form a chain of them. Nor am I such a fool as to believe all you say on the spot and without hesitation.[226]

Thus he proved his doctrine by works, not by words.[227] "Nor will he be long-winded and voluble, but speaks little and rarely like Pyrrho the Sceptic . . ."[228] "It is not . . . by eloquence but by remedies that diseases are treated. A man of few words who learns by practice to discern well would make an altogether better practitioner than he who, unpractised, overcultivates his tongue."[229] They disputed the Rationalists by actions rather than by counter-arguments. To a Rationalist arguing that the Empirical *tekhne* did not exist, the Empiric replied:

> If you persist in such an attitude, you will force me to mention the words of Diogenes, who said, on an Athenian setting him the riddle by which motion is eliminated, the sum and substance of his argument being that there is no such thing as motion: "I am surprised at these miserable seafarers who annoy us all day long with their cries of: Who is going to Rhodes, who to Cnidos, to Cos, to Lesbos?"[230]

When one Empiric was preparing to operate on a patient, a frivolous physician of some other school approached the family and argued that his own treatment would be superior. Thereupon the Empiric threatened to retire from the case, and the frightened family immediately dismissed the interloper.[231]

The Sociology of Empiricism

Empirical medicine is identical with the doctrine of the Group I Hippocratic writings in being a set of rules for practice, not a theory of the organism.[y] The physician studied the rules and mastered them in order to acquire skill.[232] The doctrine focusses on the skilful practitioner—not on physiological theory. The "master of the art" was the physician of experience.[233]

> One must hold fast to facts even from beginning to end, and occupy oneself with facts persistently if one is to acquire that ready and infallible *habit* which we call the art of medicine.
>
> (*Precepts*, cap. II: Jones, I, 315)

[y] Just as Scepticism was a code of conduct and not a metaphysical doctrine.

> [Quacks neglect] the irreproachable *methods* of the *tekhne*, wherewith a good physician, a "brother of the art" as he is called, would be at his best.
> (*Precepts*, cap. VII: Jones, I, 321)
>
> I urge that experience is useful, the learning of opinions coming far after. For who is desirous and ambitious of learning truly subtle diversities of opinion, to the neglect of calm and practised *skill*?
> (*Precepts*, cap. XIII: Jones, I, 329)

This view of the *tekhne* and of the physician presupposes a particular attitude toward society and the patient.

These physicians saw themselves as craftsmen.[z] Medicine to them was a trade whose aim was: "to endeavor to cure all things which are against the *physis* and through works to extend assurance."[234] Menodotos stated that the physician practices medicine to earn a living.[235]

The Empirics were not researchers, and their books were guides to practice rather than physiological investigations.[236] As has been discussed above, their practical attitude toward medicine led to a particular epistemology—proceeding from practice to theory, from the cure to knowledge of the organism.

This utilitarian view of medicine had an impact also on the physician's relations with the patient and with society.

Instead of interposing a tissue of speculation between himself and the patient, the Empiric accepted unmediated sensory observation as the source of his knowledge. The symptoms told him all he needed to know and were the direct criteria of therapy. Since the therapeutic symptoms were determining, even semeiotics was subordinated to therapeutics.[237a] The whole of medicine was oriented toward the pragmatic and practical task of curing.

According to Deichgraeber, they did not view themselves as a sociological unity but called themselves a "trend" in

[z]The word, "craftsman" (*demiourgos*), is used in *Precepts*, cap. II (Jones, I, 315).

[a]Deichgraeber observes that this is a parallel with homoeopathic medicine (*op. cit.*, p. 308).

medicine.[238] Thus their relationship to the patient was unmediated in another sense: they were not the conscious followers of some man or some school. They said that "other physicians are called followers of Hippocrates or Erasistratos or Praxagoras or Asclepiades or of some other man; they themselves, however, were not made by Akron, or by Timon or Philinos or Serapion who were later than Akron, or by others who preceded him."[239]

Much of their energy was directed at "dissolving" and refuting the doctrines of others.[240] They saw themselves as following the *physis* and experience, not the opinions of some teacher. Their theorems seemed self-evident, being founded in experience, and they were wrathful against others who attempted to refute them by logic. Galen accuses them of prescribing their rules "like tyrants," without proving them to be correct.[241] And Menodotos, in particular, was endlessly insulting other physicians, "barking like a dog and using gutter vituperation."[242] One may assume that their drive to individualize made them individualists and iconoclasts themselves.

Empirical medicine was thus democratic and egalitarian.[b] The physician was a workman. He used only visible signs which are reliable because they mean the same to all men.[243] His procedures could be verified by anyone who could use his five senses. He did not claim ability to see what others could not see, and he did not justify his acts by the *ipse dixit* of some teacher or master.

This egalitarian instinct, together with the holism of Empirical medicine which kept the physician mindful that he was always treating not a disease but a person, promoted an attitude of charity and forbearance toward the patient:

> You [Rationalists] are dull of heart and blind of eye by reason of your anxiety to give good reasons for your opinions.[244]

[b]"The patient must cooperate with the physician in combating the disease" (*Epidemics I,* Second Constitution, cap. XI: Jones, I, 165). "The physician must be ready, not only to do his duty himself, but also to secure the cooperation of the patient, of the attendants, and of externals" (*Aphorisms* I: 1: Jones, IV, 99).

> Sometimes give your services for nothing, calling to mind a previous benefaction or present satisfaction. And if there be an opportunity of serving one who is a stranger in financial straits, give full assistance to all such. For where there is love of man, there is also love of the *tekhne*. For some patients, though conscious that their condition is perilous, recover their health simply through their contentment with the goodness of the physician.[245]
>
> [A surgeon should be] filled with pity, so that he wishes to cure his patient, yet is not moved by his cries to go too fast, or cut less than is necessary; but he does everything just as if the cries of pain cause him no emotion.[246]

In this they were only following the example of the Hippocratic writings which they accepted:

> As to diseases, make a habit of two things—to help, or at least to do no harm.
>
> (*Epidemics I*, Second Constitution, cap. XI: Jones, I, 165)
>
> Not by daring but by judgment, not by violence but by gentleness.
>
> (*The Art*, cap. XI: Jones, II, 211)

The tie between the stress on visibility ("blind of eye") and the charity of the physician is not accidental. Rationalist involvement with abstractly conceived entities predisposed to a more hard-hearted attitude toward the patient.

The author of *Precepts* even urges postponing discussion of the fee while the patient is still sick: "it is better to reproach a patient you have saved than to extort money from those who are at death's door."[247]

This ultimately moral approach to medicine underlay the Empirical rejection of vivisection:

> Now the matters just referred to they deem to be superfluous; but what remains cruel as well, to cut into the belly and chest of a man whilst still alive, and to impose upon the art which presides over human safety someone's death, and that too in the most atrocious way.
>
> (Celsus, *Prooemium*, 40)

Some Empirics even held that dissecting the dead was unnecessary: "although not cruel, it is none the less nasty; but all that is possible to come to know in the living, the actual treatment exhibits."[248] Celsus finally concludes that what cannot be learned from corpses and "can only be learned from the living, actual practice will demonstrate in the course of treating the wounded in a somewhat slower yet much milder way."[249]

Just as the Empirical physician respected the patient's body, he also respected him as a codiscoverer and developer of the art. For the layman as well as the physician can contribute to an art founded on sensory knowledge.[c]

> Do not hesitate to inquire of laymen if thereby there seems likely to result any improvement in treatment.
>
> (*Precepts*, cap. II: Jones, I, 315)
>
> Since this remedy has considerable popular authority, and cannot possibly be a danger, although I have not read of it in medical authorities, yet I thought that it should be inserted here in my work.
>
> (Celsus, IV, 7: 5)
>
> Although these are the doctrines of the physicians, it has been found out by the experience of some country folk that anyone with a bad struma may be freed from it by eating a snake.
>
> (Celsus, V, 28: 7B)
>
> These are the remedies recognized by medical practitioners, but country people have found out by experience that if a tooth aches, cat-mint should be pulled up with its roots, and put into a pot, and water thrown over it, and placed beside the patient as he sits all covered by clothes; then red-hot stones are thrown in so as to be covered by the water; the patient inhales the steam with his mouth open, whilst, as stated above, he is completely covered over. For profuse sweating follows, and also a

[c]"That it is not commonly considered a *tekhne* is not unnatural, for it is inappropriate to call anyone a [technician] in a craft in which none are laymen, but all possess knowledge through being compelled to use it." (*Ancient Medicine*, cap. IV: Jones, 1, 21).

steady stream of phlegm flows from the mouth, and this ensures good health always for a year, and often for longer.

(Celsus, VI, 9: 7)

* * * * * *

In contrast to Rationalist doctrine, which isolated the organism from the environment, the physician from the patient, the medical profession from society, and medicine from history,[d] Empiricism brought all of these together.

It bound the organism to the environment by incorporating the exciting cause in the *tekhne* and making it an indication of treatment equal in value to the patient's symptoms.[e]

Its view of disease as *process* required a historical approach to the medical *tekhne.* Far from maintaining that medicine was discovered once and for all by Hippocrates, they held that each generation had its own contribution to make to the improvement of practice.[f]

Empiricism bound the physician to the patient by basing treatment on the *physis.* The efforts of the physician were always guided by, and subordinate to, those of the patient's natural healing power.

And Empiricism bound the medical profession to society by its stress on the *visible*—that which means the same to everyone. This generated a democratic relationship between physician and patient. The Empiric respected the layman as object of medical practice, as partner in the therapeutic process, and as codiscoverer of the *tekhne.* He agreed with the author of *Ancient Medicine* that "it is particularly necessary . . . for one who discusses this art to discuss things familiar to ordinary folk. For the subject of inquiry and discussion is simply and solely the sufferings of these same ordinary folk when they are sick or in pain" (cap. II: Jones, I, 15-17).

[d]See above, p. 235.

[e]See above, p. 252.

[f]See above, pp. 265, 267-268.

NOTES

[1] Max Neuburger, "The Doctrine of the Healing Power of Nature Throughout the Course of Time," p. 867.

[2] Deichgraeber, *op. cit.*, pp. 220-249, 408-410.

[3] Deichgraeber stresses the parallels between *Precepts* and Empiricism but, accepting a fourth-century dating, assumes the work to be pre-Empirical (Deichgraeber, *Die Griechische Empirikerschule*, pp. 277-278). Jones calls for a much later dating (Jones, I, 305-310), and Edelstein writes that it must be "late Hellenistic" ("The Professional Ethics of the Greek Physician," p. 402, note 20). The parallels with Empirical doctrine are indeed striking, and there is no reason not to accept this as a work of that school. Jones thinks that the writer's native language was not Greek but Latin, suggesting that *Precepts* was produced by an Empirical physician in Rome.

[4] Celsus, *De Medicina*, II, 8: 21. See *ibid.*, 8: 29.

[5] *Ibid.*, III, 1: 4.

[6] Deichgraeber, *op. cit.*, Fr. 361.

[7] *Ibid.*, Fr. 165.

[8] Celsus, *De Medicina*, I, 1: 4.

[9] *Precepts*, cap. XIV (Jones, I, 331).

[10] Celsus, *Prooemium*, 20.

[11] *Ibid.*, 39.

[12] Diocles, Fr. 22. Cf. with Celsus, *Prooemium*, 20.

[13] Deichgraeber, *op. cit.*, p. 337.

[14] *Ibid.*, p. 336.

[15] Caelius Aurelianus, *m.a.*, I: 113.

[16] Celsus, V, 11.

[17] Celsus, II, 14: 4 and III, 4: 4.

[18] Celsus, III, 4: 17.

[19] Celsus, II, 18ff.

[20] Celsus, II, 11: 6, 12: 2C, and 17: 2.

[21] Celsus, III, 15: 6.

[22] Pliny, *Natural History*, XX, 220.

[23] Deichgraeber, *op. cit.*, Fr. 268.

[24] Caelius Aurelianus, *m.a.*, I, 17: 181-183.

[25] K X 655.

[26] K XIV 677.

[27] Celsus, *Prooemium*, 27.

[28] Walzer, *Galen on Medical Experience*, p. 103. Celsus. *Prooemium*, 28.

[29] Celsus, *Prooemium*, 30.

[30] *Ibid.*, 31.

[31] *Loc. cit.* See also K I 76; K X 169, 181; K XIV 678.

[32] K XIX 353. K X 126. K XIII 122.

[33] K X 209.

[34] K X 387.

[35] Diogenes Laertius IX 106.

[36] Deichgraeber, *op. cit.*, Fr. 131. Cf. Robert M. Green, *Galen's Hygiene* (Springfield: Thomas, 1951), pp. 122-123.

[37] K VII 555. Deichgraeber, *op. cit.*, p. 60 (*De Subf. Emp.*)

[38] Deichgraeber, *op. cit.*, Fr. 340.

[39] K X 195.

[40] K I 77. K X 126.

[41] Sextus Empiricus, *Against the Logicians* II 203, 191, 188. Celsus, *Prooemium*, 27-28. Walzer, *Galen on Medical Experience*, pp. 104, 133.

[42] Celsus, *Prooemium*, 60.

[43] K VII 557. K X 181.

[44] Walzer, *op. cit.*, p. 131.

[45] *Ibid.*, p. 128.

[46] K X 128.

[47] Deichgraeber, *op. cit.*, p. 60 (*De Subf. Emp.*). K X 100-101. Walzer, *op. cit.*, pp. 133-134.

[48] K X 152.

[49] K VII 557. K XIV 678.

[50] Walzer, *op. cit.*, pp. 129, 150.

[51] K X 460-461. Deichgraeber, *op. cit.*, p. 57 (*De Subf. Emp.*).

[52] K XIX 396.

[53] K X 181. Deichgraeber, *op. cit.*, p. 59 (*De Subf. Emp.*). Celsus, *Prooemium*, 68-73.

[54] Celsus, *Prooemium*, 66.

[55] K X 207-208

[56] K XVIIIB 645 (this very important passage is not included in Deichgraeber).

[57] K X 181, 209. Sextus Empiricus, *Outlines of Pyrrhonism* I 81. K XV 454.

[58] Deichgraeber, *op. cit.*, Fr. 117.

[59] K XVIIIA 249.

[60] Deichgraeber, *op. cit.*, pp. 63-64 (*De Subf. Emp.*).

[61] Celsus, *Prooemium*, 74.

[62] Deichgraeber, *op. cit.*, Fr. 87.

[63] *Ibid.*, Fr. 184. K X 247. Celsus, *Prooemium*, 52-53. K VI 361.

[64] Celsus, *Prooemium*, 69.

[65] Walzer, *Galen on Medical Experience*, p. 141.

[66] Deichgraeber, *op. cit.*, Fr. 66.

[67] K II 288.

[68] Celsus, *Prooemium*, 74.

[69] K VIII 143-144.

[70] Celsus, II, 2: 1.

[71] K X 100. K XIX 357. K II 224, 288-289.

[72] Deichgraeber, *op. cit.*, pp. 83 and 85 (*De Subf. Emp.*) and Fr. 176, 177, 277.

[73] *Ibid.*, Fr. 175, 266, 276, 282. Celsus, Book VIII.

[74] *Ibid.*, p. 85 (*De Subf. Emp.*) and p. 269, note 1.

[75] *Precepts*, cap. III (Jones, I, 317).

[76] K VII 554-555. K XVIIB 663. Deichgraeber, *op. cit.*, p. 58 (*De Subf. Emp.*) and Fr. 39, 40.

[77] K X 460-461. Deichgraeber, *op. cit.*, p. 310.

[78] K XVIIIB 663. Deichgraeber, *op. cit.*, pp. 52, 58, 60, 83 (*De Subf. Emp.*).

[79] Celsus, II, 8: 15 (cf. *Aphorisms* VI: 21)

[80] *Ibid.*, I, 8: 12.

[81] *Ibid.*, II, 8: 14.

[82] *Ibid.*, II, 8: 15.

[83] *Ibid.*, II, 8: 16.

[84] *Ibid.*, II, 8: 16.

[85] *Ibid.*, II, 8: 16.

[86] *Ibid.*, II, 7: 7.

[87] *Ibid.*, II, 3: 6 (cf. *Prognosis*, cap. XVIII).

[88] *Ibid.*, II, 3: 6 (cf. *Prognosis*, cap. XI).

[89] *Ibid.*, VI, 18.

[90] Deichgraeber, *op. cit.*, Fr. 128.

[91] Celsus, III, 12-17.

[92] *Ibid.*, II, 8: 36, 7: 22, 27-36. V, 18: 7. VI, 16.

[93] *Ibid.*, II, 8: 36.

[94] *Ibid.*, V, 28: 4C.

[95] *Ibid.*, II, 8: 16, 40. Cf. *Prognosis*, cap. XIX.

[96] Deichgraeber, *op. cit.*, Fr. 359c.

[97] Celsus, *Prooemium*, 71 and VI, 6: 8E.

[98] Celsus, II, 18ff.

[99] *Ibid.*, I, 3: 22, 25. II 12. V, 3, 4, 18: 7.

[100] *Galeni in Hippocratis De Officina*, pp. 73, 79.

[101] Caelius Aurelianus, *m.a.*, II 24 137.

[102] Celsus, III, 6: 1-4, 9; 9: 2-4; 14: 1.

[103] *Ibid.*, IV, 12: 1-4.

[104] *Ibid.*, IV, 12: 6.

[105] *Galeni in Hippocratis De Officina*, p. 81.

[106] *Ibid.*, p. 73.

[107] Celsus, Vol. II (Loeb Edition), p. xiii.

[108] Celsus, II, 12: 1B.

[109] *Ibid.*, V, 18: 7B.

[110] *Ibid.*, IV, 16: 3.

[111] *Ibid.*, V, 26: 35C.

[112] *Ibid.*, V, 27: 5.

[113] *Ibid.*, VI, 7: 1D, 5.

[114] *Ibid.*, V, 27: 1C.

[115] Caelius Aurelianus, *m.a.*, III 4 40.

[116] Caelius Aurelianus, *m. chr.*, I 4 137-138.

[117] Caelius Aurelianus, *m.a.*, II 24 135. See, also, Deichgraeber, *op. cit.*, Fr. 147, 148, 179, 180.

[118] Caelius Aurelianus, *m. chr.*, I 2 50. Deichgraeber, *op. cit.*, p. 71 (*De Subf. Emp.*). *Galeni in Hippocratis De Officina*, p. 75. Celsus, *Prooemium*, 71.

[119] Celsus, III, 7: 2 and *Prooemium*, 69.

[120] Deichgraeber, *op. cit.*, Fr. 187, 262, 268.

[121] Celsus, V *passim.*

[122] Celsus, *De Medicina*, Vol. I, p. x.

[123] K X 271. K XI 431.

[124] Celsus, V, 2, 26. Deichgraeber, *op. cit.*, Fr. 241.

[125] *Outlines of Pyrrhonism* I 129-132.

[126] Deichgraeber, *op. cit.*, p. 72 (*De Subf. Emp.*)

[127] K I 119. K X 164, 182, 271. K XI 431, 476.
[128] K XIV 679.
[129] Celsus, *De Medicina*, V, *Prooemium*.
[130] *Ibid.*, Vol. I, p. ix.
[131] Celsus, II, 18ff. Walzer, *op. cit.*, p. 103.
[132] Deichgraeber, *op. cit.*, Fr. 120, 123, 184, 188, 190, 294, 295.
[133] K XVIIA 955.
[134] Deichgraeber, *op. cit.*, Fr. 294.
[135] Celsus, II, 10. Deichgraeber, *op. cit.*, p. 61 (*De Subf. Emp.*).
[136] K X 181-182, 204.
[137] K X 181, 207. K XV 454. Deichgraeber, *op. cit.*, pp. 58-59 (*De Subf. Emp.*).
[138] Deichgraeber, *op. cit.*, pp. 46, 58, 59 (*De Subf. Emp.*).
[139] *Ibid.*, p. 311 and Fr. 29, 114.
[140] Celsus, *Prooemium*, 30.
[141] K X 165-166. K XIII 366. Caelius Aurelianus, *m.a.*, I 170. Deichgraeber, *op. cit.*, p. 72 (*De Subf. Emp.*).
[142] K X 221-226.
[143] Walzer, *op. cit.*, p. 100.
[144] *Rhetoric* 1356b 29-32.
[145] Walzer, *op. cit.* pp. 88-89, 98.
[146] Deichgraeber, *op. cit.*, p. 43 (*De Subf. Emp.*).
[147] Walzer, *op. cit.*, pp. 103-104.
[148] Celsus, *Prooemium*, 36.
[149] *Ibid.*, *Prooemium*, 30.
[150] K I 77.
[151] K X 126. Deichgraeber, *op. cit.*, pp. 43, 46-47, 48, 49, 54 (*De Subf. Emp.*).
[152] *Ibid.*, p. 51 (*De Subf. Emp.*).
[153] *Ibid.*, pp. 43, 46-47, 50, 58, 63 (*De Subf. Emp.*). K I 67.
[154] *Ibid.*, pp. 288-297.
[155] *Ibid.*, Fr. 12 and pp. 44, 70, 80 (*De Subf. Emp.*). Caelius Aurelianus, *m.a.*, I 17 170.
[156] *Ibid.*, p. 44 (*De Subf. Emp.*).
[157] *Loc. cit.*
[158] *Ibid.*, Fr. 43a and 43b.
[159] *Ibid.*, p. 45 (*De Subf. Emp.*).
[160] *Ibid.* pp. 76-77 (*De Subf. Emp.*).
[161] *Loc. cit.*
[162] K VIII 142.
[163] K X 164-165. K XIII 366.
[164] K I 67-68.
[165] K I 142-143. See, also, Deichgraeber, *op. cit.*, p. 64 (*De Subf. Emp.*).
[166] *Ibid.*, p. 54 (*De Subf. Emp.*).
[167] *Ibid.*, pp. 65-69 (*De Subf. Emp.*) and K I 142-148.
[168] *Ibid.*, pp. 49-51, 69-74 (*De Subf. Emp.*). K I 68. K XIV 679.
[169] *Loc. cit.* and Fr. 12.
[170] K XIV 679.
[171] Deichgraeber, *op. cit.*, pp. 50, 70, 71 (*De Subf. Emp.*).
[172] *Ibid.*, pp. 44-49, 71 (*De Subf. Emp.*). K I 68.
[173] *Ibid.* pp. 65-66 (*De Subf. Emp.*). K XIII 188-189.
[174] *Ibid.*, p. 46 (*De Subf. Emp.*).

[175] *Ibid.*, p. 45 (*De Subf. Emp.*).

[176] *Loc. cit.*

[177] K I 68.

[178] Deichgraeber, *op. cit.*, pp. 46, 65 (*De Subf. Emp.*).

[179] Albert Favier, *Menodote de Nicomedie, passim*. Deichgraeber, *op. cit.*, pp. 296, 391.

[180] Deichgraeber, *op. cit.*, pp. 42, 63 (*De Subf. Emp.*) and Fr. 172.

[181] K VIII 720.

[182] Deichgraeber, *op. cit.*, p. 87 (*De Subf. Emp.*) and p. 259.

[183] *Ibid.*, p. 62 (*De Subf. Emp.*) and p. 306; Fr. 24. K XIII 366. K XIX 354. Walzer, *op. cit.*, pp. 132, 141.

[184] *Ibid.*, p. 62 (*De Subf. Emp.*) and Fr. 12. Walzer, *op. cit.*, p. 132.

[185] *Ibid.*, Fr. 304.

[186] Walzer, *op. cit.*, p. 133.

[187] *Ibid.*, p. 137.

[188] Deichgraeber, *op. cit.*, p. 87 (*De Subf. Emp.*).

[189] *Ibid.*, pp. 46, 65 (*De Subf. Emp.*).

[190] *Ibid.*, pp. 46. 64, 65 (*De Subf. Emp.*).

[191] *Ibid.*, p. 50 (*De Subf. Emp.*).

[192] K X 181, 204.

[193] *Precepts*, cap. I (Jones, I, 313).

[194] Celsus, *Prooemium*, 48, 74.

[195] Deichgraeber, *op. cit.*, pp. 45-46 (*De Subf. Emp.*) and Fr. 15. K VIII 720-722. K XIX 354.

[196] *Ibid.*, pp. 295, 297, and Fr. 15.

[197] *Ibid.*, p. 48 (*De Subf. Emp.*) and p. 297 (Greek: *teresis*. Latin: *conservatio*).

[198] *Ibid.*, pp. 51-53 (*De Subf. Emp.*) and Fr. 39 and 40. Englert, *op. cit.*, p. 25.

[199] Celsus, *Prooemium*, 44.

[200] K I 76.

[201] Deichgraeber, *op. cit.*, Fr. 23b and p. 295.

[202] *Loc. cit.* and K XVIIB 584.

[203] K XVIIB 584.

[204] Walzer, *op. cit.*, pp. 96-97.

[205] *Loc. cit.* and Deichgraeber, p. 47 (*De Subf. Emp.*).

[206] K X 169, 173. Walzer, *op. cit.*, p. 92.

[207] K VIII 145, 371.

[208] Walzer, *op. cit.*, p. 88.

[209] *Ibid.*, p. 101.

[210] *Ibid.*, p. 89.

[211] K I 134-135.

[212] K I 111-112. See, also, Walzer, *op. cit.*, pp. 101, 131.

[213] K I 138. Walzer, *op. cit.*, pp. 89-91.

[214] K I 144.

[215] Walzer, *op. cit.*, pp. 91-92.

[216] *Ibid.*, p. 124.

[217] *Ibid.*, p. 119.

[218] K X 36. Deichgraeber, *op. cit.*, Fr. 12 and p. 63 (*De Subf. Emp.*).

[219] Walzer, *op. cit.*, p. 127.

[220] K XVIIB 354.

[221] Deichgraeber, *op. cit.*, p. 63 (*De Subf. Emp.*).
[222] K X 36.
[223] Walzer, *op. cit.*, p. 127.
[224] Deichgraeber, p. 82 (*De Subf. Emp.*).
[225] *Ibid.*, pp. 102, 152-153 (*De Subf. Emp.*).
[226] *Ibid.*, p. 121.
[227] *Ibid.*, p. 82 (*De Subf. Emp.*).
[228] *Loc. cit.*
[229] Celsus, *Prooemium*, 39.
[230] Walzer, *op. cit.*, p. 128.
[231] Deichgraeber, *op. cit.*, p. 85 (*De Subf. Emp.*).
[232] *Ibid.*, pp. 48-49 (*De Subf. Emp.*).
[233] *Ibid.*, p. 45 (*De Subf. Emp.*).
[234] *Ibid.*, pp. 80-81 (*De Subf. Emp.*).
[235] K V 751.
[236] Deichgraeber, *op. cit.*, p. 269.
[237] *Ibid.*, Fr. 40 and p. 308.
[238] *Ibid.*, Fr. 10a, p. 53 (*De Subf. Emp.*), and p. 253.
[239] *Ibid.*, pp. 42-43 (*De Subf. Emp.*).
[240] *Ibid.*, p. 86 (*De Subf. Emp.*).
[241] K X 111.
[242] Deichgraeber, *op. cit.*, p. 84 (*De Subf. Emp.*).
[243] *Ibid.*, p. 68 (*De Subf. Emp.*).
[244] Walzer, *op. cit.*, p. 110.
[245] *Precepts*, cap. VI (Jones, I, 319).
[246] Celsus, VII, 4.
[247] *Precepts*, cap. IV (Jones, I, 317).
[248] Celsus, *Prooemium*, 44.
[249] Celsus, *Prooemium*, 75.

CHAPTER VIII

THE METHODIST SCHOOL

The third prominent school of Galen's time arose much later than the other two, in the first century B.C.—the invention of a Greek immigrant rhetorician-turned-physician named Asclepiades and his disciples.

Methodism always retained the mark of its rhetorical origins, since the balance between reason and observation was heavily weighted in favor of the former. The school's doctrines were developed by Themison of Laodicea (*circa* 50 B.C. to 20 A.D.), Thessalos of Tralles (late first century A.D.), and Soranus of Ephesus (*circa* 50-130 A.D.).

Historically this school is very important, since it apparently displaced Rationalism and Empiricism and became the most prominent medical sect of the later Roman Empire.

The Methodist contribution to medical thought was the "doctrine of apparent communities," meaning the visible common elements of disease.[1] They held that treatment should be based exclusively on these "communities."

Asclepiades laid the groundwork for this doctrine (which was brought to its culmination by Thessalos) by reintroducing the atomic theory into physiology.[a] He hypothesized that the body is a porous membraneous solid through which the fluids flow. This porous solid is matter composed of atoms which are not perceptible to the senses; nor are the pores themselves sense-perceptible. In health the fluids flow

[a]This was, of course, only a revival of the theory of Erasistratos. Galen's *On the Natural Faculties* is directed against both the Methodists and the Erasistrateans of his time. Since the remaining Methodist doctrines flow necessarily from the atomic hypothesis, Asclepiades must be considered the founder of this school rather than his pupil, Themison.

at a normal rate through the solid. If the pores are too wide open, i.e., if the atoms are moving too fast in the solid parts of the body, the fluids will flow too freely. By the same token, when the atoms are not moving fast enough, but are too close together, the fluids do not move rapidly enough through the pores.[2] The first of these diseased states was known as *status laxus* (or *fluxus*), the second as *status strictus*, and there was a third state in which the atoms were thought to be moving sometimes too rapidly and sometimes too slowly; this was called the "mixed" state (*permixtus*).[3]

Consistently with these definitions, Asclepiades considered phrenitis (brain fever) to be a "stoppage or obstruction of the [small] corpuscles of the membranes of the brain."[4] Fever, in his view, was caused by a narrowing of the pores, so that the atoms had difficulty getting through; the resulting friction caused the patient's high temperature.[5] Pain in general was caused by the "blocking of the larger corpuscles."[6] Epilepsy was due to a blocking of the large corpuscles in the brain.[7]

In this manner the Methodists abandoned the humoral doctrine for a mechanistic theory of causation.[8] They denied that the body has any natural functions, and even the very idea of function, since what appeared to be functions were viewed by them as the product of the chance interaction of atoms. They denied the existence of a spontaneous *physis* in the body and alleged that such organs as the liver and spleen were superfluous.[9] They rejected the digestive process, maintaining that the food is ground up mechanically in the stomach and distributed in the form of fine particles, ultimately as *pneuma*, to the various parts of the body where it is absorbed.[10] They even denied that the body possesses a reasoning power, attributing mental activity also to the random movements of atoms.[11] Hence Asclepiades could maintain that the young are wiser than the old—the movement of atoms is more rapid in the young.[12]

The Methodists regarded their medicine as entirely "scientific" (i.e., as a *tekhnike methodos*), not only in its theory, but in its practice.[13]

This brings us to their therapy. The therapeutic indication was furnished by the physician's determination whether the pores were too constricted or too relaxed, in other words, whether the bodily secretions and excretions: sweat, urine, stool, menstrual blood, etc.—were coming out in the proper quantities. The remedy was through opposites—a blocked flow was to be stimulated, and an excessive flow to be reduced.[14]

Status laxus was treated by maintaining the patient in a cool dark room and feeding him thick porridge and soft-boiled eggs; exercise was to be avoided in this *status*.[15] *Status strictus* was treated by keeping the patient in a warm well-lighted room, discouraging him from sleeping too much, and feeding him laxative foods.[16] If the two conditions were combined, they were treated simultaneously. A case marked by constipation and sweating was treated by administering cold foods against the sweating (caused by looseness) and sweet olive oil against the stricture (sweet foods relax).[17] One remedy for severe stricture was venesection,[18] and bloodletting was indicated generally in diseases characterized by pain, since in this way the larger corpuscles, whose blockage causes the pain, were drawn off.[19]

The Methodists admitted that the properties of drugs were revealed by experience, but they held that only the *logos* could determine when and where the remedy was to be applied.[20]

The Methodists claimed to have progressed beyond Rationalism in refusing to base medicine on "conjecture about hidden things."[21] Sextus Empiricus was taken in by their claim, writing that Methodism "alone of all the medical systems appears to avoid rash treatment of things non-evident by arbitrary assertions as to their apprehensibility or non-apprehensibility, and, following appearances, derives from them what seems beneficial."[22]

This was an error, however, as Methodism was nothing more than a simplification of Rationalism for purposes of facilitating treatment. Pliny was closer to the mark when he wrote that "Methodism, reducing the whole of medicine to the discovery of causes, made it a matter of guesswork."[23]

The two schools were at one in basing therapy on speculation about causes. But where the Rationalists maintained that the causes of disease were numerous, and that treatment had to be directed against the cause, the Methodists, who also admitted that the causes of disease are multiple,[24] insisted that these causes were unimportant for treatment because the effects of all possible causes were either *status laxus* or *status strictus*. As Celsus put it, the followers of Themison "contend that there is no cause whatever the knowledge of which has any bearing on treatment."[25] Their whole medical doctrine was permeated with the idea of the proximate cause; but, relying on a purely mechanical connection between this cause and the external symptoms, they considered the cause incorporated in the effect. Hence treating the effect was equivalent to treating the cause.

Soranus rejected anatomy as of no value for medical practice because he felt that he already knew whatever anatomy had to teach him—not because (as with the Empirics) he distrusted the reliability of this knowledge.[26b]

The Methodist "communities" (*communitates*) were only an outgrowth of the Rationalist *communia*, a reduction of these "common symptoms" to the level of absurdity. And the purpose of the "communities" was identical with that of the *communia*—to curtail the variety of disease. "Now the Greeks [that is, the leaders of other sects] hold that different types of [dropsy] should be indicated by different names . . . But, in accordance with the principles of our sect, we Methodists reject these distinctions. For a flow or suffusion of fluid is the common element of this disease, and we consider it wrong to make distinctions on the basis of the various antecedent causes."[27] "Some physicians of the [Rationalist] school have raised the question, as a topic for discussion, whether hydrophobia is a new disease; for if they found it to be new, they would also seek a new cause and treatment. But such an inquiry seems strange to us. For,

[b]Temkin writes: "one often wonders how Soranus could know that a part was constricted, dense, and compact, or loose, lax, etc. . . . one has the impression that Soranus often slips into an assumed knowledge of the physical condition of an organ" (*Soranus' Gynecology*, p. xxxiii).

while it may be that certain particular or special diseases are new, the general and leading types of disease to which all the special diseases are subordinate can never be new. And we treat diseases of the same general type in similar fashion by the application of customary and suitable remedies."[28]

Curtailing the variety of diseases made it possible to curtail the variety of treatments. Celsus criticizes Themison, who

> took into account not when the fever began, but when it ceased, or at any rate was alleviated; and awaiting the third day from that time, if there was no return of the fever, gave food at once; if fever recurred, he gave food when it ceased, or if it obstinately persisted, he certainly gave it if the fever abated. But on none of these matters is there actually an invariable precept. For it may be that the first food should be given on the first day, it may be on the second, it may be on the third, it may not be until the fourth or fifth day; it may be after one paroxysm, it may be after two, it may be after several. For it all depends upon the kind of disease, the patient's body, the climate, his age, and the time of year; where circumstances differ so greatly, there cannot be an invariable rule of time by any means.
>
> (*Celsus,* III, 4: 7-8)

The debasement of medical theory and practice by the Methodists was noted and remarked upon by their contemporaries. Pliny described Asclepiades as "a professor of rhetoric, who found his gains in that profession too small, but had a brain brilliant enough for success in other professions . . . a man who neither had practiced medicine nor knew anything of remedies that call for sharp eyes and personal experience, but could attract by his eloquent and daily-practiced oratory."[29] Celsus observed that they were only an inferior offshoot of Rationalism: "for if a man does not hold all the tenets that another Rationalist approves, he does not forthwith have to assume a different name for his art if (and this is the essential point) he relies not only on memory but also upon *ratio* . . . nor has there been anything added to what the Empirics profess, but something taken away; for Empirics gaze about over a multiplicity of matters, [the followers of Themison] look to circumstances the most simple, and nothing more than commonplaces."[30] The Empiric in Galen's *Medical Experience* states that "mention of atoms, pores, and position in the cerebral membrane . . . is a view concerning invisible things . . . [and] I must regard it as an *analogismos*."[31] Menodotos "unanswerably confuted the tenets of Asclepiades, drawing his attention to their opposition to the phenomena and to each other."[32] He charged that "everything taught by Asclepiades is false."[33]

Galen wrote that "neither Hippocrates nor Diocles nor Pleistonikos nor Praxagoras nor Mnesitheos nor Phylotimos nor Erasistratos nor Herophilos have ever heard of the communities of Thessalos."[34] He accused Asclepiades of ignoring the crisis and the critical days, and of disregarding the protective role of the *physis.*[35] Thessalos (he claimed) localizes treatment excessively, using one medicine for all parts of the body even though they may suffer from different ailments.[36] The Methodists try to reason like Rationalists but follow their own logic so consistently as to fly in the face of the facts and commit obvious errors.[37]

The Methodists, for their part, attacked the tenets of Rationalism and Empiricism, especially the latter. Asclepiades called it an indefinite mass of experience devoid of any structure.[38]

It is clear that the spectrum of medical thought runs from Empiricism through Rationalism to Methodism. Just as the categories of speculation are affected by the opposed assumptions of the Rationalists and Empirics about the nature of "reliable" medical knowledge, so in Methodism the categories of thought are again transvalued by the atomic hypothesis. A few examples will make this clear.

On the category of "experience." To the Empirics it was all-important. To the Rationalists it still had a certain role, but to the Methodists "experience" was non-existent, since nothing can appear twice or thrice in the same way; in any case, they said, experience is "utterly unreliable" without *logos*.[39] Experience was actually assimilated to *logos*, as is seen from Asclepiades' view that young men are more intelligent than old men because the atoms are circulating more freely.

While the Empirics rejected all causal theories, the Rationalists accepted a doctrine of humoral causes, and the Methodists froze this into a rigidly determined mechanical theory of causation. Replacement of the humors by atoms starts with Asclepiades who called the humors the "exciting" causes, the atoms the proximate causes.[40]

Thus Methodism attributed the same status to the humors that Rationalism did to environmental influences. As "exciting" (procatarctic) causes they were considered to fall outside a doctrinal structure whose components were the proximate causes. Just as, in Rationalism, environmental influences became "scientific" when translated into (humoral) proximate causes, so in Methodism humoral influences became "scientific" when translated into (atomic) proximate causes. This symbolizes the increasing isolation of the organism from its environment in Methodist doctrine.

And where the Empirics hypothesized an infinite number of proximate causes and the Rationalists a finite number, the Methodists reduced all proximate causes to two: those which constrict and those which relax:

> Some say that different types of phrenitis must be distinguished by the symptoms peculiar to them. Thus they say that in one type the loss of reason is manifested by laughter and childish dancing, in another type by madness, crying out, silence, or fear. But we hold that there are two types, one involving a state of stricture, the other a combination of stricture and looseness. For it is proper to make distinctions in such a way that different types of a disease are shown not by differences in symptoms but by a general and invariable indication. Such an indication will be obtained . . . from the leading types of disease, and it is on this indication that our system of treatment also depends.[41]

Like the Rationalists, the Methodists defined disease as a deviation from the "normal"; the greater the deviation, the more serious the disease.[42] In this they are both to be contrasted with Empiricism which held that no physiological norm is applicable to all persons alike.

As therapeutic categories became more abstract (logically determined) the physician's status was increasingly elevated over that of the patient. This took the form of a progressive reduction of the autonomous protective power of the *physis*. While the *physis* was the foundation of the whole Empirical therapeutic doctrine, the Rationalists had largely subordinated it to a humoral theory resting on a clash of contrary qualities. The Methodists dissolved the *physis* completely into its atomic components. Asclepiades said that it is nothing other than the body or its movements and does nothing for the preservation of the body.[43] Often, in fact, it is harmful.[44] The body has no "forces" or "powers" other than the atoms.[45]

Soranus wrote that the theory of the *physis* is useless for practice, "although it enhances learning."[46] This is an amusing parallel to Celsus' opinion that medicine ought to "draw instruction from evident causes, all obscure ones being rejected from the art although not from the practitioner's thoughts."[47] But while Celsus rejects such causes from practice because they are unknowable, Soranus rejects them because they are known to the physician in the form of the movement of atoms.

On the question of prognosis. This was a keystone of Empirical theory. In Rationalism it is largely reduced to diagnosis. In Methodism it disappears altogether. Asclepiades diluted the doctrine of prognosis by contending that the signs point only to what is probable, not to what is inevitable. Thessalos and Soranus, however, went further. The former denied the very existence of prognostic signs, since, if such exist, all who manifest the same signs should become sick with the same disease. The latter maintained that prognostic signs have no basis in logic and rest only on opinion. He transformed them into diagnostic signs—"signs of a present condition that is apt to pass into [something else]."[48]

In other respects as well the Methodist doctrine represents the extreme development of therapeutic theory away from the ideas of Empiricism. For instance, they rejected the indication from the patient's habits and mode of life—one of the most important therapeutic indications for the Empiric.[49] The Empirics had claimed that diseases and modes of treatment vary from one country to another. This was restricted and weakened by the Rationalist classification of diseased states into discrete entities. The Rationalist view was then carried to its logical conclusion by Soranus who used against his (still partially Rationalist) mentor, Asclepiades, the same argument that a Rationalist might have used against an Empiric.

> We must ask why it is that Asclepiades believes that in a given region venesection is harmful in cases of pleurisy. Is it because of the nature of the region or the nature of the disease? If his reason is the former—that is, the nature of the region—then venesection performed in that region should be harmful in all cases, not merely in cases of pleurisy, but in those of synanche, which are treated by venesection, and in those of epilepsy too, for which Asclepiades very properly prescribes venesection. But if his reason is the second one—that is, the nature of the disease—he should conclude that harm results from the treatment of pleurisy by venesection not only at Rome but elsewhere.[50]

In Methodism logic took on a life of its own and overwhelmed the remaining experiential component of Rationalist doctrine.

Naturally, the Methodists found the theory of coction very distasteful. Asclepiades described Hippocratic medicine as the "management of death."[51] Thessalos wrote to Nero that he had attacked the "noxious precepts" of Hippocrates and emerged the victor.[52]

NOTES

[1] K XIX 353. Celsus, *Prooemium,* 57.
[2] K XIV 680. Caelius Aurelianus, *m.a.,* I 105-106.
[3] K XIX 353. Celsus, *Prooemium,* 55.
[4] Caelius Aurelianus, *m.a.,* I 7.
[5] *Ibid.,* I 18.
[6] *Ibid.,* I 119.
[7] *Ibid.,* I 20.
[8] K X 8.
[9] K II 47, 28. Caelius Aurelianus, *m.a.,* I 115.
[10] *Ibid.,* I 113. Celsus, *Prooemium,* 21.
[11] K II 29.
[12] Sextus Empiricus, *Against the Logicians,* I, 323.
[13] Walzer, *op. cit.,* p. 87. K XIV 684.
[14] K I 80-81. Caelius Aurelianus, *m.a.,* I 68-69.
[15] *Ibid.,* I 60.
[16] *Loc. cit.*
[17] *Ibid.,* I 68.
[18] *Ibid.,* I 28, 70.
[19] *Ibid.,* I 119.
[20] K I 119. K X 163, 180.
[21] Celsus, *Prooemium,* 57.
[22] *Outlines of Pyrrhonism,* I 237.
[23] *Natural History,* XXVI, vii.
[24] Caelius Aurelianus, *m.a.,* I 32-33.
[25] Celsus, *Prooemium,* 54.
[26] O. Temkin, ed., *Soranus' Gynecology,* pp. 4, 7.
[27] Caelius Aurelianus, *m. chr.,* III 98.
[28] Caelius Aurelianus, *m.a.,* III, 118.
[29] *Natural History,* XXVI, vii. Sir Clifford Allbutt, who had a high opinion of Methodism, calls this a "spiteful legend" (*Greek Medicine in Rome* [London, 1921], p. 180) but adduces no evidence for his view. Pliny's testimony is accepted by others (e.g., "Asklepiades," *Pauly-Wissowa,* Vol. II, col. 1632).
[30] Celsus, *Prooemium,* 62-65 (my translation). The Spencer translation of this passage contains several errors.
[31] Walzer, *op. cit.,* p. 136.
[32] K II 52. K IV 475.
[33] Deichgraeber, *op. cit.,* p. 84 (*De Subf. Emp.*)
[34] K XVIIIA 270.
[35] K II 47.
[36] K X 210, 272.
[37] K II 47, 51-52. K XI 98.
[38] Deichgraeber, *op. cit.,* p. 88 (*De Subf. Emp.*). See, also, Walzer, *op. cit.,* p. 86.

[39] Walzer, *op. cit.*, p. 85.
[40] Caelius Aurelianus, *m.a.*, I 112.
[41] *Ibid.*, I 52.
[42] *Ibid.*, I 41.
[43] K II 28, 47.
[44] Caelius Aurelianus, *m.a.*, I 115.
[45] K VII 515.
[46] Temkin, *Soranus' Gynecology*, p. 4.
[47] Celsus, *Prooemium*, 74.
[48] Caelius Aurelianus, *m.a.*, I 22-30.
[49] K X 655.
[50] Caelius Aurelianus, *m.a.*, II 131.
[51] K XI 163.
[52] K X 8.

CHAPTER IX

GALEN AND THE CLOSE OF GREEK MEDICAL SPECULATION

"Exhausted by centuries of endeavor, often moving in a circle, Greek medicine looked at last for a definitive system which should collect the scattered stones of thought and experience and incorporate them into a single edifice."[a] The man who accomplished this task was Galen, a Greek physician residing in Rome and, after Hippocrates and Aristotle, the most important figure in the history of ancient medical thought.

Galen was one of the most influential intellectuals the world has ever produced, as his system lasted, unchanged in any essential respect, for more than 1400 years. The reason lies not in the author's originality or scientific capacity, but in his ability to crystallize in logical form the inchoate strivings of ancient Rationalism and to structure the resulting doctrine in a way which exactly suited the practical needs of the physicians of his own and later generations. He was an ingenious and encyclopedic thinker rather than a profound one, and his many writings provided an acceptable explanation of every theoretical problem which the practitioner was likely to encounter.

Acceptable metaphysical explanations of disease and reasons for particular modes of therapy are indispensable to the practicing physician, and these the Galenic system supplied in abundance. Hence the continuing popularity of his name and doctrines for a millenium and a half after his death.

Galen claimed to follow the dictates of none of the schools: "I call slaves those who designate themselves

[a]Max Neuburger, *History of Medicine* (London: Frowde, 1910), p. 240.

followers of Hippocrates or of Praxagoras or generally speaking of any man . . ."[1] He viewed his own writings as a crystallization of the best from the corpus of Greek medical thought.

For he was extremely learned in the doctrines of his own and earlier times. He knew the Hippocratic writings thoroughly and wrote commentaries on very many of them. He had studied with Empirics and was well versed in their ideas.[2] He set himself the task of reconciling the conflict between this school and Rationalism, of extracting from the medical thought of his predecessors and contemporaries a single universal architectonic structure which should serve as a guide to physicians in perpetuity.

Biography

Galen was born to one of the richest families of Pergamon, in Asia Minor, in the year 129 A.D.[3] His father, a mathematician and architect whom Galen admired extravagantly, saw to it that he received a complete philosophical education.[4] At the age of fourteen he was sent to study with representatives of all the philosophical schools—Platonic, Stoic, Epicurean, and Aristotelian. He commenced the study of medicine at sixteen and was trained thoroughly in both the Empirical and Rationalist methods.[5] "By the age of seventeen I was as learned in philosophy as in medicine."[6]

At twenty, after his father's death, Galen went away to Alexandria for more study, returning eight years later to a job as physician to the Pergamon gladiators. He later boasted of losing only two of his charges, whereas his predecessor had lost twenty-eight.[7]

He eventually grew tired of the provinces and at age thirty-two came to seek his fortune in Rome. His quarrelsome nature, boastfulness, and disdain for all other physicians immediately made him a host of enemies, but despite these defects of character—or perhaps because of them—he rapidly forged his way to the top of Roman medicine and Roman society, becoming the physician and confidant of Marcus Aurelius, Commodus, and Septimius Severus.[8]

Even during his lifetime he was revered and idolized as a virtually superhuman physician and intellectual.[9]

Except for a trip to Pergamon in the years 166-169 to escape an outbreak of plague in Rome, he spent the rest of his life in the Imperial City and died there in about 199.

A Psychological Conflict

The twenty-odd surviving volumes of Galen's writings represent about two-thirds of his total production, as a number of his books are known to have been lost. Any man stimulated to such a gigantic literary output while carrying on an active medical practice must have had some overwhelming motive, and Galen's is not difficult to ascertain.

His phenomenal production reflects a compulsion to bring unity out of multiplicity, to determine which of the doctrines in which he had been educated was correct. "If then the two parties but agreed with each other that both roads to discovery were true ones, there would be no further need for discussion."[10]

In his youth Galen leaned very far in the direction of Empiricism. He had studied with the famous Empiric, Aeschrion of Pergamon, and had the profoundest respect for him.[11] "I have no hatred for the Empirics, in whose doctrines I was raised, nor for the Dogmatists."[12] "When I hear the Empirics reasoning in this way, at first I consider their arguments very convincing, and I do not find the objections of the Dogmatists very convincing."[13] Before the age of twenty-one he had written a work, *On Medical Experience,* which sets forth an argument between his Rationalist teacher, Pelops, and the Empiric, Philippos.[b] In it the arguments for Empiricism are very convincing and are not successfully refuted by Pelops. About fifteen years later he wrote the *De Subfiguratione Empirica,* again a faithful presentation of the Empirical viewpoint but this time with a concluding chapter giving his own Rationalist criticisms.

[b]The Greek original of this work was lost, and it has been preserved only in an Arabic translation, rendered into English by Richard Walzer: *Galen on Medical Experience* (Oxford: University Press, 1947).

He made massive use of the Empirical Hippocratic exegesis in his commentaries on the Hippocratic works.

He was saved for Rationalism by his grounding in mathematics and philosophy, writing that only the former had preserved him from Pyrrhonic doubt.[14] All his life, he states, he pursued medicine and (idealist) philosophy together.[15]

He concludes that Rationalism is superior to Empiricism because the physician who relies on *logos* will err less frequently than the one who does not.[16]

Even so, he did not admire the intellectual accomplishments of many "so-called Dogmatists who do not know the bases of the *physis* and of medicine."[17] "Truly the majority of physicians neither apply themselves to experience, as good physicians could do using the institutions of the Empirics, but desirous of reasoning more perfectly, they either believe things which are stated without [logical] demonstration or they demonstrate defectively, and thus not only devise nothing good but even vitiate those things which they know from experience."[18]

But his contempt was directed most forcefully against the Methodists. "As Rationalism is superior to Empiricism, so is Empiricism superior to Methodism."[19] His writings on the medical sects have nothing good to say about the Methodists.

While he sympathized generally with the Rationalists and felt that their approach to medicine was in principle correct, many of them, in his view, were uneducated, and the doctrine itself was incomplete.[c] His solution was to return to the principles of Hippocrates, who discovered all things by *logos* and experience.[20]

By treating the problem of "experience" in medicine along the lines first set forth by Hippocrates, Galen expected to remedy the supposed one-sidedness of Empiricism as well as the overweening reliance on *logos* of the Rationalists.

[c]We do not know enough about pre-Galenic Rationalism to distinguish it readily from the post-Galenic variety. I suspect that the former was close to the degenerate Rationalism of the *Problemata* and was restored by Galen to the principles of *Nature of Man*. Hence Chapter VI (above) probably contains a large Galenic component (the four-humor doctrine in particular).

But, while he claimed that everything he wrote was based on Hippocratic principles,[21] Galen had a particular understanding of Hippocratic medicine. He accepted the Group III therapeutic doctrine as representing the true Hippocrates and calls *Nature of Man* "one of the finest studies in medicine."[22] Hence, Aristotle and the Stoic, Chrysippos, were in the direct Hippocratic tradition. Galen writes:

> I have shown elsewhere that [their] opinions were shared by Hippocrates, who lived much earlier than Aristotle. In fact, of all those known to us who have been both physicians and philosophers, Hippocrates was the first who took in hand to demonstrate that there are, in all, four mutually interacting qualities, and that to the operation of these is due the genesis and destruction of all things that come into and pass out of being. Nay, more: Hippocrates was also the first to recognize that all these qualities undergo an intimate mingling with one another; and at least the beginnings of the proofs to which Aristotle later set his hand are to be found first in the writings of Hippocrates.[23]

The correct Hippocratic doctrine is the one perfected by Aristotle, Theophrastus, Diocles, and Mnesitheos.[24] Galen wrote a whole book demonstrating the identity of the views of Plato and Hippocrates.[25] But of all the Hippocratic commentators Galen especially admires Aristotle, calling him the "greatest interpreter."[26]

He thus attributes to Hippocrates all the distinguishing features of Rationalism. Hippocrates maintained that the hot, the cold, the wet, and the dry, as well as the surrounding air, are the causes of sickness and health.[27] "Everything which he discovered he established by rational arguments."[28] When he failed to give logical proofs, this was only for the sake of brevity–because he assumed that his listeners could supply the connecting links in the reasoning.[29] Hippocrates did not base his *Aphorisms* on observation but on the nature of the thing.[30] Hippocrates used hot medicines in cold seasons and vice-versa.[31] Hippocrates was interested in events which occur frequently (in order to deduce general rules)–not in those of rare occurrence.[32] Hippocrates cured by contraries.[33] In short, Hippocrates was a "Dogmatist in all his work."[34]

By the same token Galen rejected the Empirical interpretation of Hippocrates. Hippocrates did not derive his principles from an enumeration of particulars but, like Plato, used particular examples to explain or illustrate a general principle which had been deduced logically.[35] In *Nature of Man* Hippocrates denied that the body is an organic unity.[36] Nor was Hippocrates the founder of the Empirical School.[37]

Significantly, Galen's writings make only passing reference to *The Art*[38] and do not mention *Ancient Medicine*—these being the two works containing the most cogent arguments against his own position. His predecessors, Erotian, Celsus, and others knew of these works,[39] and it is difficult to believe that Galen had not read them. Probably Edelstein is correct in surmising that Galen rejected them as unauthentic.[40] In any case, his interpretation of Hippocrates was entirely Rationalistic. While Galen thought he was reconciling experience and *logos*, he was only producing a more consistent and streamlined version of traditional Rationalism.

The Physis

Galen states that Hippocrates opened up the true road to medical knowledge and that his own task was to smooth out the logical difficulties, just as Trajan had made smooth the roads of the Roman Empire.[41] This meant completing the work started by Diocles, Mnesitheos, and others.[42]

Galen understood this task as one of fusing all the elements of the Hippocratic writings: the *physis,* the *dynamis,* coction, prognosis, the critical days, and the four humors, into a single doctrine whose acceptance by physicians would lead to a restoration of Hippocratic medicine.

He assumed that the starting-point of such a reconstruction must be a correct theory of the *physis*—a physiology—incorporating what was correct in ancient speculation about the qualities (*poiotetes*) and powers (*dynameis*). Galen observes that the *physis* has many different meanings in the

Hippocratic writings and that it had many different meanings for the physicians of his own time.[43] "Since *physis* is used in many ways, it is here to be understood as meaning what it means in the book, *Nature of Man,* wherein Hippocrates calls '*physis*' that which is generated from the first elements."[44] The problem was to develop a logical doctrine on this basis: "While the statements which the Ancients made on these points were correct, they yet omitted to defend their arguments with logical proofs . . . For this reason I have attempted to put together my arguments in the way in which it seems to me the Ancients, had any of them been still alive, would have done, in opposition to those [sc. the Empirics and Methodists] who would overturn the finest doctrines of our *tekhne.*"[45]

Galen undertook this task in his seminal work, *On the Dynameis of the Physis* [*"On the Natural Faculties"*].[46] It begins with a general eulogy of the *physis:* "Hippocrates . . . was the first to recognize what the *physis* effects, expressing his admiration of her, and is constantly singing her praises and calling her 'just'."[47] But at the same time he accepts Aristotle's interpretation of the human physiology—that it is a mixture of the four elements or qualities:

> . . . the one starting point of all this is a thoroughgoing inquiry into the question of the Hot, Cold, Dry, and Moist; this Aristotle carried out in the second of his books *On Genesis and Destruction,* where he shows that all the transmutations and alterations throughout the body take place as a result of these principles.[48]
>
> . . . bodies act upon and are acted upon by each other in virtue of the Hot, Cold, Moist, and Dry. And if one is speaking of any activity, whether it be exercised by the veins, liver, arteries, heart, alimentary canal, or any part, one will be inevitably compelled to acknowledge that this activity depends upon the way in which the four qualities are blended.[49]

Galen's problem is to reconcile the autonomous and spontaneous *physis* of the Group I writings with his own Rationalist conviction that the organism is subject to causal analysis in terms of the elements, qualities, and powers. He attempts to solve this problem through an analysis of the *physis* in terms of its *dynameis* and by dissolving the *dynameis*, in turn, into their constituent elements or qualities.

First he reduces the *physis* to its component *dynameis*. The organism contains a blood-making *dynamis* in the veins, a digestive *dynamis* in the stomach, a pulsatile *dynamis* in the heart, etc.[50] And the organs (liver, spleen, heart, brain, etc.) themselves possess four special *dynameis:* the attractive, the retentive, the alterative, and the expulsive—which are the result of the blend (*krasis*), in each organ, of the four elements (*stoicheia*) or qualities (*poiotetes*).[51]

In this way the organs, and the body as a whole, accomplish the coction and evacuation of matters which give rise to disease.[52] Galen follows Aristotle in viewing digestion as one of the forms of coction.[53]

Galen thus takes doctrinal elements from all of his predecessors and uses them to fashion a new theory of the *physis.* It is perhaps closest to *Nature of Man* where the *physis* also consists of four corporeal humors or elements (*stoicheia*) possessing *dynameis;* but Galen has made this formulation more specific by interposing a new category—the organs—between the *physis* and the humors. This new category is modelled on Aristotle's doctrine of the three levels of composition of the body. The *diadosis* (assimilation) and *anadosis* (distribution) of Erasistratos find a place (of sorts) in Galen's "attractive" and "retentive" *dynameis*.

The following comments may be made on Galen's new formulation. Although modelled on Aristotle's, it is far more Rationalist than the latter. Aristotle stressed the importance of the *heterogeneous* parts of the organism (made up of various combinations of homogeneous parts) and wrote: "to say what are the ultimate substances out of which an animal is formed, to state, for instance, that it is made of fire or earth, is not more sufficient than would be a similar account in the case of a couch or the like."[d] The heterogeneous parts, equivalent to Galen's organs, operate by their own laws

[d]*Parts of Animals* 640b 21-23. See above, p. 140.

which must be discovered. Aristotle would not have agreed with Galen's explanation of the action of the heterogeneous parts in terms of the four elements.

Galen's theory is not even logically adequate, since the same combination of qualities or elements at the level of the organ cannot logically yield the different and even opposed *dynameis* which each organ is said to possess.[e] Galen tries to argue that the same elemental components of the organ can cause it to attract, retain, and expel, but the argument is unsuccessful.[54]

Unhappy with the idea that the *physis* acts autonomously, Galen has tried to eliminate it, but he only succeeds in attaching the spontaneity of the *physis* to the organs. He would have done better to leave it where it was.

He also tries to dispose of the vitality of the *physis* by confining it to the "pulsatile *dynamis* of the heart [which] has its source in its own substance"—this last being proven by the fact that "the heart, removed from the thorax, can be seen to move for a considerable time."[55]

Galen thus attempted to abolish the Empirical-Rationalist polarity of the Hippocratic Corpus and, at the same time, to efface the difference between these two schools. But he was not equal to the task. He could give a relatively adequate verbal explanation of the fundamental Hippocratic and Empirical doctrine of the organism's vitality but only by sacrificing the spirit of this doctrine. He was a philosopher far more than a physician and doubtless viewed his verbal resolutions as genuine solutions of medical problems. Even as a logical exercise, however, his doctrine of the *physis* was not successful.

The Tekhne

Just as Galen aimed to reconcile *logos* and experience in his new theory of the *physis*, so he hoped to achieve the same end in his definition of the medical *tekhne*.

[e]A similar conclusion is reached by O. Temkin in "A Galenic Model for Quantitative Physiological Reasoning," *Bulletin of the History of Medicine* XXV (1961), 470-475, at p. 474. See, also, Sprengel, Vol. II, p. 116, and Kovner, p. 837.

He was fully aware of the Empirical reliance on experience as the basis of their *tekhne* and gave much thought to the true meaning of experience for medicine. His writings are full of exhortations to the physician to rely on experience as well as on the *logos.*[56]

The problem, however, is to know precisely what this means.

For on the fundamental issue of the connection between theory and practice Galen is squarely in the Rationalist tradition. Medical practice is based upon preexisting theory.[57] The best physician is the one who does everything by right reasoning.[58] The *logos* enables the physician to distinguish true theories from false.[59]

Although not always consistent, he seems to elevate medical theory to the status of an *episteme,* while the practice—the *tekhne*—is lowered to the level of conjecture. In the *Ars Medica* he states that the physician must distinguish between the *episteme* and the practice, that is, between the theoretical and the practical parts of medicine; theory is the *episteme* of healthy, unhealthy, and neutral causes, bodies, and symptoms, while the practice is based upon the ability to ascertain causes through the signs and symptoms.[60f] In another work he states: "I discovered some diseases which presented a scientific [according to *episteme*] diagnosis and others which fall under the sort of conjecture called *tekhne* and in which, consequently, the diagnosis had to be rectified frequently, since such is the strength of the conjecture according to *tekhne.*"[61]

He wrote many books on logical demonstration and considered these of primary importance to the physician's training.[62] His work, *On Examining Physicians,* states that anatomical knowledge is the most important subject, then the functions and uses of each organ. The examiner should

[f]In another writing he makes the following distinctions: The Rationalists say that the knowledge of causes and observation of the *physis* is scientific, symptoms and therapeutics conjectural. The Methodists say that both are scientific. But both schools are in error. For science (*episteme*) is knowledge which never departs from *logos,* and this is never found in a natural science, least of all in medicine which is, therefore, only a *tekhne* (K XIV 684).

ascertain if the candidate applies the science of reasoning in the selection of foods, drugs, and other forms of treatment. He must also be familiar with the works of the ancients. But if he proves to have neglected this learning and shows no experience or skill in these other matters, it is not necessary to examine him on clinical cases.[63]

Thus, clinical practice came last, after anatomy, physiology, and logic. "No one can cure diseases who does not know the primary elements of the body."[64] Unstructured experience is not accepted by Galen as a guide to the application of theory. The most learned physician must necessarily be the best practitioner. He goes even further, however, and denies that experience has a role to play even in the *formulation* of the theory. The key to his thought here is the statement that "those who have never learned the *tekhne* will gain nothing by experience."[65] "Since future physicians do not want to become acquainted with geometry, astronomy, dialectics, music, and other branches of the fine arts . . . they will never desire to obtain experience . . ."[66] "Logos *is needed for observation . . . observation is impossible without* logos."[67]

Theory was thus formed on the basis of logic and dialectic and tested against experience.[68] If the anticipated results were not forthcoming, this might mean that the particular practitioner was an incompetent logician but could not mean that the whole idea of a logic-based medicine was defective.[69] Hence Galen objected to Herodotos' account of the origins of the medical *tekhne*. The historian had claimed that it was developed by exposing sick people at a crossroads, so that passers-by could suggest appropriate remedies: "In this way, from the use and experience of many things, medicine was put together."[70] Galen comments that this is "experience devoid of reason and not yet a rational experience."[71]

For the same reason he rejected the Empirical procedure of arriving at general principles through the accumulation of particulars.[72] Instead, he says, precepts are discovered by reason, and their validity is tested by experience. Reason alone leads to accurate knowledge of the organism.[73]

Experience only provides examples which demonstrate the validity of the precept or theorem:

> Where an example can usefully be employed is when we are addressing someone who cannot understand, and we produce an example which will lead him to grasp what we want. But there are some men [*sc.* the Empirics] who think that we use examples to verify what needs to be established. But they are mistaken in this opinion, which lies far from the truth. The same is true of those who claim that Plato makes most of his proofs rest on a rehearsal of particulars, since we ourselves have shown that Plato was also in the habit of quoting particulars only in order to make his meaning clear.[74]

In only one area of medical theory does Galen seem to allow greater latitude to unstructured experience than was customary among his Rationalist contemporaries. This was in regard to the method of determining the medicinal powers of foods and drugs, Galen advocating trials of new drugs on the sick and the healthy. He agreed with the other Rationalists[g] that the first step in determining the power of a simple drug is sensory observation: "For by the Gods, how is it that we know that fire is hot? And how do we know that ice is cold except from the senses?"[75] But from this point, accepted by most of his Rationalist colleagues, he proceeded to tests on the sick and the healthy "of unmixed drugs in which there is no adventitious *dynamis;* this is first to be done in a person of optimum health, then in one whose health is slightly disturbed, and finally in one with a simple disease, in order to distinguish by the *logos* what is the main effect of the drug and what is accidental."[76] Thus, the powers of remedies are discovered by a mixture of reason and experience.[77] Many experiments like the above are needed to know the best medicine for each disease and for each part of the body.[78] In compounding medicines the exact proportion of each ingredient and the total strength of the compound can be determined only through experience.[79] "The proper proportions in the mixture we shall find out conjecturally before

[g]See above, pp. 221-222.

the experiment, scientifically [by *episteme*] after the experiment."[80] And he expresses a general preference for the compounds of those physicians who have the most experience.[81]

He notes, furthermore, that according to many physicians the *dynameis* of foods are discovered only by experience.[82]

The most important role for experience in Galen's pharmacology, however, was in connection with drugs which act through their "whole substance."[83] This class of drugs in Galen's doctrine echoes the Empirical idea that all medicines are unanalyzable and act as wholes. These were substances with no particularly evident primary qualities but which nonetheless had an effect on the organism, or substances such as snake poisons whose apparent primary qualities were very different from what seemed to be their secondary qualities. The effects of these substances were known only by experience.[84] Each one attracts the humor appropriate to it, and the appropriate humor can be determined only by examining the excretions or secretions produced by exhibition of the drug.[85] When Pelops explained that the ashes of river crabs are better for the bite of a mad dog than the ashes of fresh-water crabs because river crabs contain more salt and are thus more warming and drying, Galen disagreed, stating that salt-water crabs possess some peculiar property or occult virtue inherent in the whole substance, and this effects the cure.[86][h]

Some physicians claim (says Galen) that these substances act through their atoms, others say they act through their indivisible parts, and others say they are similars.[87] He himself started to write a book on remedies which act by their whole substance but never completed it.[88]

It is doubtful that Galen ever could have written a work on this class of drugs, since their recognition is a concession to unanalyzable experience. Just as he analyzed the *physis* down to its component organs but had to allow a degree of spontaneity to the organs, so his analysis of medicinal substances also runs up against the Empirical tenet that all

[h]But scorpion venom is cold (K X 245).

drugs must ultimately be considered to act as whole entities. At this point he abandoned the argument. Drugs which cure by their "whole substance" never found a logical niche in his system.

Therapeutics

Galen's therapeutics is a confused and inconsistent mixture of the practices of all his predecessors—as was to be expected of such an encyclopedic thinker. His fundamental pathology is that of the Rationalist school, involving an upsetting of the humoral balance and the predominance of one or two of the four qualities or elements. However, he also espouses the theory of coction: that disease is a process with a gradual buildup, a peak or crisis, and a decline, ending in a general resolution with evacuation or empyema.[89] In evaluating this process Galen relies on critical days, and he notes the significance of such symptoms as hemorrhage, glandular inflammation, and skin disorders denoting the various stages of the disease process.[90] He also attributes many inflammations to the penetration of blood into an unsuitable place (Erasistratos' *error loci*).[91]

The key to this confusion is, of course, Galen's reinterpretation of the theory of coction in terms of contraries, enabling him to accept the *physis,* coction, crisis, and evacuation, since they all represent nothing more than the clash and interaction of opposed elements. For, despite his theoretical acceptance of Hippocratic medicine, Galen insists that therapeutics is based upon contraries.

Thus, while he speaks the language of the Group I Hippocratic works, his words have a different meaning and lead to a different medical *practice.*

He is loud in his praise of the *physis:* "For in truth the *physies,* as [Hippocrates] himself writes somewhere, are the physicians of diseases. Now, if the *physis* does everything for the preservation of living creatures, this too is reasonable, that she should be the first to heal diseases, either by causing many sweats, or by emptying out the troublesome humors, [that is] by emission of urine or clearing the stomach or causing vomiting."[92] The physician watches for the signs of coction and crisis, showing that the *physis* has conquered the *materies morbi.*[93] And his medicines cannot themselves eliminate disease causes; the *physis* must help. The medicines only give the stimulus and the point of departure to the *physis* which does the rest.[94]

The course of the disease can be prognosed from the pulse which reveals by suitable signs when "the *physis* is awake and stirring and is about to expel from the body everything that is noxious in the humors."[95]

In one sense Galen is seen to have restored the early significance of coction—by making it a process occurring in the whole body instead of just in the stomach. But in a far more important sense he has denatured the concept completely: it is nothing more than a balancing of elements or qualities. "When I say *physis* I mean the whole substance and combination which consists of primary elements: hot, cold, wet, and dry."[96]

And Galen's espousal of the doctrine of contraries as the key to therapeutics shows that he only paid lip-service to the theory of coction. Therapeutics based on the theory of coction required the use of similars—*secunda remedia*—and Galen opposes the concept of similars both in theory and in practice.[97][i] His analysis of the organism is in terms of contraries, his analysis of the therapeutic process is in terms of contraries, and his analysis of the relations between the organism and its environment is also based upon contrariety. While he used the language of the Group I works discussed above, in therapeutic practice he was a thoroughgoing Rationalist.

Galen's doctrine of critical days shows the extent to which logic had overcome the experiential element in his view of Hippocratic medicine. The Group I writings give three mutually inconsistent series of critical days. *Prognosis* gives the series for fevers as follows: 4th day, 7th, 11th, 14th, 17th, 20th, 34th, 40th, and 60th.[98] *Epidemics I* gives two series: 1) diseases which have exacerbations on even days have crises also on even days: 4th, 6th, 8th, 10th, 14th, 20th,

[i]See discussion of Rationalist therapeutics above, pp. 224-225.

24th, 30th, 40th, 60th, 80th, and 120th; 2) diseases which have exacerbations on odd days also have crises on these odd days: 3rd, 5th, 7th, 9th, 11th, 17th, 21st, 27th, and 31st.[99] This is apparently too unstructured for Galen, and he tries to reduce them to a single series:

> Hippocrates states that the seven-day period of the critical days is more potent than the others. Next in power is the four-day period, because it is half of the seven-day period and because future crises are proclaimed from the four-day through the seven-day periods. For the four-day period is the indicator of the seven-day period, and the 11-day of the 14-day period. Hence these are the true indicators. The seven-day periods are to be estimated as follows: the first two weeks are days 1 through 7 and 8 through 14. But week three starts on day 14, so that the three-week period ends on day 20. That is why Hippocrates states that the 40th day and not the 42nd is critical, similarly the 60th and the 80th, and not the 63rd and 84th.[100]

The Hippocratic writings present this doctrine only as a general guide: "none of [the periods] can be exactly calculated in whole days," "from the first day, however, you must pay attention, and consider the question at the end of every four days, and then the issue will not escape you . . . Learning these things beforehand, you must make your conjectures at the end of each increment as the illness advances to the crisis," "one must also consider in what periods the crises occur of irregular fevers, of quartans, of quintans, of septans, and of nonans."[101] But Galen reduces it to a rigid logical formulation which can be applied in the abstract to each patient without observation of his particular characteristics.[j]

Galen is thus seen to have broken up the holistic therapeutics of the Hippocratic writers.

In the Group I and IV writings coction-evacuation is a single process: the correct remedy given at the indicated time

[j]A similar doctrine of critical days is roundly criticized by Celsus (*De Medicina*, III, 4: 11-18).

produced coction, while evacuation followed of itself. But Galen separated coction from evacuation, using separate groups of remedies for each. Coction was effected by the *contrary* remedy, and then a *new* medicine was given to produce the evacuation (*per anum, per urinas,* etc.) which the physician thought desirable. And this latter remedy was administered according to a formalized doctrine of critical days, applicable across the board to all patients.

The indiscriminate use of evacuants which characterized Rationalist therapeutics for the next millenium and a half—and which these practitioners saw as eminently Hippocratic—had little in common with the true theory of coction.

Logos and Experience in the Galenic System

Galen aimed to pursue a middle course between the Empirics, who held that medicine was based wholly on experience, and the Rationalists of his day who, like his teacher, Pelops, "claimed to be able to tell the cause of anything."[102] To him this meant giving a logical explanation of the experiential elements of therapeutic doctrine and incorporating all of them in a single all-encompassing formulation.

The theory of coction was the major experiential component of medical speculation prior to Galen, and he tried to reduce coction to an interaction among the four elements or qualities. While not successful, his reinterpretation of coction was deemed adequate by his successors for many generations. The Empirical idea of the wholeness of the remedy was isolated by him in the sub-class of medicines which act by their "whole substance" and did not affect his major thesis that remedies also can be analyzed in terms of the four qualities.

But in other ways Galen's system makes concessions to unstructured experience and its corollary that the organism is a whole entity. He admits that the human organism and its idiosyncrasy are not ultimately knowable, being perceived only by the Gods, Apollo and Aesculapius, who are the true knowers of medicine.[103] He cannot understand how the sensations, taste and smell, can be produced by combinations of the four qualities: "But how each one of these tastes originates I wish I could explain, and I would gladly listen to such information . . ."[104] The word, *dynamis,* is used to characterize such processes as digestion and blood-production "because we are ignorant of the true essence of the cause which is operating."[105] The substance (*ousia*) of the *dynamis* is some form of the *pneuma* and also the "temper [*krasis*] of the solid parts."[k] Ultimately he seems to decide that such knowledge is not needed for acquiring health or moral virtue.[106]

He states that the physician can treat better the patient whom he knows when healthy than the one whom he sees only when ill.[107] He claims that the physician must sometimes take a curative indication from the patient's own specific *physis.*[108] He invokes the idea of the variety of healthy constitutions: "if ever the perfect constitution existed, it would not remain unchanged for an instant. So that it occurs to me to wonder at the opinion of those who consider that health and the good constitution are one and invariable, and who say that whatever departs in the least from this is not health."[109]

Such ideas, while unobjectionable in themselves, are incompatible with the Rationalist assumptions. What is the patient's "specific *physis*" other than a mixture of humors, and if one humor predominates in the mixture, causing ill health, how can the indication taken from the "specific *physis*" differ from the indication taken from the peccant humor? By the same token, if a variety of different humoral combinations may all be considered equally healthy, what methodological grounds does the physician have for deciding if a person is sick and in what way he is sick? If the physician should know the patient in health in order to be able to tell when he is sick, what is the value of the whole Rationalist analytical method?

[k]K X 838. Galen, like many of his predecessors, thus yields to the temptation to bring in the *pneuma* to close a logical gap. Galen's ideas on the *pneuma* are discussed in O. Temkin, "Galen's Pneumatology," *Gesnerus,* VIII (1950), 180-189. See, also, Sprengel, *op. cit.,* Vol. II, p. 113.

Hence the Galenic system was forced to revert to unstructured experience at the most crucial points in the analysis. But here the Rationalist played into the hands of the Empiric who claimed that the Rationalist *tekhne* consisted, on one hand, of a logical doctrine which was specious because divorced from experience, and, on the other, of a crude and unstructured experience, one lacking the various tests and checks which the Empirics themselves had devised. Why claim validity for logical doctrines, they demanded, only to admit their inadequacy when put to the test of practice? Is it proper procedure to invoke unsystematic "experience" at the point where the philosopher's ingenuity exhausts itself?

Indeed, the failure of Galen's system to reduce medical experience to logical categories is evidence in favor of the Empirical argument. However many treatises he composed, Galen could not construct a thoroughly logical and consistent system, and he was always compelled to allow a role to unstructured and unsystematic experience.

Hence the theoretical effort of Rationalism ended in failure, and the Empirical criticism must be accepted. The arid logic which has been so well satirized by Moliere,[1] was

[1]In the scene from *Le Malade Imaginaire* where the would-be physician is being examined for entry into the profession (end of Act Three):

Primus Doctor: *Si mihi licentiam dat Dominus Praeses,*
Et tanti docti Doctores
Et assistantes illustres,
Tres scavanti Bacheliero
Quem estimo et honoro
Domandabo causam et rationem quare
Opium facit dormire

Bachelierus: *Mihi a docto doctore*
Domandatur causam et rationem quare
Opium facit dormire
A quoi respondeo
Quia est in eo
Virtus dormitiva
Cujus est natura
Sensus assoupire

Chorus: *Bene, bene, bene, bene respondere*
Dignus, dignus est entrare
In nostro docto corpore.

combined with ultimate reliance on experience. This was inevitable, since Galen was pursuing opposed aims. He wanted to complete the logical analysis of medicine commenced by Aristotle, Diocles, Praxagoras, and Mnesitheos, supplying the connecting links in the reasoning, but he tried to do this by restoring the theory of coction (forgotten by contemporary Rationalism) to its rightful place. The theory of coction, however, is the embodiment of the Empirical approach to therapeutics, and its necessary corollaries are the impossibility of achieving *a priori* knowledge of the organism and the requirement that therapeutics be founded in experience.

Galen's gigantic literary production is a barrier to analysis. His many inconsistencies are lost to sight in the tremendous flow of words, being buried here and there in scores of long-winded treatises.

While one is forced to respect Galen for his heroic undertaking, the effect was ultimately baneful for medical theory and practice, since it disguised the real differences between the Empirical and the Rationalist methods.

Medical thought is mankind's earliest confrontation with "science." The Greek physicists and astronomers were isolated individuals. But medicine had a broad social base, being practiced by thousands of physicians. This was the front upon which a scientific breakthrough might have been anticipated. The Empirical method, with its technique for dealing with negative instances and conducting "expert experiments," might have moved the dawn of scientific speculation a thousand years back in history. Galen aborted this effort. His monument of literary production was the gravestone of Empiricism. After his time "empiric" became a derogatory term, denoting inability to apply intellect to medical problems.[m] The victory of Galenism was a defeat for humanity.

[m]Some very early scholia on manuscripts in the Vatican library may represent the beginning of the debasement of the term, "empiric": "those doctors are empirics who provide treatment for patients without giving an account of it [*logos*], for they understand that a particular drug is able to treat a particular wound; but if someone were to ask them why it is effective for this, they could not answer" (Deichgraeber, *op. cit.,* Fr. 55. See, also, Fr. 52, 53, 54).

The Sociology of Rationalism

How are we to account for the triumph of Rationalism? Why did Galen's system, despite its logical inconsistency and lack of therapeutic value, become the orthodoxy of the corporate body of physicians in the Middle Ages and early modern times?

To put the question in a different way, why has the corporate body of physicians followed Galen in accepting unstructured experience as a last resort but rejected the Empirical demand that the *whole method* be founded in experience? Or, in yet another way, why did the Empirics attribute major importance to phenomena which, in the Rationalist view, were nothing more than exceptions to otherwise valid rules?

Explanations drawn from intellectual tradition—the fact, for instance, that the Rationalists held Aristotle in high esteem and followed his lead—are inadequate, for we would than have to ask why the Rationalists followed Aristotle rather than some other figure or, for that matter, why Aristotle himself identified his logic and metaphysic with the physical world.

One explanation popular with historians sympathetic to the Rationalist and Methodist traditions has been that the Empirics were less well educated than the Rationalists. Clifford Allbutt, a pillar of the British medical establishment of his time, called the Empirics "the philistines of medicine" who were "guided by a crude and rather barren sort of common sense."[110] George Sarton writes, "the weaknesses of Empiricism were too much respect for old remedies and a fondness for pharmaceutical experiments which sometimes verged on dilettantism or charlatanism."[111] As though every educated man in the ancient world must necessarily have subscribed to the Aristotelian or Stoic philosophies.

There is no evidence that the Empirics were less well educated than the Rationalists, and they were probably far better educated than the Methodists. They were the ancient world's leading pharmacologists, the leading commentators on the Hippocratic Corpus, and the most prominent surgeons. Galen himself never calls them uneducated, although he is puzzled at their refusal to accept his logic.

We have hinted above, at various points in the narrative, that the conflict between Empiricism and Rationalism is not to be understood solely, or even primarily, as a clash of ideas. The ideological conflict was not the cause, but the effect, of professional competition between the two bodies of medical practitioners. Ideological competition reflects socio-economic competition, and its roots lie in the realm of medical practice.

To understand the appeal of Rationalist doctrine for generations of physicians, to appreciate the reasons why it ultimately became the orthodoxy of the schools, one must look to the benefits which this doctrine conferred upon the physicians espousing it. Their acceptance of Rationalism was not determined by its value as a therapeutic instrument but because it enhanced the professional pride and prestige of the physician, made it easier for him to earn a living in the practice of medicine, and demarcated the physician from the layman.

The whole discussion of Rationalism and Empiricism makes clear the former's superiority for earning a living. It enabled the practitioner to act quickly and thus to treat more patients in a given period of time: "The Rationalist elicits the signs of diseases more rapidly and in greater number, together with the *propria* and the *communia;* nor, like the Empiric, does he take a long time, for he does not delay a day or even an hour."[112] And the Empirical method was not only slow, but arduous as well. In commenting on *Aphorisms* I: 1, "judgment is difficult," Galen observes that, while the Rationalists equate "judgment" with *logos*, the Empirics take it to mean the selection of those things which are given by experience. "But truly this is difficult and hard to discover."[113]

The Empirical method took time and demanded attention to detail, since the *propria,* and not the easily ascertained *communia,* were the key to correct treatment. Rationalism's stress on the *communia,* and the restricted number of disease categories offered by the four humors, facilitated rapid treatment and thus conferred an economic advantage. By the same token, Methodism's reduction of all disease categories to two or three made treatment even more rapid, and one of these practitioners claimed to be capable of treating the whole city of Rome by himself. Some of the Methodists, in fact, made fabulous incomes, and this system was the road to economic success in the later Roman Empire.

The income-producing potential of Methodism, as an inverse function of the time these physicians spent with their patients, was noted by the perceptive Celsus:

> It is not possible for many patients to be cared for by one practitioner, and provided that he is skilled in the art, he is a suitable one who does not much absent himself from the patient. But they who are slaves to gain [*sc.* the Methodists], since more is to be got out of a crowd, are glad to adopt those precepts which do not exact a sedulous attendance, as in this very instance. For even those who see the patient but seldom find it easy to count days or paroxysms; a physician must be always at hand, if he is to see the one thing that matters, the point when the patient is about to become too weak unless he gets food.
>
> (Celsus, III, 4: 10)

The simplicity of the Methodist system was also a source of political strength. Galen observes: "They announce that they will teach the arts in a minimum of time, and they gather together a host of disciples; from these also they acquire power in the cities where they live."[114]

On economic and political grounds, therefore, Rationalism and, *a fortiori*, Methodism were likely to be favored over Empiricism by the physicians of the Roman Empire. A high income, however, is not the only factor of importance to the medical practitioner. Equally significant is the degree to which a therapeutic doctrine ministers to his feelings of professional pride and thereby sets him apart from the mass of laymen. Here again, Rationalism possessed major advantages over Empiricism.

The metaphysical Rationalist theorem had immense appeal for the physician, since medical knowledge was thus distinguished from the knowledge possessed by laymen. *This was the principal Rationalist objection to the sense-based epistemology of Empiricism.* "The perception of the theorem must not be within the domain of the layman [*idiotes*] but only that of the professional [*tekhnites*]. Thus we declare to be in error those who say that the phenomena are the principle of the *tekhne.*"[115] "If someone called the visible phenomena the principle of the *tekhne,* he would be denying a difference between *tekhne* and absence of *tekhne;* since perception of the phenomena would be the same for the layman and the professional, the professional would in no way be elevated above the layman."[116] "The principles of the *tekhne* are taught, the apparent is not taught."[117] "How do we recognize which phenomena to observe and which not to observe? The phenomena themselves, as phenomena, do not yield this knowledge. Otherwise the layman would know as well as the physician which phenomena to observe, and *our experience would be no different from their inexperience.* But since it is not everyone who can know at first glance which phenomena to observe, and since only professionals know how to observe rationally, the determination of treatment is not based on observation of the phenomena."[118]

Basing the *tekhne* on proximate causes, and not on sensory data, serves to demarcate the professional physician from the layman. This instinctive feeling of the Rationalists that the medical profession should be set apart from the lay public is to be contrasted with the sense-based epistemology of Empiricism with its corollaries: 1) a democratic and egalitarian relationship between the physician and the patient, 2) the willingness to accept contributions to medical knowledge from lay sources.

Galen was very concerned with the professional dignity of the physician, as the above passages indicate. He remarks with some complacence: "people admired me for the dignity of my life, as well as for my professional attainments."[119] He notes that the squabbling among physicians, the same remedies being called beneficial by some and harmful by others, makes the public calumniate the profession.[120] "Hence the finest aspects of these arts are neglected, and what is chiefly practiced is how to shine before the crowd, to speak and act with a view to pleasure, to flatter and address the rich and powerful day by day, to accompany them, escort them home, act as menials at their feasts, and play generally the buffoon . . ."[121]

The physician would elevate himself from this ignoble position only by acquiring a thorough knowledge of the causes of disease and health. Such knowledge was metaphysical knowledge which the layman did not possess. Armed with it the physician could give explanations of diseases and of his therapeutic procedures. He could give names to diseases, thus satisfying the perennial desire of the patient to know what he was suffering from: "to ascribe illness to some innate or congenital weakness of the stomach, intestines, liver, eyes, or some other part of the body is to know no more than the layman."[122]

It was undignified to admit ignorance of the causes of disease and health: "You have often seen the Empirics changing from one medicine to another, without giving any reason for it, just because they have seen it work somewhere before. They hope to stumble on the remedy by accident. But such a cure would rather be attributed to good luck than to the *logos.*"[123]

Galen wanted physicians to be philosophers: "It is true that philosophy is necessary for medicine . . . we must be philosophers if we are to be real disciples of Hippocrates, and if we do so, nothing can prevent us from being his equals or his superiors."[124]

Many of Galen's views reflect his concern for professional dignity. This is why he disapproved of Menodotos, who practiced medicine only to earn a living. It conditioned his feelings about the Methodists, who not only based medicine on sense-perceptible phenomena but wanted to teach the *tekhne* in *six months.*[125] "To the Methodists the Rationalist observes that since the communities indicate treatment, and the notion of treatment presents itself at the same time as the indicative phenomena, the communities yield indications to the layman, and you in no way differ from them."[126] "Shoemakers, carpenters, and blacksmiths are jumping into medicine, abandoning their ancient trades."[127]

He wanted to restrict entry into the profession to persons of suitably aristocratic background. He himself was from one of the prominent families of Pergamon, and he derides the Methodist leader: "Insolent Thessalos, do not make the fellow-craftsmen of your father [a weaver] judges of physicians."[128] "For it is true, and Plato has said it himself, that it is a matter of testing the intellects of all those who would study the *tekhne.* But this cannot be done with a book, but by many conversations, and those who would study it must be suited to it. For Hippocrates in *The Surgery* shows that not everyone is suited to medicine, only those who have the time and the disposition."[129]

He complains that people only see the utilitarian side of medicine, not its philosophical side. "As Plato says, if children or witless people had to judge between a physician and a cook, the cook would come off best by a long way."[130] Considering that medicine had its origins in cooking, that cooking is the basis of the theory of coction which Galen claims to uphold, and that even Diocles and Praxagoras wrote books on diet and cookery, the denigration of cooks by Galen is inappropriate. But the contrast between Rationalism and Empiricism is very close to that between the philosopher and the cook.

Galen's desire to elevate the status of the physician above that of the layman has its corollary in his attitude toward the *physis.* For the physician's attitude toward the innate healing power is intimately connected with his views on professional dignity. If the *physis* can do the work, what need is there for the physician? The decline in the role of the *physis,* its reinterpretation in terms of contraries in the Rationalist tradition, reflect the conflict with the physician's professional pride. Galen, who wants to revive the *physis,* has to explain his position carefully lest his fellow-practitioners take offense. Thus, while the *physis* is in principle capable of doing the work of healing, sometimes it acts wrongly and must then be corrected by the physician.[131] Sometimes it is too weak and must then be strengthened by the physician.[132] If the crisis is perfect, the physician need not do anything, but if it is less than perfect, the physician must step in and help the *physis.*[133]

In commenting on "the *physies* are the physicians of diseases" (*Epidemics* VI, 5: V, 315, L.) Galen proffers the following: *"Perhaps someone will suspect that the medical* tekhne *is abolished by this saying.* But the words are not to be taken at face value, since they bear a higher sense, requiring an accurate explanation . . . . It seems better to us to say that the *physis* heals diseases, but the medical *tekhne* also, as well as the physician, and also the physician's assistant and also venesection and also the flow of blood which this induces. Perhaps someone will also think that the cook contributes something as well, and the weaver and the builder and the blacksmith, and certain other technicians whose works we use in ministering to the patients . . ." The question is which of these is first in dignity, which second, and which third. It is necessary to distinguish them from one another.

Now wine is a remedy when administered at the right time and harmful when given at the wrong time. But the physician decides when to give it. So he is more important than the wine in producing health. The physician finds the occasion through his knowledge of the *tekhne* of distinguishing healthy and unhealthy things. Hence the physician is subordinate to the *tekhne* itself. And the *tekhne* is subordinate to the *physis.*

But Galen throws a sop to the physician in two ways. First, the *physis* usually needs the assistance of the physician. And secondly, the physician is the head of a whole hierarchy: "last in dignity are the ones who produce for us clysters, scalpels, probes, forceps, and other medical instruments, herbalists and root-gatherers, metallurgists, and others of this sort; above them are the *tekhne's* which they pursue; above these are the physician's assistants; then come the physicians, the medical *tekhne,* and the *physis.*"[134]

All in all, the physician's dignity was safe in Rationalism. He was above the layman in possessing philosophical knowledge of proximate causes. He was in theory subordinate to the *physis*, but in practice he was elevated above the *physis*. Not only was he permitted to interfere with the latter's operations, but the scientific validity of such interference could never be verified by the patient or by any non-professional. Being outside ordinary sense-perception, the justification for the physician's procedures was within the sole purview of the corporate body of the profession.

Methodism, also, was a metaphysical theory of disease causes, despite its reliance on sensory data, since the causes were incorporated in their effects. The physician's recognition of the *status laxus* or *status strictus* was equivalent to a recognition of the causes operating within the organism to produce the *status*. Pliny was correct in observing that Methodism "reduced the whole of medicine to the discovery of causes." And, as we have noted, the Methodists carried to its logical culmination the incipient Rationalist denigration of the *physis*.

Methodism was thus a short-cut to Rationalist metaphysical knowledge. It could be learned in only six months, and at the end of this period its adherents could claim total familiarity with causal knowledge of the organism to the extent that this was needed for medical practice. They knew better than the *physis* itself how to produce health.

The ascendancy of Methodism in the later Roman Empire, and the ultimate triumph of Rationalism over Empiricism, are due to the socio-economic and psychological advantages of a metaphysically based medicine and the drawbacks of a medicine which relies on sensory data.

Empiricism was the medicine of the countryside and of villages and small towns where the physician could come to know his patients well: "it is more useful to have in the practitioner a friend rather than a stranger."[135] These physicians were craftsmen who lived in democratic equality with their patients and made a living by their technical skill in curing. Their acts were based upon sensory knowledge accessible to all, and they were consequently in potential competition with every layman—being distinguished from them only by *possession of greater skill.* Every layman was considered to possess the rudiments of medical ability, and only the highly competent physician would be clearly preferred to a non-professional.

Rationalism in its early years was probably the medicine of the larger cities with a more transient population where the practitioner was in economic competition with others and survived by his ability to diagnose and treat a large number of patients rapidly.

The two systems coexisted for centuries until confronted with the dynamic social changes accompanying the urbanization of the Roman Empire in the early Christian era. The population movement to the cities, and the growth of the latter, introduced new stresses into the previously static relations between Empiricism and Rationalism, bringing to the fore the socio-economic and psychological advantages of the latter.

These advantages led to the offshoot of Methodism—a system of medicine preeminently adapted to the treatment of patients in an overpopulated urban environment. Celsus writes that the Methodists, "who take charge of large hospitals, because they cannot pay full attention to individuals, resort to these *communia.*"[136]

And while the economic benefit of a Rationalist or Methodist practice was important enough, the other—social or psychological—rewards of a metaphysical medicine were even more telling advantages in the competition with Empiricism. In urban practice the physician could not have extensive personal knowledge of his patients, and the patients could not come to know their physician well. Hence the latter could not defend himself by his reputation, skill, and economic strength alone, but sought protection as well from his status as member of the corporate body of physicians.

The relationship between physician and patient, after all, is not always one of trust and confidence. Frequently it is one of mistrust and hostility. Many patients cannot be saved by even the best physician, and even the best physicians make errors of judgment. In the intimate setting of a small town or village, where the physician is known personally to all, mistakes in treatment are judged against the background of the physician's whole life. But this factor is absent in the socially mobile city. Here the physician looks to his own economic power for protection against irate patients but, even more, to the support of his fellow-practitioners. The elements in a medical ideology which contribute to the strength and cohesiveness of the corporate body of physicians become paramount.

These are precisely the elements which, as mentioned earlier, minister to his sense of professional dignity and demarcate him from the layman. It may be postulated that the more abstract and metaphysical the therapeutic doctrine, the more suitable an instrument it is for binding the medical profession into a cohesive group. By the same token, the more a therapeutic doctrine relies on sensory data and observation, the less suitable it is as an instrument of professional cohesiveness.

This seems paradoxical in the light of Empirical reliance on sensory data because "it means the same to all," in opposition to the proximate causes which have a different significance for each observer. However, it is not more paradoxical than is the survival through the ages of the therapeutically worthless Galenism while Empiricism, which was scientific because it individualized treatment, should have perished.

Empiricism was a body of rules for practice whose application demanded a high degree of skill and conscientiousness. The correctness of their application could be verified by all, since it was based upon sensory data. The stresses inherent in this mode of practice served to fragment its adherents, not to unify them.[n]

Rationalism, on the contrary, was abstract. It was a metaphysical doctrine whose truth or falsity could not be verified by reference to any sensory data. All of its adherents could swear by the word of the same master while inter-

[n]As noted earlier, Deichgraeber states that the Empirics did not form a "sociological unity" (*op. cit.*, p. 253).

preting the word differently. All could profess allegiance to the same abstract ideology while applying it differently to the individual case. Hence, the Rationalist *tekhne* served to unite medical practitioners, not to divide them.

But the abstract nature of the Rationalist doctrine—the factor which made it alluring to the physician—was precisely the factor which made it an unscientific mode of practice. Methodism, being even more abstract, was even less scientific. Rationalism and Methodism could not be compared with Empiricism for scientific insight and therapeutic potential. Juvenal satirizes the medicine of Themison, "how many patients he could kill in one autumn."[137] Galen states the same.[138] But the Empirics "could heal fractures and wounds and ulcers and conditions which others could not cure, foretelling those things which would occur in the future, and sometimes telling some of the things from which the patient was suffering even before interrogating him, and, similarly, some of the things which had already befallen him" so that "men are amazed at his art."[139]

Even without this testimony, however, it would be clear that the Empirics were better physicians than the Rationalists and the Methodists. Caution, careful observation, and individualization of treatment have always been the hallmarks of the good physician.

Hence there is a conflict between the interests of the patient and those of the corporate body of physicians. The elements of a medical ideology which predispose to scientific treatment are the very ones which detract from the professional cohesiveness of the corporate body of physicians. This conflict of interests was noted and satirized by Moliere in *L'Amour Medecin* where one of the pompous physicians declares: "It is better to die according to the rules than to recover against the rules" (Act II, Scene V). Or, in the same play (Act II, Scene III), where two physicians are discussing a recent case:

Tomes: But, by the way, what position do you take in the quarrel between the two physicians, Theophrastus and Artemius? It is an affair which has split the whole corporate body.

Desfonandres: Me? I am for Artemius.

Tomes: I am too. It's not that his opinion, as we saw, did not kill the patient, while that of Theophrastus was much better. But he was wrong under the circumstances and should not have had a different opinion from that of his elder.

Desfonandres: Absolutely. The formalities must always be preserved, whatever happens . . .

Tomes: A dead man is only a dead man and is of no consequence; but a formality neglected is severely prejudicial to the whole corporate body.

The medical student examined in *Le Malade Imaginaire* (end of Act III) swears never to use any remedy not sanctioned by the profession, even if the patient dies.[o]

This is the tragedy of medical history. The curative potential of a therapeutic doctrine has only marginal relevance to its socio-economic viability. In the clash of competing systems the elements of a doctrine which afford it a political or economic advantage are determining. These, in turn, are necessarily the elements which detract from the doctrine's scientific potential. A scientific therapeutics must strive for individualization and must be able to deal methodically with the variety of different diseases and different constitutions. This sort of doctrine, however, is inadequate support for the professional body of physicians. Such a body will always seek a doctrine which is abstract. Allegiance is professed to abstract principles, and the correctness of their application can be decided only by the corporate body itself. In this way the physician is shielded from society and cannot be called to account for his errors.

[o]In Moliere's hilarious dog-Latin:

De non jamais te servire
De remediis aucunis
Quam de ceux seulement doctae facultatis,
Maladus dût-il crevare
Et mori de suo malo.

NOTES

[1] K XIX 13.
[2] K VIII 142. K XIX 16-17, 38.
[3] K V 49-50.
[4] K XIX 59.
[5] K VII 558. K VIII 143-144.
[6] K XIX 59.
[7] Max Meyerhoff, "Autobiographische Bruchstuecke Galens aus Arabischen Quellen," *Sudhoffs Archiv,* XXII (1929), 72-86, at p. 77.
[8] K XIV 657-669.
[9] K XIV 660.
[10] K I 74. See, also, K V 860.
[11] K XII 356-357.
[12] K VIII 144.
[13] K VIII 142-143.
[14] K XIX 40.
[15] K XIX 59.
[16] K X 210. K XVIIIB 315.
[17] K X 170.
[18] K X 122.
[19] K X 210.
[20] K XV 67. K XVI 82-83. K XIX 34. K XVIIB 608.
[21] K XIX 34.
[22] K II 132.
[23] K II 5.
[24] K X 108, 118. K XVIIB 608.
[25] K V 1-914.
[26] K X 15.
[27] K XVIIA 506.
[28] K XVIIIA 525.
[29] K X 274.
[30] K XVIIB 584.
[31] K X 213.
[32] K IX 896.
[33] *Galeni In Hippocratis De Officina,* p. 79. K XVIIIB 906.
[34] K XVIIB 347.
[35] *Galeni In Hippocratis De Officina,* p. 83. K XVIIA 14. K XVIIIB 909.
[36] K XV 67.
[37] K XVIIIA 524-525. K XVIIA 507.
[38] K XIX 350.
[39] See Jones, *Hippocrates* (Loeb Edition), Vol. I, pp. xxxviii-xxxix, xlii.
[40] See his article, "Hippokrates," in *Pauly-Wissowa,* Supplementband VI, col. 1316.
[41] K X 633.
[42] K X 5. K XVIIB 608.

[43] K V 703-707. K XV 570-571. K XVIIB 529-532.
[44] K XVIIB 529.
[45] K II 178.
[46] K II 1-214.
[47] K II 38. See, also, K XVIIB 222-223.
[48] K II 167-168.
[49] K II 126.
[50] K II 7-15.
[51] K II 12-13, 182-186.
[52] See the discussion in S. Kovner, *Istoriya Meditsiny* (Kiev, 1888), pp. 936ff.
[53] K II 89-90, 200-201. K X 97.
[54] K II 196-197.
[55] K II 614.
[56] K IX 842. K XIII 116-117. K XVIIB 353-354. Walzer, *op. cit.*, p. 85.
[57] K XIX 351.
[58] K XIX 355.
[59] K XIX 53, 59.
[60] K I 308. See K XVIIB 349.
[61] K VIII 144-145.
[62] K XIX 43, 53.
[63] A. Z. Iskander, "Galen and Rhazes on Examining Physicians," *Bulletin of the History of Medicine,* XXXVI (1962), 362-365, at p. 365.
[64] K X 460.
[65] A. Z. Iskander, *op. cit.*, p. 364.
[66] K X 5.
[67] K I 134.
[68] K I 58.
[69] K XV 454-455.
[70] K XIV 675-676.
[71] *Loc. cit.*
[72] K XVIIA 13.
[73] K VI 363-364.
[74] *Galeni in Hippocratis De Officina,* p. 83. See also K XVIIIB 909.
[75] K XI 434-435. See, also, K XIV 220 and, in general, Lynn Thorndike, *A History of Magic and Experimental Science,* Vol. I (New York, 1923), pp. 154-165, for a discussion of the role of experience in the Galenic system.
[76] K XVI 86-87.
[77] K X 896. K XVI 83.
[78] K XII 350. K XIV 82.
[79] K XIII 467, 700-701, 706-707.
[80] K XIII 867.
[81] K XII 968, 988.
[82] K VI 453.
[83] K IV 760-761. K XII 358-359.
[84] K VI 395. K X 244, 895.
[85] K I 356. K II 44.
[86] K XII 358-359.
[87] K IV 761.
[88] K XII 357-358
[89] K I 195. K XVIIB 726.
[90] Kovner, *op. cit.*, pp. 931-933.

[91] K VII 707-714. K IX 690-695.

[92] K XV 310-311.

[93] K I 365. K XI 34. K XVIIB 225-226, 437-439. Deichgraeber, *op. cit.*, Fr. 128.

[94] K I 207-208.

[95] K XIV 617. K XI 8, 10-11. K I 334-337.

[96] K I 675.

[97] *Galeni In Hippocratis De Officina*, pp. 73-75.

[98] *Prognosis*, cap. XX (Jones, II, 43-45).

[99] *Epidemics I*, cap. XXVI (Jones, I, 185).

[100] K XVI 273-274.

[101] *Prognosis*, cap. XX and *Epidemics I*, cap. XXVI (Jones I, 185 and II, 43-45). See also, Jones' discussion in *Hippocrates* (Loeb Edition), Vol. I, pp. liv-lv.

[102] K XII 359.

[103] K X 209.

[104] K XI 455.

[105] K II 9-10.

[106] K IV 762.

[107] *Galeni In Hippocratis De Officina*, p. 103.

[108] K I 70. See, also, K X 180, 205; K XVIIB 381-382.

[109] K VI 28.

[110] *Greek Medicine in Rome*, p. 116. Allbutt was very sympathetic to Methodism, as has been noted, defending Asclepiades against Pliny (*Ibid.*, p. 180).

[111] *Galen of Pergamon* (Lawrence, 1954), p. 33.

[112] K XVIIIB 645.

[113] K XVIIB 354.

[114] K XIV 600.

[115] K I 110.

[116] K I 111.

[117] K I 112.

[118] K I 124.

[119] K XIV 614.

[120] K XVI 87.

[121] K XIV 600.

[122] K X 460.

[123] K X 169.

[124] K I 59-60, 62-63.

[125] K X 5, 37-38, 204, 208.

[126] K I 125. See, also, K I 158, 204.

[127] K X 5.

[128] K X 8, 10. K IX 657.

[129] K XVIIB 351.

[130] K XIV 605.

[131] K XVIIB 440.

[132] K XVIIB 442.

[133] K XVIIB 437.

[134] K XVIIB 222-230.

[135] Celsus, *Prooemium*, 73.

[136] Celsus, *Prooemium*, 65.

[137] *Satire X*.

[138] K X 915.

[139] Deichgraeber, *op. cit.*, p. 83 (*De Subf. Emp.*).

PART FOUR

THE PARACELSAN REVOLUTION

PART FOUR

THE PARACELSAN REVOLUTION

The main substance of the art lies in experience and also love.[1]

Galen's system—or the Arabic imitations by Avicenna (Ibn Sina, 980-1036), Rhazes (860-932), and Averroes (1126-1198)—dominated the European schools for 1400 years[a], and the influence of Galenic thought is felt in medicine to this very day.[2]

The first massive assault on this citadel of learning came at the hands of Theophrastus Bombast von Hohenheim (1493-1541), known as Paracelsus.

Paracelsus is an extremely original and profound thinker, and his philosophy thus presents great inherent difficulties. What is more, he wrote a tremendous amount—on theological themes as well as medical, the very volume of his output increasing the burden on the reader. And his style—verbose, ungrammatical, and often unintelligible—adds a final obstacle.

He led a disorderly, drunken, peripatetic life, many of his works being dictated to his disciples and followers during drinking bouts and only published posthumously. Despite the heroic efforts of his principal editor, Johannes Huser, who brought out four editions of Paracelsus' works in the late sixteenth and early seventeenth centuries, many passages remain obscure.[b]

[a]Except Salerno and Montpellier (See below, p. 484, note).

[b]The most useful edition of Paracelsus' works is Karl Sudhoff and Wilhelm Matthiessen, *Theophrastus von Hohenheim, genannt Paracelsus: Saemtliche Werke. I. Abteilung: Medizinische, naturwissenschaftliche, und philosophische Schriften* (Munich and Berlin, 1922-1925, 1928-1933); *II. Abteilung: Die theologischen und religionsphilosophischen Schriften* (Munich, Berlin, Wiesbaden,

Paracelsus was an encyclopedic writer who brought together and reinterpreted a number of the strands in the intellectual life of his time. He was familiar with Galen and, through him, with the Empirical School. He was well versed in theology. He was apparently acquainted with neo-Platonism and the works of its contemporary exponents, Marsilio Ficino (1433-1499), Pico della Mirandola (1463-1494), and Agrippa von Nettesheim (1487-1535). He knew the ideas, vocabulary, and practices of the alchemists who for centuries had been delving into the physical nature of matter (the tradition goes back to ancient times, but the active practice of alchemy on a large scale started in the Middle Ages). And he accepted astrology.

Finally, he knew and admired the Hippocratic works—then being translated into Latin by Niccolo Leoniceno (1428-1524), professor of medicine at Padua, Bologna, and Ferrara, and Thomas Linacre (1460-1524), physician to Henry VII and Henry VIII.

The fall of Constantinople in 1453 had brought a flood of refugee scholars to Western Europe, and among them were many who knew and loved the Hippocratic writings—at this time almost unknown outside the Greek-speaking world. Paracelsus was one of the first to appreciate them at their true value, and his writings are a major conduit of the Empirical Hippocratic ideas into Renaissance medicine.

1923-1955). The first part contains 14 volumes, the second part, when completed, will be approximately 10 volumes.

Very little of Paracelsus has been translated into English: the two-volume translation by Arthur Edward Waite, *The Hermetic and Alchemical Writings of Paracelsus the Great* (2 vols., London, 1894); Kurt Leidecker's translation of the *Volumen Medicinae Paramirum* which appeared as a Supplement to the *Bulletin of the History of Medicine* (Baltimore, 1949); a selection of four of his more important minor works, *Four Treatises,* ed. Henry Sigerist (Baltimore, 1941); and a valuable book of selections edited by Carl Jung's associate, Jolande Jacobi, *Paracelsus: Selected Writings* (2nd ed. rev.; New York: Bollingen Series, XXVIII, 1958).

Another extremely valuable book of selections (untranslated), with comments in Dutch, is R.A.B. Oosterhuis, *Paracelsus en Hahnemann: Een Renaissance der Geneeskunst* (Leiden, 1937).

The literature on Paracelsus himself is very extensive. The most important are Walter Pagel's two books: *Paracelsus: An Introduction to Philosophical Medicine in the Era of the Renaissance* (New York and Basel, 1958) and *Das*

All of these materials were fused by him into a new *weltanschauung* which had its justification in his observations and experience as a practicing physician. Traditional ideas were revalued by him and reoriented—the outcome being a completely new and sharply original doctrine.

The problem is to find the key to this system, the organizing principle which brings its elements into focus. Since he was a philosopher, a mystic, an alchemist, a deeply religious man, a social revolutionary, a scientist, and an astrologer, these aspects of his thought have all offered points of departure for Paracelsan exegesis.

But in our view the correct approach is to stress his experience as a practicing physician. His religious, mystical, alchemical, and other ideas must be interpreted for their relevance to the physician's primary task of curing sick people. The main source of his inspiration was his experience as a physician, as is proved by his repeated statements that medical theory grows out of medical practice: *"Ex cura nascitur theoria, non contra,"*[3] *"Die theorik vom microcosmo, die allein ist praxis und nit theorica."*[4] His many mutually contradictory doctrines can be understood only as a series of rationalizations of his medical experience— a family of theories rising out of his practice. The ties between them are not to be sought on the logical plane. They are interconnected only by their common relationship to his practice. They are the different facets of a single *weltanschauung* formed and forged during Paracelsus' years in the metal mines and smelting establishments treating the diseases of the workers who toiled there.

Only in this way can the disparate aspects of his thought be made coherent and internally consistent—by relating them to his practice. Any other approach generates confusion and falls short of offering a key to Paracelsus as a whole.

Medizinische Weltbild des Paracelsus, Seine Zusammenhaenge mit Neuplatonismus und Gnosis (Wiesbaden, 1962); C. G. Jung's two studies: *Paracelsus* (St. Gallen, 1952), and *Paracelsica: Zwei Vorlesungen ueber den Arzt und Philosophen Theophrastus* (Zurich and Leipsig, 1942); and Oswald Croll, *Philosophy Reformed and Improved in Four Profound Tractates* (London, 1657). A recent popular account of Paracelsus by Henry Pachter, *Paracelsus, Magic Into Science* (New York, 1951), has valuable biographical detail.

A great part of the difficulty of the Paracelsan texts stems from this—he was attempting to give expression to perceptions and discoveries for which the language of the time was not prepared and to which the thought patterns of his contemporaries were not accustomed. He had to invent new words and concepts to express these insights. He deliberately contrasts what is learned from books with what is learned from patients.[5] He laments the difficulty of putting into words what he has experienced and justifies thereby his resort to parables, similes, and figures of speech:

> It is good to learn from that which can teach, that is, from examples. For what cannot be described nor interpreted can be shown. And what the speaker does not want everyone to understand will, by parables and similes, be clear to him for whom it is intended. Thus philosophy uses parables to teach us through figures, forms, virtues, and similes, so that through these we will learn that which need demands that we learn. For thus Christ has spoken, in a way not understood by all, but only by those who were meant to understand. Thus also medicine is not an art of each and all, but only for him who understands it.
>
> (S-M I/X 544-545. *Von Oeffnung der Haut, Liber Primus, Caput III.*)

His invocation of "magic" is another metaphorical way of describing his experience: magic reveals unseen influences, the Magus brings celestial forces down to earth and uses the powers of heaven for healing. This in no way means that the physician invokes occult, spiritual, or daemonic forces. It is an effort to conceptualize the process of healing, to put into words Paracelsus' vision of how the physician uses his perception and knowledge to alleviate suffering.[c] Any other interpretation would make him into a trickster and charlatan.

Our analysis stresses the link between Paracelsus and the Empirical School. He greatly amplified and reorganized the

[c]The following account is thus an expansion of the two essays by Carl Jung noted above. The same view of Paracelsus underlies the work by Oosterhuis.

ancient teachings, however, and justified them on Christian grounds: medicine is founded in experience and love. Paracelsus at many points adduces a religious justification for procedures which the Empirics had been content to leave without doctrinal support.

Although he has often been called an "empiric," no attempt has been made to bring out the very intimate relation between his ideas and those of the Empirical School. Such an attempt must center on Paracelsus' practice. Our analysis is thus confined to his therapeutics and does not explore his theology, his astrology, or his alchemy, beyond their immediate connection with medical practice. We are confident, however, that it will throw light on the non-medical sides of his thought. Paracelsus was above all a practicing physician, and his whole philosophy was formed by this seminal experience.

This interpretation provides an answer to one of the puzzles of Paracelsan criticism—namely, the apparent ambiguity of his position vis-a-vis other Renaissance figures. Like them, he emphasized the importance of the individual but seemed to do so on the basis of a philosophy and cosmology which were Christian, and not classical, in inspiration and which were apparently opposed to the classical tradition.[6] While not underestimating the significance of Christian doctrine for Paracelsus, we may point out that there were, in fact, two classical traditions. Paracelsus, too, was familiar with the ideas of antiquity, but the tradition to which he reverted was that of the Empirical School. His opposition to Galenism, which had a valid classical basis, has been mistakenly taken as opposition to the classics generally.

NOTES

[1] S-M I/VII 369. *Spital-Buch (erster teil). Doctor Theophrastus allen aerzten seinen gruss.*

[2] The only complete translation of Avicenna into a modern language (Russian) is the one recently issued by the Academy of Sciences of Uzbekistan (Abnali Ibn Sina, *Kanon Vrachebnoi Nauki.* Tashkent: Izd. Akad. Nauk Uzbek. S.S.R., 1954. Four Volumes). An excellent history of the Galenic doctrine is Owsei Temkin, *Galenism: Rise and Decline of a Medical Philosophy* (Ithaca and London: Cornell University Press, 1973).

[3] S-M I/IV 120. *Nachschriften und Notizen aus der Vorlesung de Gradibus. In caput septimum libri quinti.*

[4] S-M I/VIII 340. *Von den hinfallenden Siechtagen der Mutter. Par. IV.*

[5] S-M I/XI 176. *Labyrinthus medicorum errantium. Das ander capitel.*

[6] Pagel, *Paracelsus*, p. 36.

CHAPTER X

PARACELSUS THE MAN

Biography

Paracelsus' biography is of prime significance for his medical teachings. He was born in 1493 in Einsiedeln, Canton Schwyz, about forty miles from Zurich. This village had for centuries been a place of pilgrimage, and the religious character of his boyhood surroundings must have left a stamp upon Paracelsus. His peasant mother, moreover, who is reputed to have been very devout, was a bondswoman in the Benedictine Abbey of the village. Paracelsus' father, the illegitimate son of a Swabian noble family, was a physician, but the family was poor.

Paracelsus' mother died when he was nine years old, and the father and son moved to Villach where the former accepted an appointment as physician in the metal mines of Sigismond Fueger.[1] Paracelsus worked as a young man in the mines and, from his twentieth to his twenty-fifth year, in a smelting plant in the Tyrol.[2]

These were the determining influences on Paracelsus' character and outlook: his devoutly religious mother, his physician father, their poverty, the stigma of his father's illegitimacy, and, finally, his intimate involvement early in life with the diseases of miners and metal workers.

Paracelsus entered the study of medicine at a comparatively early age and seems to have attended several universities: Vienna, Ferrara, and possibly elsewhere—particularly in northern Italy. He knew the necessary Latin of the times and probably some Greek, although he must have learned them with reluctance. "I tell you it is much easier to learn the stars and herbs than those intricate Latin and Greek grammars. It would be much better to learn medicine first and Latin later."[3] He claimed to have been awarded the medical degree at Ferrara in 1515, but this has never been proven.

When he took the name, Paracelsus, is unknown. Some scholars have even denied that he used it at all, but his signet ring has on it the initials "THP."[4] The name must be considered both a Latinization of Hohenheim and a boast that the bearer was greater even than the Empirical physician, Celsus.

After leaving the university he practiced medicine along traditional lines but gave it up in disgust after discovering that he was only harming his patients:

> I found that the medicine which I had learned was faulty, and that those who had written about it neither knew nor understood it. They all tried to teach what they did not know. They are vainglorious babblers in all their wealth and pomp, and there is not more in them than in a worm-eaten coffin. So I had to look for a different approach.
>
> (S-M I/X 20. *Das Erste Buch der Grossen Wundarznei. Vorred in den ersten tractat.* See also S-M I/VIII 200. *Das Buch Paragranum. Der dritte tractat.*)

The search for a "different approach" stamped his life with the erratic character which has become so famous. From 1515 until his death in 1541 he had difficulty remaining longer than a few months in one place and soon became a polemical antagonist of all the medical doctrines of the schools, attacking ferociously whatever did not accord with his own vision.

One of his longer sojourns in a single place was from 1526 to 1528 in Basel. He was appointed municipal physician after curing one of the town's prominent citizens, the publisher Froben, of an ulcer on the leg. The appointment carried with it the right to lecture at the university, and he availed himself of it. The announcement of his course is worth quoting *in extenso,* since it gives an excellent resumé of his medical beliefs:

Of all disciplines medicine, alone, through the Grace of God, and according to the opinion of authors divine and profane, is recognized as a sacred art. Yet, few doctors today practice it with success and therefore the time has come to bring it back to its former dignity, to cleanse it from the dregs of the barbarians and to purge their errors. We shall do so not by strictly adhering to the rules of the ancients, but exclusively by studying nature and using the experience which we have gained in long years of practice. Who does not know that most contemporary doctors fail because they slavishly abide by the precepts of Avicenna, Galen, and Hippocrates, as though these were Apollo's oracles from which it is not allowed to digress by a finger's breadth. If it pleases God, this way may lead to splendid titles, but does not make a true doctor. What a doctor needs is not eloquence or knowledge of language and of books, illustrious though they be, but profound knowledge of nature and her works. The task of the rhetorician is to bring the judge over to his opinion. The doctor must know the causes and symptoms of the disease and use his judgment to prescribe the right medicine . . . . I do not compile [my textbooks] from the excerpts of Hippocrates or Galen. In ceaseless toil I created them anew upon the foundation of experience, the supreme teacher of all things. If I want to prove anything, I shall not do so by quoting authorities but by experiment and by reasoning thereupon . . . . I do not believe in the ancient doctrine of complexions and humors . . . . It is because of these doctrines that so few physicians have correct views of disease, its origins and its course . . . . Farewell and come with a good will to study our attempt to reform medicine.

(S-M I/IV 3-4. *Intimatio, Basileae, 5 Juni 1527: das "Baseler Programm"*)

In Basel he became acquainted with some of the leading persons of the Humanist movement: Erasmus, Holbein, Oecolampadius. He was surrounded by admirers, and the future seemed to lie clear before him. However, his quarrelsome nature soon had him at odds with everyone. He was supposed to supervise the town apothecaries, but he had already decided that the customary lengthy prescriptions of the day were not only valueless but poisonous—better suited to increasing the income of the apothecaries than improving the health of the patient:

> The longer the recipes the less virtue in them.
>
> (S-M I/VI 148. *Bertheonei. Beschlussrede*)

> It is better to know and understand one remedy than to rummage through the great libraries of the monasteries, where of a thousand pages, barely one is understood . . . The Nature does not call for long recipes.
>
> (S-M I/VI 144. *Drei Buecher der Wundarznei. Bk. II., Cap. VII.*)

> I write short prescriptions, not forty to sixty ingredients. I prescribe little and seldom. I do not empty their boxes for them. I do not bring much money into their kitchens. Yet this is the business for which they calumniate me. Now judge for yourselves to whom do I owe most? Or to whom have I pledged myself as *Doctor*? To help the apothecary empty the bags in the kitchen, or the patient from the kitchen to his benefit?
>
> (S-M I/XI 154-155. *Sieben Defensiones.* Sixth Defense)

What is more, he violated professional ethics by charging, in a letter to the aldermen of Basel, that the physicians and pharmacists were in a conspiracy with one another to milk the public.[5]

His university lectures were a focus of controversy, as the above announcement reveals. He attacked the ordinary and accepted medical ideas. He lectured in German instead of the customary Latin. And, in culmination, he burned some of the sacrosanct medical texts of Galen and Avicenna in the students' bonfire on St. John's Day "so that all of this misery should go up in the air with the smoke."[6] [a]

[a] We have only Paracelsus' word for this escapade, and scholars have attempted to prove that it did not happen.

His stay in Basel ended abruptly in consequence of a lawsuit which he brought against one of the town dignitaries for a 100-guilder fee. The patient had offered this reward to anyone who could rid him of an incurable disease.[b] After being cured by some of Paracelsus' laudanum pills he offered to settle for three guilders, which itself was generous remuneration, but Paracelsus insisted on the full amount (probably a year's income for the average physician). He took the case to court but lost, and since his protector, Froben, had meanwhile died of a stroke, Paracelsus had no one to rely on for assistance. Furthermore, the town's other physicians blamed the stroke on the medicines which Paracelsus had given Froben for his ulcer.

In desperation he posted a public notice attacking the city administration. This was a serious offence, and the whole town rose against him. Warned by a friend, Paracelsus escaped a few minutes ahead of the sheriff.

The Basel episode, which may be viewed as the turning point in Paracelsus' life, his one and only attempt to lead a respectable existence, is typical and revealing. Doctors, apothecaries, and the high and wellborn were always on the opposite side of the barricade from Paracelsus. He came as a liberating force—to free medicine from the shackles of Galenism and liberate the bodies and spirits of men from bondage. In 1525 he had participated in the peasant rebellion in Salzburg, escaping with his life only thanks to his physician's gown. He was proud of his complicity:

> . . . I made the peasants rebellious so that they no longer pay tithes to you or care for what you say. Mind, if my sermon were inspired by the devil, they would follow you, not me. However, what I said has been inspired by the Holy Spirit; ergo it was the Gospel.[7]

The peasant's son and the miner's friend identified with the lower orders of society. Although during his life he doctored princes and nobles, he relaxed only in the company of artisans and teamsters.

[b] This may have been a deliberate plot to humiliate Paracelsus. Pachter, *op. cit.,* p. 170.

Another of his storied quarrels (which authorities today feel is probably fictional but which is perfectly typical of Paracelsus) was with the Fugger family over their cure for syphilis. This disease had appeared in Europe at the end of the fifteenth century, apparently the gift of the New World to the Old. The frantic search for remedies soon uncovered guaiac wood, which took on additional luster by being expensive and also from the New World. The astute Fuggers secured a monopoly on this remedy and, to ensure a favorable medical press, sold shares in their cargo ships to the leading physicians of the day.

Paracelsus had a different idea and espoused the use of mercury—the competing, minority medication for syphilis. He published a short pamphlet on the subject and, furthermore, urged physicians to reduce their doses, as they were killing patients with mercury more quickly than even the syphilis could do it. "You know that *argentum vivum* is nothing but poison and daily experience proves it . . . [but] you anoint patients with it more thickly than a cobbler anoints leather with grease."[8]

He planned a larger work on the subject, the *Eight Books on the French Disease,* and actually published a part of it in 1529. The appearance of further installments, however, was abruptly halted by a decree of censorship from the Leipzig medical faculty and its dean, Heinrich Stromer, who himself had a considerable investment in the guaiac ships of the Fuggers. The complete text of this work was not published in Paracelsus' lifetime.[9]

Paracelsus is best remembered today for introducing or popularizing a number of mineral remedies. Many were already known to the profession: iron, saltpeter, ammonia of sulfur (liver of sulfur), bicarbonate of soda, sulphuric acid, and red and black *pulvis solaris* (mercurial and antimonial compounds). Paracelsus appears to have added several new ones: flower of sulphur, calomel, blue vitriol, and other zinc, copper, arsenic, and lead compounds.[10] He was himself a good chemist and worked to discover preparations of the mineral compounds which would be less poisonous than those in common use. And, as with mercury, he tried to persuade his colleagues to give smaller doses:

> Where in all your books is a *purgatio* that is not poison or serves not death, or can be used without annoyance? if *dosis* is not given its proper weight? . . . What is there that is not poison? All things are poison, and nothing is without poison: the *dosis* alone makes a thing not poison. For example, every food and every drink, if taken beyond its dose, is poison: the result proves it.
>
> (S-M I/XI 138. *Sieben Defensiones.* Third Defense)

But he did not rely exclusively on mineral remedies. He shared fully the Empiric's love for the pharmacological side of medicine. "Nature is so excellent in its gifts that . . . it better befits a man to know one herb in the meadow, but to know it thoroughly, than to see the whole meadow without knowing what grows on it."[11] And, like the Empirics, he did not hesitate to seek knowledge of remedies from non-professionals:

> The physician does not learn everything he must know and master at high colleges alone; from time to time he must consult old women, gypsies, magicians, wayfarers, and all manner of peasant folk and random people, and learn from them; for these have more knowledge about such things than all the high colleges.
>
> (S-M I/XIV 541. *De occulta philosophia*)

He thus offended against the caste interests of the medical profession which, like the ancient Rationalists, was suspicious of lay contributions to medicine—especially when the remedy could not be explained according to doctrine. A lampoon issued in Basel ridicules him for using the folk remedies, onion and garlic.[12]

Paracelsus traveled incessantly, especially after his Basel sojourn, claiming to have covered all of Europe from England to Russia and from Sweden to Alexandria and Constantinople. His wanderings came to an end in September, 1541, when he died in Salzburg from a presumed atrophy of the kidneys or liver cancer.[13c] His will, drawn up in the last days before his death, is a model of charity and Christian resignation. In it he commends "his life, and death, and his poor soul to the shield and protection of Almighty God, in the steadfast hope that the eternal mercy of God will not allow the bitter sufferings, the martyrdom, and death of Our Savior, Hallowed Lord Jesus Christ, to be fruitless and of no avail to him, a miserable man." He appointed as his legatee "the poor, the wretched, and the needy people who have no stipend or other provision made for them" and was buried next to the town paupers in the cemetery of St. Sebastian in Salzburg.[14]

Psychological Traits: "Alterius non sit qui suus esse potest"

Paracelsus' most pronounced psychological trait is alienation. Throughout his life he avoided sustained contact with any other human. Never married, he seems to have felt a repugnance for the opposite sex.[d]

Nor had he friends of his own sex. He felt closest of all to God. "Happy is he who walks in the ways of the Apostles, takes neither office nor wife, and has no possessions."[15] Pachter has noted with insight that he was unable to be an equal among equals but was always a king or a beggar. He could communicate only through the printing press.[16] He made mounting demands on the loyalty of his friends and seemed to feel relief when, being only human, they eventually turned against him.

[c]It is commonly thought that his death was due indirectly to his undoubted alcoholism, but kidney damage is one of the common sequelae of lead poisoning, and it is not wildly presumptuous to hold that Paracelsus ultimately paid with his life for his knowledge of the metals.

[d]Van Helmont attributed this to the fact that "a sow, in a place where three ways meet, had gelded him" (*Oriatrike, or Physick Refined* [London, 1662], p. 230) but gives no source for his observation. Paracelsus' disciple, Johannes Oporinus, stated that he had never had sexual relations. The long sword which Paracelsus carried, and in whose hilt he kept his most powerful medicine, laudanum, seems an obvious compensatory symbol for sexual incapacity.

His alienation from human contact explains the extremely blunt language he used in his professional controversies:

> I am said to be a strange fellow with an uncivil answer. I do not wash up to the satisfaction of everyone. I do not answer everyone's contention in humility.
>
> (S-M I/XI 151. *Sieben Defensiones.* Sixth Defense)

> I have thus far used simple language, and I cannot boast of any rhetoric or subtleties; I speak in the language of my birth and my country, for I am from Einsiedeln, of Swiss nationality, and let no one find fault with me for my rough speech. My writings must not be judged by my language, but by my art and experience, which I offer the whole world, and which I hope will be useful to the whole world.
>
> (S-M I/X 199. *Das erste Buch der Grossen Wundarznei. Beschlussred*)

> By nature I am not subtly spun, nor is it the custom of my native land to accomplish anything by spinning silk. Nor are we raised on figs, nor on mead, nor on wheaten bread, but on cheese, milk, and oatcakes, which cannot give one a subtle disposition. Moreover, a man clings all his days to what he received in his youth; and my youth was coarse as compared to that of the subtle, pampered, and over-refined. For those who are raised in soft clothes and in women's apartments, and we who are brought up among the pine cones, have trouble in understanding one another well.
>
> (S-M I/XI 151-152. *Sieben Defensiones.* Sixth Defense)

In compensation for his inability to be on good terms with professional equals or the highly placed of the world, Paracelsus possessed a generalized and diffuse love for all of humanity, especially for the sick:

> We have warred for a long time. They drove me out of Lithuania and Prussia and from Poland, and still it was not enough for them. The Dutch did not like me either,

> nor the schools, neither Jews nor Monks—but, thank God, the patients liked me.
>
> (S-M I/VI 180. *Entwuerfe, Notizen und Ausarbeitungen zur Bertheonea. Excusatio ad lectorem.*)

> This is my vow: . . . to love the sick, each and all of them, more than if my own body were at stake . . . not to trust any apothecary, nor to do violence to any child.
>
> (S-M I/VI 181. *Entwuerfe, Notizen und Ausarbeitungen zur Bertheonea. Jus jurandum*)

He identifies with the maltreated patient, claiming that the physicians who attack his ideas are the same who torture and maim their patients.[17]

The exhortation to love the patient is extended by him to all physicians:

> The difference between a physician and the rest of men is this, that the others need think only of themselves, while the physician must care not only for himself but also for others. His office consists of nothing but compassion for others. But his compassion does not originate in him any more than the efficacy of the remedy emanates from him. And because there is nothing that comes from him—although he accomplishes it as though it were his work—his office is not to murder and injure, to strangle and cripple, but to cure the patient by the charity and love with which God has endowed man. A physician is uncharitable if he does not understand the nature of his office here below and does not live up to the responsibilities of his office. What is the meaning of an office to which one is appointed by God, if not to carry out and fulfill the will of God?
>
> (S-M VIII 264-265. *Von den hinfallenden Siechtagen. Der erste paragraphus*)

Thus the absolutely indispensable quality with which the physician must be endowed is love:

> The art of medicine is rooted in the heart. If your heart is false, you will also be a false physician; if your heart is just, you will also be a true physician.

> (S-M I/VIII 266. *Von den hinfallenden Siechtagen. Der erste paragraphus*)
>
> No one requires greater love of the heart than the physician. For him the ultimate instance is man's distress. Privilege and lineage pale to nothingness—only distress has meaning.
>
> (S-M I/VIII 322. *Von den hinfallenden Siechtagen der Mutter. Par. I.*)

Paracelsus even introduces this idea into his commentary on Hippocrates. He interprets *Aphorisms* I: 1 ("... It is not enough for the physician to do what is necessary, but the patient and the attendants must do their part as well, and the circumstances must be favorable .... ") to mean that "all the attendants of the sick man must be of the same heart as he .... The reason: love thy neighbor as thyself. Then he will get well."[18]

There is another story about Paracelsus—perhaps apocryphal but nonetheless characteristic—that while a student he belonged to the Brethren of the Common Life, a lay group which held man's existence to be justified by charity rather than faith. The members lived together in fraternal communities and performed works of charity for the poor.

This polarity in Paracelsus' character—the striving for solitude vs. the strong urge to charity and love—is reflected in many ways in his writings. The holism of his philosophy may be viewed as the corollary of his desire for oneness and solitude:

> There is one single number that should determine our life on earth, and this number is One. . . . It is true that the Godhead is Three, but the Three is again comprised in the One. And because God transforms Himself into the One, we men on earth must also strive for the One, devote ourselves to the One, and live in it. In this number is rest and peace, and in no other. What goes beyond it is unrest and conflict, struggle of one against another. For if a calculator sets down a number and counts further than one, who can say at what number he will stop? But this

> question is the difficulty that gnaws at us and worries us. How much more pleasant and better it would be if we always walked in the path of the One.
>
> (S-M I/X 581. *Die Prognostikation auf 24 zukuenftige Jahre. Vorred*)

His motto—*Omne donum perfectum a Deo, imperfectum a Diabolo*—reflects this holistic approach to medicine. What is partial or incomplete is tainted with evil. "The art of medicine is true, just, certain, perfect, and whole."[19]

His philosophy regards the organism as a unique entity which can only be understood as a whole, and the medicine, in turn, as a specific and inimitable, unanalyzable, substance. "As little as the sun is divided up, one part to the flowers, one part to the trees, one part to the stones, etc., that little we may divide the strength of the medicine."[20][e]

The feeling of alienation accounts for Paracelsus' conviction that he was selected by God for a special mission. He viewed himself as the precursor of a new medicine. "I here in this work introduce a new *theorica,* also *physica,* together with new concepts."[21] He sees himself as another Christ—who came to rid the world of Pagan doctrines, was persecuted and suffered, but whose word would triumph one day. The Christian doctrine based on love would oust the false, pagan, Galenic, and Arabic teachings of the schools.[22]

The idea that medicine shall be rooted in love has several corollaries. In the first place, this is the touchstone for distinguishing the good physician from the bad one, the physician who assumes the full responsibility of the profession from the one who merely exploits its privileges:

> If now Christ had to suffer Himself to be sold and betrayed for the sake of selfish gain, how much more do the false physicians make man lame and crooked, strangle and kill him, in order that their profit be increased and

[e]For this reason Pagel denies that Paracelsus' thought can be considered scientific, since "Paracelsus is concerned not with measurable quantities and the mathematical laws underlying phenomena, but with individual objects determined by intrinsic divine virtues which defy scientific analysis" (*Paracelsus,* p. 39). The question of scientific method in Paracelsus is discussed below, pp. 467-471.

> not hindered. For as soon as the love of one's neighbor grows cold, it can bear him good fruit no more; and such fruit as is borne is for selfish gain. Thus should we know that there are two kinds of physician, those who act for love, and for profit, and by their works are they both known . . . the physician should sell what he has and heal the sick . . . . In consideration of their own profit [physicians] accept everything that comes to them. Thus too come all the lazy and profligate rascals into medicine and sell their medicine, whether it makes sense or not. Now he who can fill sacks with gold, he is praised, he is a good physician . . . .
>
> (S-M I/XI 146. *Sieben Defensiones.* Fifth Defense)

> There are two kinds of physicians—those who work for love and those who work for their own profit. They are both known by their works; the true and just physician is known by his love and by his unfailing love for his neighbor. The unjust physicians are known by their transgressions against the commandment; for they reap, although they have not sown, and they are like ravening wolves; they reap because they want to reap, in order to increase their profit, and they are heedless of the commandment of love.
>
> (S-M I/XI 147. *Sieben Defensiones.* Fifth Defense)

Paracelsus expresses his contempt for the false physician—who heals by books, without love—in his usual brutal and overbearing manner:

> Avicenna, Galen, Rhazes, Montagnana, Mesue, and others, after me and not I after you! Ye of Paris, ye of Montpellier, ye of Swabia, ye of Meissen, ye of Cologne, ye of Vienna, and those who dwell on the Danube and the Rhine, ye islands on the sea, thou Italy, thou Dalmatia, thou Sarmatia, thou Athens, ye Greeks, ye Arabs, ye Israelites, after me, and not I after you! Even in the remotest corners there will be none of you on whom the dogs will not piss. But I shall be monarch and mine

> will be the monarchy, and I shall lead the monarchy; gird your loins . . . .
>
> (S-M I/VIII 56. *Paragranum. Vorrede und erste zwei Buecher. Entwuerfe und I. Ausarbeitung in Berezhausen. Vorred*)

> I am Theophrastus, and greater than those to whom you liken me; I am Theophrastus, and in addition I am *monarcha medicorum,* monarch of physicians, and I can prove to you what you cannot prove. I will let Luther defend his cause, and I will defend my cause, and I will defeat those of my colleagues who turn against me, this I shall do with the help of the *arcana* . . . . It was not the constellations that made me a physician: God made me . . . . I need not don a coat of mail or a buckler against you, for you are not learned or experienced enough to refute even one word of mine. I wish I could protect my bald head against the flies as effectively as I can defend my monarchy . . . . I will not defend my monarchy with empty talk but with *arcana.* And I do not take my medicines from the apothecaries; their shops are but foul sculleries, from which comes nothing but foul broths. As for you, you defend your kingdom with belly-crawling and flattery. How long do you think this will last? . . . Let me tell you this: every little hair on my neck knows more than you and all your scribes, and my shoebuckles are more learned than your Galen and Avicenna, and my beard has more experience than all your high colleges.
>
> (S-M I/VIII 63-65. *Paragranum. Vorrede und erste zwei Buecher. Entwuerfe und I. Ausarbeitung in Berezhausen. Vorred*)

The physician learns not from books but from people. The common man is beloved of God—hence he is the prime source of medical knowledge.

> The above-mentioned *Doctores* of medicine should consider better what they plainly see, that for instance an

unlettered peasant heals more than all of them with all their books and red gowns.

(S-M I/XI 136. *Sieben Defensiones.* Second Defense)

A common peasant knows more than they. Also a Jew . . . . Isn't it vicious and disgraceful that a municipal doctor with a salary should run away from the patients, cannot help them, must leave them lying, whereas others, who have not studied medicine, help the patients?

(S-M I/IX 153-154. *Die drei (vier) Buecher des Opus Paramirum. Tractatus quartus et tartarus quartus*)

Paracelsus justified his incessant travels by the need for contact with common people of all nations:

For many years I studied at the universities of Germany, Italy, and France, seeking to discover the foundations of medicine. However, I did not content myself with their teachings and writings and books, but continued my travels to Granada and Lisbon, through Spain and England, through Brandenburg, Prussia, Lithuania, Poland, Hungary, Wallachia, Transylvania, Croatia, the Wendian Mark, and yet other countries which there is no need to mention here, and wherever I went, I eagerly and diligently investigated and sought after the tested and reliable arts of medicine. I went not only to the doctors, but also to barbers, bathkeepers, learned physicians, women, and magicians who pursue the art of healing; I went to alchemists, to monasteries, to nobles and common folk, to the experts and the simple . . . . .

(S-M I/X 19-20. *Das erste Buch der Grossen Wundarznei. Vorred in den ersten tractat*)

This was why he taught and lectured in German instead of the traditional Latin—to separate medicine from school learning, which he identified with the professional hubris of the physician—and restore its lost contact with the layman:[23 f]

[f]Some of the German commentators, especially during the Nazi era, have regarded this as a streak of nationalism in Paracelsus, but Paracelsus of course aligned himself with the people as a class and not as a nation.

> I have here to explain philosophy, firstly as an introduction to medicine . . . and I am doing this in German to make it less strange and to bring science to the common people.
>
> (S-M I/VIII 144. *Das Buch Paragranum. Der erste tractat, von der philosophia*)

It may be noted parenthetically that Paracelsus' effort to bring medicine within the grasp of the uneducated people was viewed with resentment by medical authorities and perceived as a threat to their positions. A contemporary, Winter von Andernach (1505-1574), wrote that Paracelsus "prefers to work for the common people than for honest men."[24]

Finally, the idea that love is the basis of medicine has a direct influence on therapeutic doctrine. The Pagan physicians who are devoid of love work against the patient in their medication, that is, they work against the natural healing power in every organism.[25]

The leveller who sided with the peasants' efforts to tear down the structure of authority and prepare the way for a flowering of the human spirit is, in his medical role, a believer in the beneficent influence of the natural healing power. Conviction of the innate goodness of man becomes belief in his natural self-healing capacity.

NOTES

[1] Pachter, *op. cit.*, p. 22.

[2] Pagel, *Paracelsus*, p. 10; Sigerist, *op. cit.*, p. 46.

[3] S-M I/XIV 624. *De pestilitate.* Regarded as spurious by Sudhoff.

[4] For a picture see Jacobi, *op. cit.*, p. 9.

[5] S-M I/IV 142. *Zwei Eingaben an der Rat der Stadt Basel, Sommer, 1527.*

[6] S-M I/VIII 58. *Paragranum. Vorrede und erste zwei Buecher. Entwuerfe und I. Ausarbeitung in Berezhausen. Vorrede.*

[7] Pachter, *op. cit.*, p. 103. Translated from Sudhoff, *Versuch einer Kritik der Echtheit der Paracelsischen Schriften,* II (Berlin, 1898-1899), p. 333.

[8] S-M I/XI 138. *Sieben Defensiones.* Third Defense.

[9] Pachter, *op. cit.*, pp. 179ff. Pagel, *Paracelsus,* p. 24. The publishing history of this work is discussed in S-M I/VII, pp. 7-28. See also, R. Toellner, "Matthaeus Kardinal Lang von Wellenburg und Paracelsus; zur Polemik des Paracelsus gegen Kardinal Lang und die Fugger," *Current Problems in the History of Medicine* (Proceedings of the XIX International Congress for the History of Medicine), Basel and New York: S. Karger, 1966, pp. 489-497.

[10] Robert Multhauf, "Medical Chemistry and 'the Paracelsans,'" *Bulletin of the History of Medicine,* XXVIII (1954), 101-126.

[11] S-M I/VI 289. *Von allen offenen Schaeden. Beschlussrede.*

[12] Pachter, *op. cit.*, p. 164.

[13] Jacobi, *op. cit.*, p. lx.

[14] *Ibid.*, pp. lx-lxi.

[15] Quoted in Karl Bittel, *Paracelsus. Leben und Lebensweisheit im Selbstzeugnissen* (Leipzig, Reclam, 1945), p. 11.

[16] Pachter, *op. cit.*, p. 194.

[17] S-M I/VIII 145. *Das Buch Paragranum. Der erste tractat.*

[18] S-M I/IV 498. *Deutsche Kommentare zu den Aphorismen des Hippokrates. Aphorismus I. Oportet autem se ipsum etc.*

[19] S-M I/X 20. *Das erste Buch der Grossen Wundarznei. Vorred in den ersten tractat.*

[20] S-M I/VII 269. *Vom Ursprung und Herkommen der Franzosen. V. capitel.*

[21] S-M I/XI 127. *Sieben Defensiones.* First Defense.

[22] S-M I/I 176. *Volumen medicinae Paramirum, Bk. II* of *Prologues: Prologue VI.* Cf. *Ibid.*, pp. 232-233. *Bk. V, Particle* II.

[23] Pagel, *Paracelsus,* p. 244, n. 122.

[24] Quoted in Sprengel, *Histoire de la Medecine,* III (Paris, 1815), 284.

[25] S-M I/I 232. *Volumen Medicinae Paramirum. Bk. V, Particle II.*

CHAPTER XI

MEDICINE'S RETURN TO EXPERIENCE

Paracelsus' course announcement promised to "cleanse [medicine] from the dregs of the barbarians and purge their errors . . . not by strictly adhering to the rules of the ancients but exclusively by studying nature and using the experience which we have gained in long years of practice."

Paracelsus contrasts "experience" and the "return to nature" with the lifeless logic of the schools. What is more, "nature" and "experience" are largely identified with one another:

> Nature is that which points to the causes . . . what nature points to is reason [*ratio*] . . . nature gives the ground; understanding [*verstand*] comes from the ground. Since then [it] comes out of nature, what is nature? Experience [*experientia*]. Experience comes from Almighty God; this, and no other, must be the origin of the physician. For we are not our own schoolmaster; the one which shows us the force of nature is the one which describes the ground for us.
>
> (S-M I/VI 178-179. *Entwuerfe, Notizen und Ausarbeitungen zur Bertheonea. Argumentum II.*)

This is because the physician's experience (*experientia* or *erfahrenheit*) reflects or crystallizes the operations (i.e., the "experience") of nature.

"Nature" (*die natur*) has the same dual meaning for Paracelsus that *physis* had in Greek medicine—encompassing both the external physical world and the vital force of the organism. For Paracelsus, as for the Empirical physicians, acceptance of the *physis* requires founding medicine in experience.

"Nature" as the body's self-healing potential is discussed below.[a] Here we need only note that "nature" in both senses is intimately associated with the concept of "experience." Hence "experience" is of pervasive significance for Paracelsan medicine, and his treatment of this concept is identical with its development by the Empirical School.

Paracelsus contrasts the taciturn and businesslike physician, who knows how to heal, with the glib and garrulous one who lacks experience and can only give explanations:

> Now in order to consider the welfare of the miners so that they can be protected from the aforementioned miners' sickness, it is no longer meet to speak with learned men and philosophers, but with experienced men; for it is the manner and the innate custom of any experienced man not to confront another experienced man with idle talk. The health of the patient is considered in few and short words by the experienced, since the words of idle talk cannot cure. They cannot please the patients either, nor can the latter love these words. Experience is so constituted that an understanding of its works makes itself known to everyone without much gab. For this reason, more attention should be paid to practice to determine what it is. It should be left alone, and this experience should defend itself, and the results which should move every unbeliever to believe in physic should be examined. For the results are so clear that they are not in need of any disputation . . . .
>
> (S-M I/IX 483. *Von der Bergsucht und anderen Bergkrankheiten drei Buecher. Das erste Buch. Der viert tractat. Das erst capitel.*)

But pay heed further how I justify myself in this accusation that I give a rough answer. The other physicians know little of the arts; they resort to friendly, pleasing, charming words. They advise people with breeding and fine words; they set forth all things at length, delightfully, with distinct differentiations, and say: "Come again soon, my dear sir; my dear wife, go and

[a] See Chapter XVI.

> accompany the gentleman," etc. I say thus: "What wilt thou? I have no time now; it is not so urgent." Now I have upset the applecart! They have made such fools of the patients that they are completely of the belief that a friendly affectionate manner, ceremony, ingratiating ways, much ado, constitute art and medicine. They call him "Young sir," who only comes from the shopkeeper's. They call another, "Sir, wise Sir" who is a cobbler and a dullard, where I say "Thou"; but with this I throw away my resources. My intention is to gain nothing with my tongue, but only with works. As they, however, are not of this opinion, they can well say in their way that I am a strange, queer-headed fellow, that I give little good advice. I do not believe in feeding myself on friendly caresses, wherefore I cannot use what befits me not, nor what I have not learned. For it is not necessary to use such flattery and to deal tenderly with every boor who is not fit to be carried in a dung-barrow. Medicine should be such, that the physician may answer according to his flesh and blood, his country's customs and his own nature: rough, rude, stern, gentle, mild, virtuous, friendly, delightful—according to how he is by nature and by acquired habit. But let this not be his art, but only the briefest answer! And on with the works! That's the way to oil the wheels.
>
> (S-M I/XI 152. *Sieben Defensiones*. Sixth Defense)

Experience is important in another way: the validity of book-learning and received doctrines must be continually tested in practice:

> It is a perversion that ye let Machaon, Apollo, Aristotle, Galen, Averroes, Rhazes be answerable. Instead ye must first test [*probiren*] whether they have lied or not.
>
> (S-M I/IX 229. *Die drei (vier) Buecher des Opus Paramirum. Liber quartus de matrice*)
>
> Now the question is whether the doctrine of the physicians of the universities is the art of medicine or whether mine is. This will be proved through works.
>
> (S-M I/XI 128. *Sieben Defensiones*. First Defense)

Hence the art is learned not from books but from experience:

> The art of medicine cannot be inherited, nor can it be copied from books; it must be digested many times and many times spat out; one must always rechew it and knead it thoroughly, and one must be alert while learning it, one must not doze like peasants turning over pears in the sun.
>
> (S-M I/X 225. *Das zweite Buch der Grossen Wundarznei. Vorred in das ander Buch*)
>
> The right path does not consist in speculation, but leads deep into experience. From experience the physician receives his help, and upon it rests all his skill. He must have rich knowledge based on experience, for he is born blind, and book knowledge has never made a single physician. For this purpose he needs not human, but divine things, and therefore he should not treat truth lightheadedly. He does not act for himself but for God, and God bestows His grace upon him so that he may come to the assistance of his fellow men in their needs. Medicine does not serve man's self-conceit but his pressing needs.
>
> (S-M I/VII 202. *Vom Ursprung and Herkommen der Franzosen. Capitel XIV.*)
>
> Many arts come to us through random experience. A patient tries something and gets better. The light of nature has pointed out to him something which he himself disdained and regarded as of no value.[b]
>
> (S-M I/VIII 292. *Von den hinfallenden Siechtagen. Der drit paragraphus*)

This was another argument justifying his continual travels:

> He who would explore nature must tread her books with his feet. Holy Scripture is explored through its letters, but nature is explored from country to country; it has as many pages as there are countries. This is the code of nature and thus must her leaves be turned.
>
> (S-M I/XI 145-146. *Sieben Defensiones.* Fourth Defense)

[b]For definition and discussion of the "light of nature" see *infra,* pp. 372-373.

> How can a man become a good geographer or cosmographer if he always sits by the fireside? Does not the sight of a thing give the eyes a true foundation? Then let the foundation be made solid. What can the roaster of pears experience in his chimney corner. . . . The diseases migrate hither and thither throughout the broad world, and do not stay in one place. If a man desires to recognize many various diseases, he must travel from place to place; if he travels far, he will experience a great deal, and he will learn to recognize many things.
>
> (S-M I/XI 142. *Sieben Defensiones*. Fourth Defense)

Paracelsus, for these reasons, propose that the separate branches of medicine and surgery be united—shocking the profession and fueling the opposition to his ideas:

> How can ye establish it as another faculty and profession? Ye wood doctor and fool! . . . In *judicando* ye are a physician, in *curando* a surgeon. . . . For the patient needs surgery and not theory [*physic*]. It is the doctor who needs the latter. That is, there can be no surgeon who is not also a physician. The latter begets the surgeon, and the surgeon tests the physician. For, unless he is also a surgeon, the physician has no way to test his own works. He is nothing but a stuffed dummy and a painted ass.
>
> (S-M I/I 342. *Liber de podagricis et suis speciebus. Cura*)

Both surgeon and physician spring from the same philosophy; they are divided only in practice.[1]

The sixteenth-century physician confined himself to diagnosis, prescription-writing, and speculation about disease, while the less educated surgeons not only performed operations and treated wounds but did virtually all the manual labor associated with medical practice—this being beneath the dignity of the learned physician. And the apothecaries prepared and dispensed medicines. Paracelsus' holism led him to propose unification of the three specialties. The physician who relies on the apothecary's prescription is like a person who knows how to drink wine but not how to raise grapes.[2]

And the true insult to the physician's dignity is that he cannot himself follow through with the cure but must leave it in the hands of the surgeon:

> The physician is of no account without works. . . . The work of physicians is not empty talk.
>
> (S-M I/XI 126. *Sieben Defensiones. Vorred*)
>
> The art of healing makes the physician, not name or school. What is the use of appearing great and making a big show if we don't know the art. What is the use of being honored by princes, lords, states, and lands . . . if we don't have the art?
>
> (S-M I/VII 370. *Spital-Buch (Erster Teil). Doctor Theophrastus allen aerzten seinen gruss*)
>
> The patients should be his book, they do not mislead.
>
> (S-M I/XI 85. *Das Buch von den tartarischen Krankheiten. Das XIII. capitel*)

Hence his books on "surgery" (*wundarznei*) are actually on therapeutics. He claims not to be a physician at all, but only a surgeon.[3] He notes that there are two kinds of surgery: from the outside and from the inside.[4] His works on surgery deal with "everything which the eyes can perceive within the body, as it is brought before the eyes with all of its signs."[5]

Thus it is clear that for Paracelsus "experience" is needed to learn the art and to practice it. But he carries the argument a step further: not only is the art learned by experience, the art *is* experience—the reflection in the physician's mind of the experience (practice) of nature:

> Philosophy is knowing through practice. It is nothing but *practica globuli* or *sphaerae*.
>
> (S-M I/VIII 39. *Paragranum. Vorrede und erste zwei Buecher. Entwuerfe und I. Ausarbeitung in Berezhausen. IV. Liber quatuor columnarum medicinae. praefatio*)

As is customary for him, Paracelsus gives this a religious underpinning. "Experience must be valid and certain, for it is from God."[6] The reason is that God, when he expelled Adam from Paradise, ordered him to earn his living by the sweat of his brow:

> What man can give an account of or explain how he learned to till the soil, to raise vines, or to make cheese? No one unless he can point to his teacher, and the teacher will in turn point to his teacher, and so on and on, until we come to the first teacher. And to whom can he point? To no one except to Him who created man; for He also gave him his knowledge. What would men do if they had not been ordained to work? The commandment was: "In the sweat of thy face shalt thou eat bread . . ." God said: "Let it be!" And there was everything, but not "art" nor the light of nature. But when Adam was driven out of Paradise, God created the light of nature for him by ordering him to gain sustenance through the toil of his hands, and He also created the light of Eve when he said: "In sorrow shalt thou bring forth children." Thus the creatures that had hitherto been like unto angels became earthly and mortal. And Eve was taught to raise her children, and thus cradles and nursing came into being. The word was sufficient to create man; it was also sufficient to create the light that man needed . . . when he was driven out of paradise. For only then did the "inner man," "the man of the second creation," come into being.
>
> (S-M I/VIII 290-292. *Von den hinfallenden Siechtagen. Der drit paragraphus*)

Hence labor is divinely ordained. Just as the laborer must earn his living through labor, so must man learn through his own experience.

> Happiness does not consist in laziness, or sensual pleasure, or riches, or chattering, or gluttony. In labor and in sweat must each man use the gifts that God conferred upon him on earth, either as peasant in the fields, as a workman in the smithy, in the mines, on the seas, in medicine, or as one who proclaims the word of God.
>
> (S-M II/I 253-254. *De honestiis utrisque divitiis*)

He is clearly influenced by the New Testament doctrine that faith must be proved through works: "For as the body without the spirit is dead, so faith without works is dead also" (*James* II:26):

> The proper way resides in work and action, in doing and producing; the perverse man does nothing, but talks a great deal. We must not judge a man by his words, but by his heart. The heart speaks through words only when they are confirmed by deeds.
>
> (S-M I/IX 223. *Die drei (vier) Buecher des Opus Paramirum. Liber quartus de matrice*)
>
> When Christ spoke and taught, his words were always accompanied by deeds. It should be the same in medicine. Those who spend their time in idle chatter and disputes and do no work speak vain words, for which they will be held to account. . . . Words and deeds should be wedded to each other. A theoretician of theology may talk about God and put the works aside, but a physician has no right to act thus; like a saint, he must prove himself by words and deeds. He whose words are efficacious is a saint. Similarly, only he whose remedies are efficacious is a physician. . . . There should be nothing in medicine except what results from both word and deed, because medicine is a true art, and truth lies only in the deed and not in idle talk. . . . Therefore study and learn that words and deeds are but one thing; if you fail to understand this, you are not a physician.
>
> (S-M I/X 281-282. *Das zweite Buch der Grossen Wundarznei. Vorred in den andern tractat*)

But he develops this idea to the conclusion that faith (i.e., knowledge) actually *arises out of works:* through his experience the physician acquires knowledge of the workings of nature:

> The works must give the things and the experience; with the inexperienced there is no faith. The faith is in the experienced. Therefore, the physician shall be experienced *so that he will know that he can believe.*
>
> (S-M I/I 57. *Elf Traktat. 3. Von farbsuchten, Andere Redaktion*)

> Works alone lead one to faith, that is to say the works of nature, her signs and marvels. And since faith is based on works, signs, and marvels, it is fitting that we philosophize as believers and not as heathens . . . we are convinced that he who wants to believe must also know; for only from knowledge, and because of knowledge, does faith arise. . . . *For first comes knowledge, then faith,* and then the fruit; this is the ground on which the philosopher must stand.
>
> (S-M I/XIII 246. *Weiteres in Konzepten und Ausarbeitungen zu den Meteoren: B. Nach Abschriften des Montanus und Anderer. Prologus in die Buecher meteororum.*)

Thus the universe has its practice and the physician has his practice. Through experience the physician can grasp the "*practica globuli* or *sphaerae*" and make it his own. He cannot learn this from books.

If we carry further the parallel between works leading to faith and experience leading to medical knowledge, we find that just as faith is knowledge of God, i.e., of what is invisible to man, so is medical knowledge the knowledge of invisible things. "For belief in medicine is not anything else but knowing the invisible things' work, course, nature, kind, property, the same way as the visible ones."[7] To perform his duties properly the physician must know what is occurring within the body. "So noble is man and so exalted is the physician's mandate, and thus so great must the art of the physician be, that none of the body's needs should be unknown to him."[8] Here Paracelsus confronts the perennial problem of how to understand the workings of the organism and the powers of medicinal substances—which are invisible to the eye but must be known if the healer is to heal.

How is the physician, through experience, to acquire knowledge of the functioning of the body and of the workings of medicine? This can be divided into (1) how knowledge in general is derived from experience, and (2) how the physician's knowledge is derived from experience.

Experience as a Source of Knowledge

Experience yields knowledge of invisible things: (1) through the five senses whereby man perceives the external world, and (2) through the "light of nature", meaning man's capacity to understand and interpret the data of sense-perception.

Paracelsus extolls sense-perception as the true source of knowledge.

> Your eyes which take delight in experience are your masters; for your own fantasies and speculations cannot advance you so far that you can boast of being a physician. Nor can you acquire the art of medicine by sophisms, or after the manner of the sophists, those pseudo-scientists, who imagine that their own wisdom reaches as far as the end of the earth and the sea and all the elements.
>
> (S-M I/XI 29. *Das Buch von den tartarischen Krankheiten. Das ander capitel*)
>
> From his own head a man cannot learn the theory of medicine, but only from that which his eyes see and his fingers touch. . . . If a man were brought up in a monastery and had never experienced anything but what takes place in the monastery, and the monastic customs and ways, he would know nothing except these very monastic customs. If he should then encounter other customs, he would not know what to do, for he knows only his own tune. . . . He would not have anything to say except what he had learned in his monastery; moreover this monastic doctrine originated only in speculation . . . and was contrived only by men. . . . Consequently, our monastic scholar remains inexperienced and can never get to the fundament of things, whence everything comes; for this can never be discovered by pure theory.
>
> (S-M I/XI 24-25. *Das Buch von den tartarischen Krankheiten. Das ander capitel*)

And he gives this the usual religious interpretation:

> If Christ says "*Perscrutamini scripturas*," why whould I not say of this, "*Perscrutamini naturas rerum.*"
>
> (S-M I/XI 130. *Sieben Defensiones.* First Defense)

> Does not the sight of a thing give the eyes a true foundation? Then let the foundation be made solid . . . what can the carpenter learn without the knowledge acquired by his eyesight? Or what can be proved without the help of the eyesight? Did not God reveal Himself to our eyes, and does He not call us to witness that our eyes have seen Him? How then should an art or anything else deprive itself of the testimony of the eyes?
>
> (S-M I/XI 142. *Sieben Defensiones.* Fourth Defense)

The data acquired by man through his senses are transformed into knowledge by the "light of nature"—Paracelsus' reinterpretation of the *logos*:

> For the light of nature is only reason [*vernunft*], and nothing else. Therefore he who wants to be a just physician must, out of his reason, that is, out of the light of nature, believe and medicate, and not without that light. For the light is that which gives the belief.
>
> (S-M I/I 300. *Ein Buechlein (Philosophia) de generatione Hominis.*)

It will be recalled that "nature" is identified by Paracelsus with "experience." The light of "nature" is thus the capacity to learn from experience, to remove the veil from the potential knowledge which lies hidden in each of us:

> We received all the members of our body at the first creation, after all other things had been created. But the knowledge that man needs was not yet in Adam but was given him only when he was expelled from Paradise. Then he received "knowledge" through the Angel; but not all knowledge. For he and his children must learn one thing after another in the light of nature, *in order to bring to light that which lies hidden in all things*. For although man was created whole as regards his body, he was not so created as regards his "art." All the arts have been given him, but not in an immediately recognizable form; he

must discover them by learning. We learn that which we already know. There is no peasant who does not already know everything by his natural light. But he overshadows it so that it does not shine forth.

(S-M I/VIII 291. *Von den hinfallenden Siechtagen. Der drit paragraphus*)

This capacity in man is exactly the same as the capacity possessed by animals to learn from experience:

A snake which gets wounded heals itself. Why? Man also seeks his healing in herbs and stones. From where does he have the reason and art? Out of the brutish kind, for that reason he seeks it. If now this is done by the snake, do not be astonished for you are the snake's son. Your father does it, and you inherit his capacity; the snake is a doctor, and therefore you, in a brutish sense, are also a doctor. . . . Now as the snake knows her help and knows the herb, there is also such an understanding in you, that you shall know by the same spirit which teaches the snake and is a brutish spirit and belongs to the brutes. Therefore do not be astonished that the snake knows medicine. She has had it for a longer time than you, and you have it from her; for you are made out of the matter of brutish nature, and therefore both of you are equal.

(S-M I/XIII 316. *De Fundamento Scientiarum Sapientiaeque, drei Traktate. Tractatus III.* Also, S-M I/VIII 328, *Von hinfallenden Siechtagen der Mutter. Par. II.* An animal understands to drink when it is thirsty through its senses and its *vernunft*)

The contrast for Paracelsus is not between the *logos* and experience, as it was for the ancients, since he has assimilated experience to the *logos* by interpreting the latter as the capacity to learn from experience. He does formulate an opposition between knowledge acquired through the light of nature and that revealed divinely: "The eternal wisdom originates directly in the light of the Holy Ghost, the other wisdom directly in the light of nature."[9] But the more important formulation of the ancient opposition between *logos* and experience is for him the opposition between true knowledge—revealed by sense perception and the light of nature—and the false and uncertain knowledge revealed by logic:

> What need have you of all this rhetorical twaddle which doesn't form a physician but breaks him. What are you seeking in your logic and your dialectic, which are all against the physician and interfere with the light of nature. These things are not given by nature but by the dark spirit . . . who delights in these illusory things.
>
> (S-M I/VIII 321. *Von hinfallenden Siechtagen der Mutter. Par. I.*)

The books of logic and dialectic are true only inasmuch as they agree with the light of nature: "that which is in disagreement with it is like a labyrinth that has neither sure entrance nor exit."[10]

The Categories of Knowledge

By employing his five senses and the light of nature, man acquires knowledge of nature. The various branches of this knowledge are called by Paracelsus: philosophy, astrology, science (*scientia*) and wisdom (*sapientia*).[c]

Sapientia is knowledge of the primal causes of all things, and this book of knowledge can be read only by God.[11] Mortal man is sometimes admitted to it by special dispensation, but for all practical purposes it may be eliminated from consideration. Philosophy and astrology are that knowledge of the outer world which man acquires through his senses and the light of nature. "We have the truths of philosophy from nature; she has taught us these without fantasizing. Just as Christ offered his person to our eyes, so we have personal

[c]Although Paracelsus in one place maintains that astrology is a part of astronomy (S-M I/XII 91. *Astronomia Magna. Bk. I. Was astrologia sei und was der astrologus. Cap. IV.*), from the point of view of the twentieth century, he means astrology when he states *astronomia.* His interest is exclusively in the effect of the stars on human events and human destiny. Hence we will translate *astronomia* as "astrology," since "astronomy" would be misleading.

teachers in nature. Philosophy is born out of seeing and touching, and not out of nonseeing. For seeing and touching beget the truth."[12]

Philosophy and astrology differ only in their subject matter. The former is knowledge of the terrestrial globe; the latter is knowledge of the heavens.[13] Both philosophy and astrology are learned through the senses and the light of nature, from observation of externals.

> A physician should first of all be an astrologer. Now necessity demands that his eyes should give him evidence, in order that he may be such; without this evidence he is only an astrological gossip.
>
> (S-M I/XI 144. *Sieben Defensiones.* Fourth Defense.)

Finally, Paracelsus introduces the concept of *scientia*—meaning the laws of the universe and differing from *philosophia* which is man's *understanding* of the universe. *Scientia* is independent of man's knowledge. However, when a physician understands the *scientia* of the universe, and insofar as he understands it, it becomes part of his philosophy.[14] *Scientia* also includes knowledge of the functioning of the organism.[15]

Knowledge of *scientia* is given by the light of nature and not by speculation.[16] In particular, the practice of medicine brings the physician to an understanding of the *scientia* of the organism.[17]

Experience as the Source of Medical Knowledge

Hence medical knowledge is part and parcel of philosophical and astrological knowledge and is acquired in the same way. Just as the author of *Ancient Medicine* denied that "clear knowledge of the *physis* can be obtained from any source other than a study of medicine," so Paracelsus maintains that medical practice is the source of knowledge of (the) nature:

> The mysteries of the firmament are revealed by the physician; to him the mysteries of nature are manifest, and he communicates them to other learned men.

> (S-M I/VIII 76. *Paragranum. Vorrede und erste zwei Buecher. Entwuerfe und I. Ausarbeitung in Berezhausen. Der erste grund der arznei, welcher ist philosophia*)

> Of all men the physician is supreme in the study and knowledge of nature and her light, and that is what enables him to be a helper of the sick.
>
> (S-M I/X 277-278. *Das zweite Buch der Grossen Wundarznei. Der erst tractat. Das XX. capitel*)

The physician obtains this knowledge of nature through his experience. And to Paracelsus this means his therapeutic experience. To Paracelsus medicine means therapeutics. Therapeutics is the beginning and end of medicine, to which all else is subordinate.

> Therapeutics is the noblest pearl and the supreme treasure, and it holds first place in medicine; and there is nothing on earth that can be valued more highly than the curing of the sick. . . . It is a commandment of God that you shall love Him, this is the supreme good, and there is nothing that man may prize above it. The next commandment says thou shalt love thy neighbor as thyself, and it follows immediately upon the first. Now by what manner on earth can greater love be shown a neighbor than when a man motivated by true love discovers the curative virtues of remedies, in order to avert the great sufferings, the diseases, and the death that threaten his neighbor?
>
> (S-M I/X 350. *Das zweite Buch der Grossen Wundarznei. Der drit tractat. Doctors Paracelsi vorred*)

> What sense would it make, or what would it benefit a physician if he discovered the origin of diseases but could not cure or alleviate them?
>
> (S-M I/X 276. *Das zweite Buch der Grossen Wundarznei. Der erst tractat. Das XX. capitel*)

Hence medical theory is based on therapeutic practice. "For the fruits govern the roots and not the roots the fruits."[18] "For the ground lies where the remedy lies; in the latter lies the recognition, understanding, knowledge, and that which leads to them."[19d] "Practice should not be based on speculative theory; theory should be derived from practice."[20]

> Theory and practice should together form one and should remain undivided. For every theory is also a kind of speculative practice, and is no more and no less than active practice. But what would you do if your speculation did not jibe with findings based on practice? Both must be true or both must be untrue. Look at the carpenter: first he builds his house in his head. But whence does he take this structure? From his active practice. And if he did not have this, he could not erect his structure in his mind; thus, both theory and practice rest upon experience.[e]
>
> (S-M I/VI 314. *Von Blattern, Laehme, Beulen, Loechern, und Zittrachten der Franzosen und ihres gleichen. Das erste Buch. Das viert capitel*)

The whole purpose and aim of medicine is its practice:

> The art is that which is effective. This is the aim—not knowledge but performance; that is the physician's art.
>
> (S-M I/VIII 173. *Das Buch Paragranum. Der ander tractat, von der astronomia*)

The relative positions of theory and practice constituted another of the issues which divided the Rationalists and the Empirics. Paracelsus realized that the Galenists of his time adhered to the opposite view: "We are also separated in that they take the *practicam* from the *theorik*, while I take the *theorik* from the *praktik*."[21] The Galenist theory was merely an arbitrary invention to cover up and justify their practice.[f]

[d] S-M I/VI 179: "For every cure gives the origin, beginning, essence, middle resolution, and end; that is the cornerstone of the physician." (*Entwuerfe, Notizen, und Ausarbeitungen zur Bertheonea, Argumentum III.*).

[e] Cf. with Aristotle, *Parts of Animals* 639b 16-640a 8 (above, p. 148).

[f] S-M I/IX 153. He adds: *"und [sie] habens dohin gebracht das al menschen die arznei fliehen und haltens fuer bueberei und bescheisserei" (Die drei (vier) Buecher des Opus Paramirum. Tractatus quartus et tartarus quartus*).

Since Paracelsus is so categorical in maintaining that practice precedes theory, we are justified in examining his practice to see what light it throws on his theory. His theory can be understood and made a consistent whole only if based on his practice. Hence the argument in the present analysis proceeds from Paracelsus' practice to his theory and attempts to make the theory intelligible in the light of his practice.

NOTES

[1] S-M I/VIII 157. *Das Buch Paragranum. Der erste tractat.*

[2] S-M I/IV 60. *De Gradibus et Compositionibus Receptorum et Naturalium Libri VII. Liber Septimus. Caput tertium.*

[3] S-M I/VIII 157. *Das Buch Paragranum. Der erste tractat.*

[4] S-M I/VI 58. *Drei Buecher der Wundarznei. Argumentum ueber dise ganze wundarznei doctoris Theophrasti.*

[5] S-M I/VI 179. *Entwuerfe, Notizen, und Ausarbeitungen zur Bertheonea. Argumentum III. in quo causam enumerat.*

[6] S-M I/IV 496. *Deutsche Kommentare zu den Aphorismen des Hippokrates. Aphorismus I. Experimentum fallax.*

[7] S-M I/I 57. *Elf Traktat. 3. Von farbsuchten, Andere Redaktion.*

[8] S-M I/VIII 339. *Von hinfallenden Siechtagen der Mutter. Par. IV.*

[9] S-M I/XII 8. *Astronomia Magna. Vorrede in die ganz sagacem philosophiam.*

[10] S-M I/XI 170. *Labyrinthus Medicorum Errantium. Theophrastus lectori Salutem.*

[11] S-M I/XI 171. *Labyrinthus Medicorum Errantium. Das erste capitel.*

[12] S-M I/VIII 306. *Von den hinfallenden Siechtagen. Von corallen.* On the light of nature as the source of astrological knowledge, see S-M I/XI 164. *Labyrinthus medicorum errantium. Theophrastus von Hohenheim sagt den Hippokratischen doctoribus seinen gruss.* Cf. also S-M I/XI 144. *Sieben Defensiones.* Fourth Defense. S-M I/XII 91. *Astronomia Magna. Bk. I. Cap. IV, Was astrologia sei und was der astrologus.*

[13] S-M I/VIII 373. *Zwei Buecher von der Pestilenz und ihren Zufaellen. Das erst Buch. Das erst Capitel.* S-M I/VIII 77. *Paragranum. Vorrede und erste zwei Buecher. Entwuerfe und I. Ausarbeitung in Berezhausen. Der erste grund der arznei, welcher ist philosophia.*

[14] S-M I/IX 93. *Die drei (vier) Buecher des Opus Paramirum. Liber secundus, caput secundum.*

[15] S-M I/VIII 71-72. *Paragranum. Vorrede und erste zwei Buecher. Entwuerfe und I. Ausarbeitung in Berezhausen. Der erste grund der arznei, welcher ist philosophia.*

[16] S-M I/I 38. *Elf Tractat. 2. Vom Schwinen oder schwintsucht. Andere Redaktion.*

[17] S-M I/XI 195. *Labyrinthus medicorum errantium. Das VI. capitel.* For further discussion of *scientia*, see below, pp. 000.

[18] S-M I/I 42. *Elf Traktat. Vom Schwinen oder Schwintsucht. Andere Redaktion.*

[19] S-M I/VIII 83-84. *Paragranum. Vorrede und erste zwei Buecher. Entwuerfe und I. Ausarbeitung in Berezhausen. Der erste grund der arznei, welcher ist philosophia.*

[20] S-M I/XI 183. *Labyrinthus Medicorum Errantium. Das IV. capitel.*

[21] S-M I/VI 211. *Von allen offenen Schaeden. Zu dem Leser.*

CHAPTER XII

PARACELSUS' PRACTICE

The Doctrine of Similars

Paracelsus' whole medical practice was based on the doctrine of similars, on the idea that the substance which causes the disease will also cure it:

> Never a hot illness has been cured by something cold, nor a cold one by something hot. But it has happened that like has cured like.
>
> (S-M I/IX 236. *Entwuerfe zu den vier Buecher des Opus Paramirum. Theophrastus Hohenheim de origine morborum et sanitatis. Tractatus II.*)
>
> It would be a wild kind of order if we should seek our salvation in the opposite; thus, when a child cries for bread to his father, he will not give him snakes for bread.
>
> (S-M I/IX 63. *Die drei (vier) Buecher des Opus Paramirum. Liber primus, Caput V.*)
>
> Now the things in nature are so created that nothing in her happens by opposition. That is, contrary things do not get together in the course of nature, only the same to the same.
>
> (S-M I/IX 528. *Von der Bergsucht und anderen Bergkrankheiten. Das drit Buch. Der drit tractat. Das ander capitel*)
>
> For man is not to be understood thus, that contrary were treated with contrary, such as fire with water, but same in same. For if it were so that only something contrary would drive away a contrary, such as the fire by water, what would there then be to drive away the water? What the air? What the earth? What the winter? What the summer?

> (S-M I/X 553-554. *Von Oeffnung der Haut, ein Fragment. Liber primus. Caput VII.*)

Just as the Empirics opposed their similars to the Rationalist contraries, so Paracelsus attacks the Galenic medicine of the schools for the same reason: "They have always but mended, hot to cold, constricting to laxative, and with such charlatanism, in which there never has been, and never may be, any ground such as behooves a physician."[1]

The only opposites are medicine and disease:

> The physician always has to use that which is ordained against [the disease]. And where that is not understood by the physician, but where he always wants to quench fire by water, then he goes astray in medicine and harms the patients.
>
> (S-M I/X 329. *Das zweite Buch der Grossen Wundarznei. Der ander tractat. Das XV. Capitel*)

> *Contraria a contrariis curantur*, that is, hot drives away what is cold, that is wrong. It has never been true in medicine, but thus: *arcanum* and illness are *contraria. Arcanum* is health, and illness is antagonistic to health; these two drive out one another, each the other. Those are the antagonists which drive out one another, and always the one drives the other out by its death, so that there is nothing any more of its antagonist, which total driving out is not the case with the cold and the hot.
>
> (S-M I/VIII 88-89. *Paragranum. Vorrede und erste zwei Buecher. Entwuerfe und I. Ausarbeitung in Berezhausen. Der erste grund der arznei, welcher ist philosophia*)

The Galenic dietary prescriptions, also based upon contraries, are equally valueless:

> Food serves the physical body merely as does manure the field. Such food brings forth no fruit in the physical body, it does not augment the seed in it, it does nothing else but sustain the body and make it luscious as manure does the field .... Food is useful to man as if it were its fertilizer. For neither life nor reason, nor the indwelling

> spirits, nor anything in the same category comes from eating and drinking . . . . The food acts upon the body in conformity with the body's wont, yet it has no influence upon what is in the body.
>
> (S-M I/I 204. *Volumen Medicinae Paramirum, Bk. 3, Cap. III.*)

Against the Galenic contraries Paracelsus asserted the doctrine of similars in all branches of therapeutics. Some of the extensions of this doctrine would appear, *a priori*, quite indefensible. For instance, diseases which arise from wounds are cured by the infliction of wounds:

> There are many illnesses which are made to go away by wounds, namely, all those which arise through wounds: such as lethargy and paralysis. These come from wounds and, on the other hand, are healed by wounds.
>
> (S-M I/VI 100-101. *Drei Buecher der Wundarznei, Bertheonei. Cap. XV.*)

And calcareous deposits (tartar) within the body, caused by calcium in the food, can be dissolved by remedies made of calcium and calcium-like substances:

> The things which I propose are the following: crabs' eyes, *lapis iudaicus, lapis lyncis, lapis lazuli, lapis spongiae, lapis aquilae, lapis glaciei,* etc. Not that all of them should be taken together, but each one is sufficient by itself . . . you should know that, to drive out the tartar, roots, herbs, seeds, etc., are not enough, but only the equivalent stones, as indicated above, of which there are more than I have listed. In each is the power of driving away tartar.
>
> (S-M I/XI 108-109. *Das Buch von den tartarischen Krankheiten. Das XVIII. capitel*)

We have three reasons for assuming that cure by similars is rooted in Paracelsus' personal experience. In the first place, he states that his theory is derived from his practice, that is, from experience. In the second place, cure by similars is the focal point of all his medical views. And, finally, this doctrine dates from Paracelsus' early years in the metal mines.

His work on miners' diseases sets forth his understanding of cure by similars in its clearest form:

> If he [the miner] now has an illness, and takes the ore which he has been breaking and melts the silver out of it, then he finds in that which is extracted that which has made him ill. Therefore then know that the fume that goes from the ore has the same kind of poison in it that comes off the silver when it is being melted. Thus also the rose can give off a smell and make us faint by this smell, while the *corpus* of the rose is undamaged, and thus know that a power emanates from things and comes into man. This power leads men into a long illness which would be shorter if the *corpus* itself had been taken. For example, if arsenic is taken, then death comes quickly, but if the *corpus* is not taken, but only its *spiritus,* then instead of one hour, it takes a whole year; that is, what the *corpus* accomplishes in ten hours, the *spiritus* takes ten years . . . . Know then that whoever wants to understand the mine diseases with certainty, must know the symptoms of acute poisoning and death by the *corpus* of these substances. And by the same symptoms, if observed carefully, he may infer the same mine diseases–which species it is, i.e. out of which *corpus* the *spiritus* has arisen. Thus the symptoms are recognized. For example, the taking of realgar dries out the lungs, out of which dryness the breath is changed, and there is labored breathing and loss of color in the face. Also it gives rise to fissures and rifts in the liver, and with the same goes an unnatural thirst, and the folds of the stomach gnaw and grind and peel off like the bark of a tree. There are dry fits and a heavy, hard, digestion, also hot flashes, pounding, and trembling of the heart. After that a breaking out in all the members and after that quinsy and accompanying head-disease. Thus note the effects of the poison, and with which illnesses they are accompanied. Thus over the course of long years and days the same *spiritus* of the realgar gives rise to a steady illness with the same manifestations as those mentioned above. Such

infected miners are easily, depending upon the course of the outer sky, inclined to all sky-induced illnesses, as fever, consumption, madness, quinsy.

> (S-M I/IX 478-479. *Von der Bergsucht und anderen Bergkrankheiten. Das erste Buch. Der dritte tractat. Das ander capitel*)

If the poison of antimony is taken, then there is a dry, hacking cough, much stinging in the side and headache, much drying out of stools, much ulcering of the spleen, hot blood, mange, scabies, parching, and jaundice.

> (S-M I/IX 480. *Von der Bergsucht und anderen Bergkrankheiten. Das erste Buch. Der dritte tractat. Das drit capitel*)

For the good heals the evil next to it. For example, that which makes jaundice also cures jaundice, and if the good is separated from the evil, then the *arcanum* against jaundice is there . . . also gold is a medicine of all those illnesses which its ore miners contract. As also the *saturnus* has with it the *arcanum* of those illnesses which arise from lead, and thus it is to be understood with regard to others, that what may be harmful to us through our hands, the same is also again fashioned by our hands into a remedy. And what is impossible for these *arcana*, will be impossible [for anything else to cure].

> (S-M I/IX 481-482. *Von der Bergsucht und anderen Bergkrankheiten. Das erste Buch. Der dritte tractat. Das viert capitel*)

These passages contain a number of seminal ideas: (1) the diseases of metal miners are cured by the metals which cause them, (2) disease is a spiritual entity caused by an emanation from the metal, (3) the symptoms of disease may be viewed as equivalent (although in a milder form) to the symptoms of metal poisoning, (4) the remedy for a given disease is found by separating the "good" from the "evil" in the metal at the root of the disease.

These passages also reveal Paracelsus' very acute powers of observation.[a]

The remainder of Paracelsus' medical teachings, and his cosmological views as well, may be interpreted as his effort to understand why pills and medicines made from lead, gold, and other metals seemed to cure miners and smelters of the diseases arising from exposure to these metals or their fumes. He developed a series of doctrinal corollaries, discussed in detail below, each of which offers a point of departure for understanding his cosmology.

These corollaries, however, must not be regarded as causal explanations of the doctrine of similars, since that would mean understanding the ultimate causes of things, and *sapientia* (the knowledge of causes) is the province of God alone. The process of cure is a mystery: "For the medicine is such that so far no physician has yet seen in what way the illness uses it for defense and how the medicine makes one healthy."[2]

> As little as the physician may know how the plants grow out of the earth from what *materia*, but only the earth knows it, so little may he understand the disease.
>
> (S-M I/VII 270. *Vom Ursprung und Herkommen der Franzosen. Das viert Buch. Das VI. capitel*)

In any case, the great variety of theories offered, and their mutual incompatibility, rule out the possibility that Paracelsus was trying to present a physiological explanation of the doctrine of similars.

The purpose of these theories is to guide the physician's practice. They are symbolic interpretations and extrapolations from the observed facts of sickness and cure. They aim to present the *scientia* of nature, that is, its practice, in order to assist the physician in *his* practice.

[a]They were not confined to physical diseases only. He was equally sharp-sighted in observing the symptoms of mental derangement. Gregory Zilboorg writes: "Paracelsus anticipated the descriptive method in psychiatry by almost fifty years. He describes the clinical symptoms of epilepsy, mania, and hysteria . . . in the manner of an earnest observer . . . . It is indeed surprising, and rather puzzling, to find so many details, so accurately related and so well arranged, in these clinical descriptions of Paracelsus." Sigerist, *op. cit.*, p. 131.

The New Science of Medicine

Paracelsus' first interpretation of the doctrine of similars is that the mineral in the remedy "drives out" of the body the mineral which lies at the base of the disease:

> In the same manner as the devil is driven out of man, the poisonous diseases are expelled by means of such physic, just as evil expels evil and good retains good.
>
> (S-M I/IX 477. *Von der Bergsucht und anderen Bergkrankheiten. Das erste Buch. Der dritte tractat. Das erst capitel*)

> Therefore then know that the illnesses which are equivalent to the outer ones in their manifestations, come from the same matters. Hereupon, in compounding recipes, it must be known what parts are against the arsenic, what are against the *mercurius,* what against sulphur, etc., and all minerals. These shall be understood in this table, in which it is learned to remedy all minerals by minerals, for they themselves drive away one another.
>
> (S-M I/IX 242. *Entwuerfe zu den vier Buechern des Opus Paramirum*)

The second is that the various minerals have different "flavors." Hence the mineral in the remedy affects the mineral at the base of the disease by its opposed flavor:

> Against a bitter salt in medicine, its like is a sweet salt, not a bitter one! Against a sharp one, a mild one; against a dry, a damp one, and thus on and on.
>
> (S-M I/X 558. *Von Oeffnung der Haut. Ein Fragment. Liber secundus de cura ulcerum. Caput I.*)

Closely allied to this is the view that every substance contains something beneficial and something harmful. The harmful element causes disease, while the curative power of the substance comes from its beneficial component:

> That which makes the jaundice also cures the jaundice. Which, consequently, is to say that in the same thing there is the evil and the good; out of the evil grows the

jaundice, and if the good is separated from the evil, then the *arcanum* against the jaundice is there.

(S-M I/IX 481. *Von der Bergsucht und anderen Bergkrankheiten. Das erste Buch. Der dritte tractat. Das viert capitel*)

The corollary is that a technique must be found to separate the good from the bad, and here Paracelsus introduces alchemy:

> [It is said that] the prescriptions which I write are poison, corrosive, and an extraction of all that is evil and poisonous in nature . . . . [I ask] whether they knew what was poison and what not, or whether in poison there is no *mysterium* of nature . . . . What every simple is in itself, is by art made into many things, into all shapes and forms like food which stands on the table; if a man eats it, it becomes human flesh, through a dog, dog's flesh; through a cat, cat's flesh. Thus it is with medicines; they become what you make of them. If it is possible to make evil out of good, it is also possible to make good out of evil. No one should condemn a thing who knows not its transmutation, and who knows not what separation does. Though a thing is poison, it may well be turned into non-poison.
>
> (S-M I/XI 137, 139. *Sieben Defensiones.* Third Defense)
>
> The process of [alchemical] separation understand in this way: you see that nothing is so evil that it does not have some excellent good in it. Consider . . . malmsey is the highest drink and the best; on the other hand, however, it has the most corrosive vinegar in it, which is a pure *alumen.* Thus nature is so ordered that always something evil and something good together make an *arcanum,* and the poison must be in the body just as much as the balsam, the sour as well as the sweet; for in the body there are all colors, all tastes, and the like . . . . And if you wonder how the *alumen* or sal, etc. may be invisibly in the bodies, remember how vinegar lies dormant in wine

> and is never noticed, and still more how copper lies concealed in vitriol and is the vitriol itself.
>
> (S-M I/VI 129-130. *Drei Buecher der Wundarznei. Cap. V. Vom beinfresser*)

This theory and the preceding one are obvious attempts to evade the full force of the doctrine of similars by introducing the principle of contrariety.[b]

The third interpretation adopted by Paracelsus is that the disease accepts a remedy of the same "anatomy" as itself. If they were not similar in form, the disease and the remedy could not get together within the organism:

> Thus nature and man want to be fitted together in health and in disease and matched together and brought together. In this lies the way of cure and of making healthy.
>
> (S-M I/VIII 185. *Das Buch Paragranum. Alchimia der dritte grund medicinae*)
>
> Member to member, so illness and *arcanum* get together.
>
> (S-M I/VIII 88. *Paragranum. Vorrede und erste zwei Buecher. Entwuerfe und I. Ausarbeitung in Berezhausen. Der erste grund der arznei, welcher ist philosophia*)
>
> Now this anatomy is as though two are together, a teacher and a disciple; the teacher must have the same anatomy as the disciple. Otherwise the latter will not be able to learn.
>
> (S-M I/I 321. *Liber de podagricis et suis speciebus. Liber I. Anatomia*)
>
> . . . in the same way know of the medicine that it is a woman in form, as is indicated above. Therefore then learn how to recognize the spouse in all growing things [*gewechse*—natural substances], i.e. the form of the

[b]Another formulation of the law of cure in terms of contraries is the following: "if it is melancholic, then you shall for that use *contraria*. As the *melancholicus* is sad, so heal him by a medicine that is laughing. If he is laughing, then heal him by a sad medicine." S-M I/II 452. *Das siebente Buch in der Arznei, von den Krankheiten die der Vernunft berauben, de morbis amentium. Methodus secunda. Das V. capitel.*

medicine which is in the medicine and which is indicated to you by its power and the shape of its physiognomy . . . . For as the inner man of the illness lies in the man and is in the man, thus there is also such a man in the medicine, who has hands and feet, head and eyes, belly and everything, and the way the inner one is, so also is his spouse.

(S-M I/I 366. *Von den Podagrischen Krankheiten und was ihnen anhaengig (zwei Buecher). Liber secundus*)

The illnesses are forged and made in the same way as man is, in that each illness is a man, i.e. in the property and form of a man, and thus also the medicine. It thereupon follows that the illness desires its woman, that is, the medicine. Now it is necessary to bring these into concordance, i.e. a conjunction of the two into one anatomy, like man and woman. If these are found, then is the physician whole and perfect.

(S-M I/I 363. *Von den podagrischen Krankheiten und was ihnen anhaengig (zwei Buecher). Liber secundus*)

Another theory is astrological. The remedy comes together with the disease and cures it because both are governed by the same star:

All operations and virtues of medicines are governed by the sky, if it makes them concord and conjoin. If it does not make them concord, then the physician's purpose will not be accomplished. Thus in selecting and prescribing medicines, you must fit together and match the sky of the disease with the sky of the medicine.

(S-M I/VIII 170. *Das Buch Paragranum. Der ander tractat. Von der astronomia*)

It now follows that sky and earth, air and water, is one man in the science, and man is one world with sky and earth, with air and water also in the science. Thus the saturn of the microcosm accepts the saturn of the sky; thus the jupiter of the sky accepts the jupiter of the microcosm, for they are two skies and one conjunction which are not separated.

(S-M I/IX 94. *Die drei (vier) Buecher des Opus Paramirum. Liber secundus. Caput secundum*)

The final theory relies on the healing power of nature. The body's self-healing capacity (in some cases, the illness itself) seizes the remedy and uses it curatively:

> Therefore know that the illness, since it acts this way with the medicine, must itself be experienced and at least must be learned in the medicine . . . . the nature is the physician . . . . If the medicine is the right weapon, then the illness itself will strike, and you will not comprehend how the stroke was done.
>
> (S-M I/VII 239. *Vom Ursprung und Herkommen der Franzosen. Das dritte Buch. Das ander capitel*)

A corollary is that, since cure is by the innate healing power, the physician must strengthen this power. Paracelsus occasionally calls illness a process of combustion through which the sulphurous component of the body is consumed; medication must strengthen this sulphurous component.[3]

Each interpretation of cure by similars casts light on some aspect of Paracelsus' medical cosmology. The latter's apparent inconsistency and illogicality are due to the incompatibility of these interpretations with one another. For example, the idea that one mineral drives out the other by virtue of its different flavor has little in common with the idea that the mineral in the remedy strengthens its equivalent in the organism. Sometimes the interpretations are complementary, however, or can be made so by slight adjustments of doctrine: the idea that the mineral of the disease is expelled by the mineral in the remedy has a tenuous connection with expulsion of the disease by the body's innate healing power.

But none of these reconciliations of apparent contradictions (which are the despair of Paracelsan commentators) are really necessary, since they were not necessary for Paracelsus himself. For him the connections among the aspects of his medical cosmology were supplied by practice alone—by the observed fact of cure through similars.

NOTES

[1] S-M I/VIII 305. *Von den hinfallenden Siechtagen. Von Corallen.*

[2] S-M I/VII 238. *Vom Ursprung und Herkommen der Franzosen. Das dritte Buch. Das ander capitel.*

[3] S-M I/VI 107. *Drei Buecher der Wundarznei. Das erste Buch. Cap. XVIII.*

CHAPTER XIII

MINERALS DRIVE OUT THEIR EQUIVALENTS: ASTROLOGICAL CORRESPONDENCES

The expulsion of disease minerals by the minerals in remedies has as corollaries: that the components of the organism are mineralic, that the components of the remedy are also mineralic, and that disease has a mineralic origin.

This formulation of cure by similars is an effort to analyze the organism and its environment in the same terms—to find a common denominator of the two—and is Paracelsus' version of the Hippocratic concept that disease arises from the impact of morbific environmental stimuli on the organism.

The mineralic component of the environment acts on the mineralic component of the organism.

The outcome is the doctrine of microcosm and macrocosm, and the *anatomia mineralis*.

* * * * * * * * *

The concepts of microcosm and macrocosm had been current in philosophy since antiquity and were adapted by Paracelsus to his particular needs.[a]

The microcosm, man, lies in the macrocosm of the universe and is subject to its influence:

> The whole world surrounds man as a circle surrounds one point. From this it follows that all things are related to this one point, no differently from an apple seed which is surrounded and preserved by the fruit, and which draws its sustenance from it . . . . Similarly, man is a seed and the world is his apple; and just as the seed fares in the

[a]A good discussion of the historical antecedents of this doctrine may be found in Pagel's *Paracelsus*, pp. 65ff. and *Das Medizinische Weltbild, passim.*

apple, so does man fare in the world which surrounds him.

(S-M I/XII 164, 167. *Astronomia Magna. Bk. I, Das Buch der Philosophei des himlischen Firmaments. Das sibent capitel*)

The surrounding environment affects man's health in several ways: through his food and drink, the air, and the stars:

It is also well not to forget that the vessels, instruments and passages of elimination are defiled orally by the air, or by food or drink. This takes place as follows. The air which we inhale is not without poison by which we are affected considerably. In this connection remember, however, that with the multitude of foods and drinks, and the foods and drinks which cause trouble and are not attuned to the instruments of the body, even to the extent of disrupting the instruments—and that quite considerably—the alchemist cannot function and digestion becomes putrefaction and decay. The stomach and the rest of the organs in the body adjust themselves in accordance with the quality of the poison in the thing which man takes in .... For you physicians ought to remember and realize that there is only one poison which produces the disease hearth, and not several. For instance, when you eat meat, cabbage, vegetables, and seasoning, and decay sets in in the stomach after their enjoyment, not all of them are culprits; only one is the culprit. Either it is the poison of the cabbage, or it is that of the meat, that of the vegetables or that of the seasoning ... Let this, thus, be also one principle by which to recognize the mother of all diseases, of which there are many hundreds.[b]

(S-M I/I 198. *Volumen Medicinae Paramirum. Bk. II, Cap. XI.*)

... the air is the *corpus* from which the lung receives its sickness, and outside of the physical air, nothing harmful

[b]The "alchemist" is the vital force which effects digestion (and other functions). For more on coction and digestion see below, pp. 430-431.

> is added to the lung. Take an example, someone drinks, and this drinking turns out to be harmful to the lungs. This injury does not arise from the drink, but from the air that is contained in this drink . . . . The air must be discussed, and it is entirely to be understood like a food, and as it is possible that food produces diseases, thus it is also possible for the air to give birth to these things . . . . In the same manner as you see that a chaos lies between heaven and earth, which produces all the diseases of the lungs, their fevers, ulcers, consumption, plethora, cough, gasping, and oppression, together with all the other kinds. Man must nourish his lungs with this same chaos. Now the chaos is governed by the power of the stars. It is therefore subject to their rule over it, and as this species of ruled chaos is given to the air, thus does it impress itself on the lungs.
>
> (S-M I/IX 465. *Von der Bergsucht und anderen Bergkrankheiten, Bk. I, Tract. I, Cap. II.*)

The microcosm is affected by the macrocosm because both are made from the same substance:

> The Scriptures state that God took the *limus terrae,* the primordial stuff of the earth, and formed man out of this mass. Furthermore they state that man is ashes and powder, dust and earth; and this proves sufficiently that he is made of this primordial substance . . . . But *limus terrae* is also the Great World, and thus man was created from heaven and earth. *Limus terrae* is an extract of the firmament, of the universe of stars, and at the same time of all the elements.
>
> (S-M I/XII 33. *Astronomia Magna. Bk. I. Das Buch der Philosophei des himlischen firmaments. Das ander capitel*)

> For what is outside is also inside; and what is not outside man is not inside. The outer and the inner are one thing, one constellation, one influence, one concordance, one duration . . . . one fruit. For this is the *limbus,* the primordial matter which contains all creatures in germ, just as man is contained in the *limbus* of his parents. The

> *limbus* of Adam was heaven and earth, water and air; and thus man remains like the *limbus*, he too contains heaven and earth, water and air; indeed, he is nothing but these.
>
> (S-M I/VIII 180. *Das Buch Paragranum. Der ander tractat. Von der astronomia*)

> Man and the outer things are matched to one another, inasmuch as they accept each other . . . . Inasmuch as man, now, is made out of the *limbus*, and the *limbus* is the whole world, then it is to be known accordingly that anything accepts its like. For if man were not thus made out of the whole circle, from all the pieces, then he could not be the microcosm, and then he would not be capable of accepting what is in the macrocosm. But he is of it, that is, of its substance, because everything he eats is of it . . . . This link existing, as that of a son to his father, it is thus fitting that no one will help the son more appropriately than the father . . . . when we want to prescribe medicaments, we administer the whole world, that is, all virtues of the sky and earth, of the air and water.
>
> (S-M I/IX 94. *Die drei (vier) Buecher des Opus Paramirum. Liber secundus. Caput secundum*)

But Paracelsus expands the doctrine by incorporating the four Aristotelian elements. Earth and water characterize the earthly part of the macrocosm, fire and air the sidereal part (the stars). Man, however, contains all four elements—showing his extraction from both parts of the macrocosm:[1]

> For the body is twofold, of the nature of the firmament, and earthy.
>
> (S-M I/I 204. *Volumen Medicinae Paramirum. Bk. III, Cap. II.*)

> . . . the sun and the moon and all planets, as well as all the stars and the whole chaos, are in man . . . . The body attracts heaven . . . and this takes place in accordance with the great divine order. Man consists of the four elements, not only—as some hold—because he has four tempers, but also because he partakes of the nature,

essence, and properties of these elements. In him there lies the "young heaven," that is to say, all the planets are part of man's structure and they are the children of the "great heaven" which is their father. For man was created from heaven and earth, and is therefore like them.

(S-M I/VIII 163-164. *Das Buch Paragranum. Der ander tractat. Von der astronomia*)

The sidereal component is the source of man's animal life, that is, the quality of being alive which he has in common with brute creation:

For we must know that man has two kinds of life–animal life and sidereal life .... Hence man has also an animal body and a sidereal body; and both are one, and are not separated. The relations between the two are as follows. The animal body, the body of flesh and blood, is in itself always dead. Only through the action of the sidereal body does the motion of life come into the other body. The sidereal body is fire and air; but it is also bound to the animal life of man.

(S-M I/XIV 597-598. *De Pestilitate*)

After all this you should understand by *ens astrale* the following. It is something we do not see, something which sustains life in us and in everything that is alive and sentient. This something derives from the heavenly bodies. To illustrate: A fire which burns must have wood. Otherwise there would be no fire. Thus you observe that fire is a vital thing, yet it cannot live without wood. Now for the application .... The body is the wood, the life within it the fire. Now life derives its substance from the body. Consequently, the body must possess something which prevents it from being consumed by life, but, on the contrary, continues to exist. That is the thing concerning which we tell you as the *ens*. It hails from the firmament.

(S-M I/I 182. *Volumen Medicinae Paramirum. Bk. I, Cap. VI.*)

The sidereal component of man is also the source of the light of nature (since man possesses this in common with the beasts):

> The light of nature in man comes from the stars, and his flesh and blood belong to the material elements. Thus two influences operate in man. One is that of the firmamental light, which includes wisdom, art, reason. All these are the children of this father . . . . The second influence emanates from matter, and it includes concupiscence, eating, drinking, and everything that relates to the flesh and blood.
>
> (S-M I/XII 22. *Astronomia Magna. Bk. I. Das Buch der philosophei des himlischen firmaments. Das erste capitel*)
>
> Man is the child of two fathers—one father is the earth, the other is heaven . . . . From the earth he receives the material body, from heaven his character. Thus the earth moulds his shape, and then heaven endows this shape with the light of nature.
>
> (S-M I/IX 641. *Von des Bades Pfaeffers Tugenden, Kraeften, und Wirkung. Dem hochwirdigen fuersten und herren, herrn Joann Jacob Russinger*)

The soul is yet a third component of the organism. The body is endowed with soul while still in the womb but after it has received life. Hence, the soul and the principle of life are different.[2] The soul in man is the equivalent of the "virtue" or power in a stone or mineral.[3] The body decays, but the soul lasts forever—just as minerals never lose their powers.[4] The soul is the immortal part of man, with its seat in the heart.[5]

The macrocosm can provoke disease in the microcosm through five mechanisms, which Paracelsus calls the five *entia:* the *ens astrorum*, the *ens veneni*, the *ens naturale,* the *ens spirituale*, and the *ens Dei.* Each of these *entia* characterizes one of the relationships between the microcosm and the macrocosm, that is, one of the ways in which the microcosm can become ill through the influence of the macrocosm.

The *ens astrorum* is a device for fitting astrology into medicine—already foreshadowed by Paracelsus' assertion that part of man is from the stars and by his identification of this sidereal component with the Aristotelian fire and air.

We may first note his general acceptance of the principles of astrology:

> In the beginning of the examination you first judge whether or not the patient is subject to Venus. . . . If you do this thoroughly you now have the name of the illness. This is the first step in the diagnosis and gives you the general disease, which includes many species.
>
> (S-M I/VII 327. *Vom Ursprung und Herkommen der Franzosen. Das VII. Buch. Das drit capitel.* In the *Paragranum*, he calls astrology one of the four pillars of medicine S-M I/VIII 55-56. *Paragranum. Vorrede und erste zwei Buecher. Entwuerfe und erste Ausarbeitung in Berezhausen. Vorred*)
>
> We, men, have a heaven, and it lies in each of us in its entire plentitude, undivided and corresponding to each man's specificity. Thus each human life takes its own course, thus dying, death, and disease are unequally distributed, in each case according to the action of the heavens. For if the same heaven were in all of us, all men would have to be equally sick and equally healthy. But this is not so; the unity of the Great Heaven is split into our diversities by the various moments at which we are born. As soon as a child is conceived, it receives its own heaven. If all children had been born at the same moment, all of them would have had the same heaven in them, and their lives would have followed the same course. Therefore, the starry vault imprints itself on the inner heaven of a man. A miracle without equal!
>
> (S-M I/VIII 100-101. *Paragranum. Vorrede und erste zwei Buecher. Entwuerfe und I. Ausarbeitung in Berezhausen. Der ander grund der Arznei*)
>
> Those stars you need to use in the higher sky, those let be your road and your way, that way you also must go.

> (S-M I/I 37. *Elf Traktat. 2. Vom schweinen oder schwintsucht. Andere Redaktion:* also, S-M I/XI 132. *Sieben Defensiones.* Second Defense)

However, he limits the application of astrology[c]—in the first place, by assimilating astral influence to other natural influences:

> The stars do not control anything in us, they mold nothing in us, they do not irritate anything, they bias nothing; they are free by themselves and we are free by ourselves. Nevertheless, remember that we may not live without the heavenly bodies. For cold and heat and the digestive agent of the things we eat and utilize, come from them. But man does not. Nevertheless they are of use to us, and we need them as direly as we need cold and heat, eating and drinking, and air.
>
> (S-M I/I 180. *Volumen Medicinae Paramirum. Bk. I, Cap. IV.*)

Thus the astral influence is similar to an aerial or atmospheric poison:

> You should know that [the stars] surround the entire world like the shell an egg. Air penetrates through the shell and first passes through it toward the center of the world. Stars, mind you, which are poisonous, pollute the air with their poison. Accordingly, wherever the poison penetrates, on that same spot the identical diseases will crop out in conformity to the character of the star in question. To be sure, the entire air in the world is not poisoned by the star, but merely a part thereof, depending on its strength. It is likewise so with the good qualities of the stars. *Ens astrale* thus signifies the odor, vapor, exudation of the stars, as mixed with the air.
>
> (S-M I/I 184. *Volumen Medicinae Paramirum. Bk. I, Cap. VIII.*)

> The heaven is the element fire and . . . its elemental movement produces the chaos which shall be discussed

[c]Pachter, *op. cit.*, pp. 31, 68, suggests that Paracelsus opposed astrology in his youth but became increasingly reconciled to it in later years.

> here. And in the same manner as water is brought to boil by fire, the chaos is that which is boiled by the element of heaven. And just as the meat in water gives up its strength to the water, so the stars are like the meat and give their strength to the aforementioned chaos. And just as the soup from the meat is food for man, so the chaos, of which we are speaking here, is also food for man.
>
> (S-M I/IX 466. *Von der Bergsucht und anderen Bergkrankheiten. Bk. I, Tract. I, Cap. III.* "Chaos" is an alternate word for "air.")

> Our body is like a lake and its members like the fishes. If life, which resides in the body and in all its members, is being poisoned by the stars, then also the inner organs, which take up the poison, become diseased. Observe, then, that some *entia astralia* have such a poisonous nature that they will harm only the blood, as the realgar-exuding stars. Some will harm merely the head, as do the mercurial ones; some, like the salts, only the bones and vessels. A number are so constituted that they produce dropsy and tumors, as orpiment; others, again, fevers, as the bitter ones.
>
> (S-M I/I 187. *Volumen Medicinae Paramirum. Bk. I, Cap. XI.*)

A second limitation is that the stars do not foreordain the future but only indicate forces which may affect the future:

> Christ and His apostles prophesy the seasons of nations, but the [astrologer] states the seasons of natural events. This is a mighty difference; take note of it and understand it aright, ye scientists and theologians! For what God prophesies takes place and nothing can prevent it from coming true. But what the [astrologer] predicts may or may not happen. Thus prophecy springs from one source, [astrology] from another.
>
> (S-M I/XII 19. *Astronomia Magna. Bk. I, Das Buch der Philosophei des himlischen firmaments. Das I. capitel*)

In any case, since man can study the stars and understand astral influences, he can counteract them. In this sense, Paracelsus maintains that there is interaction between the macrocosm and the microcosm:

> The conjunction between heaven and man is as follows. . . . There is a double firmament, one in heaven and one in each body, and these are linked by mutual concordance, and not by unilateral dependence of the body upon the firmament.
>
> (S-M I/I 236. *Zwei Bruchstuecke zum ersten der 5 entien. Bruchstueck I: De Ente Astrali*)

> It is not true that the firmament exerts a compelling action upon man; on the contrary, man himself acts upon the world more than he is influenced by it.
>
> (S-M I/XI 241. *Deutsche Praktik auf das Jahre 1538. Vorred zum Leser*)

Furthermore, the stars only influence man's sensual nature, and thus they can be counteracted by his willpower:

> As glass filters out the light of the sun, so man's willpower can oppose and filter out some of the astral influence.
>
> (S-M I/VIII 163. *Das Buch Paragranum. Der ander tractat*)

> The stars are subject to the philosopher; they must follow him and not he them. Only the man who is still animal is governed, mastered, compelled, and driven by the stars, so that he has no choice but to follow them—just as the thief cannot escape the gallows, the murderer the wheel, the fish the fisherman, the bird the snare, or the game the hunter. But the reason for all this is that such a man does not know himself and does not know how to use the energies hidden in him, nor does he know that he carries the stars within himself, that he is the microcosm, and thus carries in him the whole firmament with all its influences.
>
> (S-M I/XI 378. *Die 9 Buecher de Natura rerum. Von den astralischen zeichen der Physionomei am menschen*)

In particular, the physician can govern and guide astral influences by his knowledge of medicine:

> Heaven makes disease: the physician drives it away again. Now just as heaven has to yield to the physician, so, too, must the devil yield through the right ordering of medicine.
>
> (S-M I/XI 134. *Sieben Defensiones,* Second Defense)

Finally, Christian doctrine provides a limitation on astrology. As the stars only influence the sensual nature of man, the Christian should overcome this influence:

> . . . this action has influence only upon the emotions and upon the heathen, sensual reason. But we are Christians and we should live like Christians.
>
> (S-M I/XI 241. *Deutsche Praktik auf das Jahre 1538. Vorred zum Leser*)

Thus the soul is not subject to astral influences but is the locus of man's freedom. And in this way astrology is superseded by the Christian religion. Astrology is subject to the will of God, and God's will can be known in various other ways—specifically, through revelation.[6]

However, Paracelsus concludes that astrology and Christian doctrine must coexist, each in its own sphere:

> Who . . . can doubt that [astrology] and its light have paled beneath the light of Christ? Nevertheless it is our duty to say that the sick need a physician, while few need an apostle; similarly, many forecasts must be made by the [astrologer] and not by the prophets. Thus each has his part—the prophet, the [astrologer], the apostle, and the physician. For this reason [astrology] has not been abolished, nor forbidden to us Christians; we have only been commanded to use it in a Christian manner. For the Father has set us in the light of nature, and the Son in the eternal light. Therefore it is indispensable that we should know them both.
>
> (S-M I/XII 496-497. *Von erkantnus des gestirns*)

Thus, although Paracelsus accepted astrology, he attempted to circumscribe it by assimilating astral influences to other environmental forces, specifically, poisonous emanations from food and air.[7]

The *ens veneni* refers to the various *earthly* (as opposed to stellar) poisons which can harm men, in particular those taken in with the nourishment:

> The body has been given us without poison, and there is no poison in it. But in what we must offer the body as food, in that there is poison. In other words, the body has been created perfect, but not the other. Now in that other animals and fruits are good for us, they may also be poison to us.
>
> (S-M I/I 189. *Volumen Medicinae Paramirum. Bk. II, Cap. I.*)

This poison is produced when the alchemist inside the body is not functioning properly: the food putrefies and decays inside the organism, giving rise to poisons which "become a hearth for those diseases which are subject to it."[8 d] Man may be injured by the *ens veneni* even when the stars are propitious.

The *ens naturae* is the *physis* of the body, its natural constitution. Paracelsus interprets this in astrological terms:

> This child's firmament incurs at birth a predestined aspect. By this is meant that when creation is accomplished perfectly in the child, his destiny is fixed at the same instant, which has reference to how long the *ens naturale* is to run. Supposing I assume that birth takes place at a certain hour. Then, along with this creation, is given the end, which, let us say, would occur in the 30th year. In this case creation and its *ens* have the capacity of being cognizant by nature and as part of nature how long the *ens naturale* is to run . . . . Hence *ens naturae* and *creati* determine, as to duration, all events which are connatural to the bodily planets in the body, so they will all be fulfilled in the time between birth and predestined end.

[d]Here Paracelsus is perhaps influenced by the Egyptian doctrine of putrefaction.

(S-M I/I 206. *Volumen Medicinae Paramirum. Bk. III, Cap. V.*)

In practice, however, the *ens naturale* would seem to refer to specific disturbances of the organism which have no easily defined connection with the environment. Some of these are attributable to man's internal stars (chronic diseases), some to the elements within the body (the acute diseases), others to the temperaments, and a fourth group to the humors.[9]

The category of the *ens spirituale* includes diseases of the spirit—meaning the mind or will.[10] It means those diseases which are not of the soul and not of the body considered in its material aspect. Individuals can affect and injure each other through the spirit. They can will each other to be sick. The individual can also make himself sick through vices such as envy. All of these fall under the *ens spirituale.*[11]

The fifth category, the *ens Dei,* includes all the diseases of the other four categories. They are referred to the *ens Dei* when they are sent directly by God rather than through one of the other *entia.* In a sense all of Christian medicine, as opposed to Pagan, is based on the *ens Dei.*[12]

A significant aspect of the *entia* is that each can cause *all* diseases. This is best exemplified, of course, by the *ens Dei*—as God can cause all diseases directly—but it is equally true of the other four *entia.* Paracelsus is led to this doctrine by the observation that there exist five methods of curing:

> Know that all diseases are cured by five different methods. Medical practice with us, thus, starts with therapy, and not with etiology, inasmuch as the therapeutic process leads to the cause.
>
> (S-M I/I 165. *Volumen Medicinae Paramirum.* Bk. I of Prologues, Prologue I.)

Thus, just as medical theory is generated by practice, so is the cause of disease revealed by its therapy. That diseases may be cured in a number of different ways indicates that they have a number of causes. The *ens naturale* is the province of the *physis*-healers (*naturales*), meaning Galen, Avicenna, Rhazes, and the like, who cured by contraries.[13e] The faith-healers (*fideles*) cure by faith.[14] The *spirituales* utilize the spiritual essences from herbs and roots—Hippocrates was of this school.[15] The *characterales* utilize astrology for recognition of disease and thus cure through the *ens astrorum.*[16] And the specificists (*specifici*), a category which includes the Empirics, treat all diseases "specifically as to form as well as essence."[17f]

Since these five modes of treatment exist, Paracelsus concludes that each disease can take five different forms. The practitioner must recognize the particular form of the disease, since "no power responds to the cure meant for another."[18] An epilepsy or syphilis must be cured by the system of practice corresponding to the *ens* which has caused the disease.

Paracelsus' invocation of the *entia* is significant: (1) for the idea that disease causes are revealed by their cures[g] and (2) as first step away from the Rationalist idea that diseases are finite in number to the Empirical view that they are infinite. By abruptly quintupling the existing disease categories he considerably complicates any possible doctrine of proximate causes.

Furthermore, the five *entia* are a blow at anatomical investigation as a method of elucidating disease causes.

Thus Paracelsus is attacking two of the fundamental postulates of school medicine—the proximate cause of disease

[e]The *ens naturale* is Paracelsus' reinterpretation of the Galenic *physis.* This *ens* is the only one which is apparently independent of external causative factors and thus corresponds to the proximate cause which plays so important a role in Galenic therapeutics. Paracelsus calls it, astrologically, the "firmament in the body" (I/I 204, Bk. III, Cap. III.). Hence Galen and Avicenna are "*naturales.*" Elsewhere he notes that Galen was not so much a *naturalis* as a *characteralis* meaning one who "believe[s] that proper recognition and proper designation heals"—a reference to the Rationalist reliance on proper definition of the disease as the preliminary to its cure (*Ibid.*, pp. 167-168, Bk. I of Prologues, Prologue III; *Ibid.*, p. 170, Bk. II of Prologues, Prologue I.).

[f]These are apparently the physicians who cure through the *ens veneni,* although Paracelsus does not say so. It will be noted that the categories of physicians correspond only roughly with the five *entia.*

[g]For further development of this idea, see below, pp. 409 ff; 446 ff.

and anatomical analysis as the technique for discovering it. In their place he hypothesizes the *anatomia essentialis* or *mineralis*—meaning that the components of the organism are mineralic.

This is merely a refinement of the view that the microcosm and macrocosm are made of the same substance:

> Thus now the microcosm is *minor mundus* and has in its body all the minerals of the world. Thereupon know that from this it follows that the body takes its medicine out of the world, for the body is the same thing as the world. Therefore it follows from that that all minerals are good for men, each one to that mineral which lies in the body of the microcosm.
>
> (S-M I/IX 210. *Die drei (vier) Buecher des Opus Paramirum. Liber quartus de matrice*)

> And the cause of all the mineralic diseases is that man stands in all minerals, and that as many species as are outside, that many there are inside. Out of that shall a physician have his knowledge, that all illnesses come from these. For that arm yourself well, for the minerals will do away with your four humors, and will expose your foolishness to the light of day.
>
> (S-M I/V 138. *Autographische Entwuerfe zu den Buechern de Tartaro. Tractatus quintus. Caput I.*)

The *anatomia essentialis* is the anatomy of the living body, while the Galenist anatomy is anatomy of the dead: "We have in mind not the anatomy of the Italians, *id est cadaverum.*"[19]

In his distinction between the two anatomies Paracelsus merely reflects the traditional Empirical distrust of anatomical investigation as a source of reliable medical knowledge:

> For although I may know local anatomy, what concern is it to jaundice? to dropsy? To which other illnesses? This anatomy is of use only to external wounds and disease origins, and not to anything inside, that is to say, the principal causes . . . . Therefore it astonishes me that you set up the dead body as a ground of knowledge of what is

useful for the living body, without considering that the essence, property, and strength, which is the highest part of anatomy, have died and become corrupted . . . . Thus I warn you that if you ever wish to preserve the living body, not to seek its benefit in the dead.

(S-M I/VI 332. *Von Blattern, Laehme, Beulen, Loechern, und Zittrachten der Franzosen und ihres gleichen. Das II. Buch. Das erste capitel*)

Anatomy tells you nothing at all: "for to learn from the inner man one must have before one's eyes the last man and the first man and all men; for in all men lie all illnesses, in one man there lies one illness."[20]

On this basis Paracelsus now approaches the problem of disease cause. We have noted that knowledge of ultimate causes falls in the domain of *sapientia* and is inaccessible to man.[21] Hence Paracelsus shifts the discussion from disease cause (*ursache*) to disease origin (*ursprung*).[22] "Thus, stick to the rule to find out that from which the disease springs, not the causes [*die ursachen*] why it is what it is."[23] The *Volumen Medicinae Paramirum* is a discussion of disease *origins,* not of causes.

And the disease origin is only the mineral, in the body's matrix, from which the disease arises. The mineral of the macrocosm provokes disease in man by stimulating the corresponding mineral in the microcosm, and this mineral generates the disease as a seed does its tree:[24]

If the *iliadus* [the matrix] lets a mineral go from its chains, then such beginnings of diseases happen.

(S-M I/VI 276. *Von allen offenen Schaeden. Das VII. Buch. Vom wilden feuer*)

Saltpeter makes a fistula as it separates out of the matrix.

(S-M I/VI 286. *Von allen offenen Schaeden. Das VII. Buch. Von den fistulen*)

[The mercury in man] . . . is attracted by the upper stars from the earth up into their regions, in the same manner as the needles of compasses are attracted in an opposite

> manner by a southerly magnet. Therefore, know now that the stars have in themselves the fleeing *mercurius* which has been driven away by the fire and which they too cooked and prepared before it existed.
>
> (S-M I/IX 495. *Von der Bergsucht und anderen Bergkrankheiten. Das ander Buch. Der erst tractat. Das viert capitel*)
>
> For the fruits [the diseases] are called minerals and are taken for minerals. Thus, when you see erysipelas, say there is vitriol. When you see cancer, say there is calcothar. If you see lupus, say there is *plumosum*. For it is such species that you shall observe and examine in what way the minerals of the outside world and those in man correspond to each other.
>
> (S-M I/IX 237. *Entwuerfe zu den vier Buechern des Opus Paramirum*)

In health no mineral is thrown up to the surface of the body out of the *iliadus*.[25]

Paracelsus does not consider minerals to be actually present in the body (as is seen from the following astrological analogy), but the observed symptoms and signs of diseases are identical with the effects of various minerals on the body:

> Just as the astrologers give the names of men and animals to the signs of the zodiac because on both sides there is an identical essence, even though in form [*die form*] they cannot be compared (one being alive with flesh and blood and the other not), but the cause of this is that the two *corpora* have the same nature and property, thus also I give names to the open lesions and compare them in origin, property, and kind to the minerals arising from the four matrices. *Not that I take such names from the forms or the corpora, but rather I take them from the identical effects which may be attributed to both.* The microcosm does not have the *corpora* or forms of the world in it, but rather its kinds and properties, from which it results that the corrosives of the microcosm may

justly and rightly be named and called after the salts, vitriols, *alumina,* arsenics, etc. For it is more suitable to medicine than to philosophy to recognize and know the properties and kinds than the forms and *corpora,* which give no strength against one another.

(S-M I/VI 234. *Von allen offenen Schaeden. Das ander Buch*)

The Aristotelian-Galenic doctrine of causes is greatly altered by Paracelsus. While Galen and the other Rationalists had not been explicit on the subject, their "proximate causes" were a mixture of the Aristotelian material, efficient, and formal causes: the material entity – the humoral dyscrasia – was the efficient cause of the "disease" and, indeed, the "disease" itself.[h] It was also equivalent to the disease "form" or entity. As with Aristotle himself, these "forms" were defined, above all, as *invisible* – inhering in the body just as the Platonic Ideas underlay the world of nature.[i]

Paracelsus aimed to eliminate from medicine all speculation about the invisible. Hence he assimilated the disease "form" to its "origin" – the mineral within the body which was known through the symptoms. He thus shifted attention away from the (hidden) internal causes to the (visible) symptoms which defined the disease "form." Invisible in Rationalism, the formal cause became visible in the philosophy of Paracelsus.

Thus the visible symptoms, which for Galen were the disease effect, are for Paracelsus identical with the formal cause. Galen's environmental causes, which he regarded as too indeterminate to be of utility for therapeutics and relegated to the realm of prevention, become for Paracelsus the efficient causes of disease: "The sky is the causer of these things through the element fire and gives birth to this illness in the microcosm."[26] "Now the igniter is in the upper sky, but the *materia* is in the lower sky."[27] In culmination,

[h]See *supra* pp. 132-133, 218 ff.

[i]This is also neo-Platonic concept and is discussed in Volume II of this work.

anatomy (*anatomia essentialis*) arises out of therapeutics instead of being its foundation.[j]

By shifting the focus of medicine to the formal causes of disease Paracelsus at a stroke abolished that invisible empire which was the exclusive preserve of the medical profession. The indignation of the latter at this blow to their interests is seen in the comments of Thomas Erastus (1523-1583) who called Paracelsus a "beast" and a "grunting swine" and said that he abolished the knowledge of the ancients, replacing sane teaching by insane delusion, the certain by the uncertain, the comprehensible by the incomprehensible, truth by false names and doctrines, the useful by the useless, and salubrious medicine by pestilential poison![28]

But, while Paracelsus' views are far from Galenism, they conform rather closely to the Group IV Hippocratic writings. Knowledge arises from therapeutics: "What the ancients wrote is erroneous, setting the origins of the disease hidden in the body and the result in the visible lesions. This is not enough for the physician, but he is brought by the cure and the healing to the lesions as well as to other illnesses."[29] The proximate causes inside the body cannot be cognized directly. Hippocrates' undefined and non-substantial humor becomes the equally non-substantial mineral—both of these concepts being operational definitions of observed processes whose scientific validity is tested only by their utility for practice.

Thus the idea that one mineral drives out the other is the starting point for a whole cosmology. The great world is able to generate disease in the little world because both are composed of the same minerals. Astrology is incorporated by assimilating astral influences to mineral poisons. Since the disease takes the form of an aroused mineral in the matrix of the organism, the curative remedy must be the one which expells the aroused mineral from the body.

[j]He shifts efficient causes outside the body in yet another way: the cause of treatment is "a man who knows what the treatment is based on." S-M I/I 169. *Volumen Medicinae Paramirum*. Bk. I of Prologues, Prologue IV.

NOTES

[1] S-M I/XIV 597-598. *De Pestilitate.*

[2] S-M I/I 270-272. *Das Buch von der Gebaerung der empfindlichen Dinge in der Vernunft. Tractatus tertius. Caput quartum.*

[3] S-M I/XIV 215-216. *De vera influentia rerum liber.*

[4] S-M I/II 47. *Herbarius.*

[5] S-M I/XII 315. *Astronomia Magna. Das ander Buch. Das ander capitel;* Also, *Ibid.*, p. 299, *Das ander Buch, Das erste capitel.*

[6] On the subordination of the stars to the Divine will, see S-M I/XII 91. *Astronomia Magna. Bk. I, cap. IV. Was astrologia sei und was der astrologus;* S-M I/IX 578. *De peste libri tres cum additionibus. Imaginatio impressionis.*

[7] S-M I/I 184. *Volumen Medicinae Paramirum. Bk. I, Cap. VIII.*

[8] *Ibid.*, p. 196. *Bk. II, Cap. IX.*

[9] *Ibid.*, p. 214., *Bk. III, Particle I.*

[10] *Ibid.*, pp. 217-218, *Bk. IV, Cap. III, IV.*

[11] *Ibid.*, p. 223, *Bk. IV, Cap. X.*

[12] *Ibid.*, pp. 225 ff, *Bk. V.*

[13] *Ibid.*, p. 167, Bk. I of Prologues, Prologue III.

[14] *Ibid.*, p. 168, Bk. I of Prologues, Prologue III.

[15] *Loc. cit.*

[16] *Loc. cit.*

[17] *Loc. cit.*

[18] *Ibid.*, p. 172, Bk. II of Prologues. Prologue III.

[19] S-M I/II 325. *Von den natuerlichen Wassern. Buch III-V. Das vierte Buch. Das dritte tractat.*

[20] S-M I/VIII 86. *Paragranum. Vorrede und erste zwei Buecher. Entwuerfe und I. Ausarbeitung in Berezhausen. Der erste grund der arznei, welcher ist philosophia.*

[21] *Ibid.*, p. 94. *Der ander grund der arznei, welcher ist astronomia.*

[22] S-M I/I 169. *Volumen Medicinae Paramirum. Bk. I of Prologues. Prologue IV.*

[23] *Ibid.*, p. 186. *Tractatus I, Cap. IX.*

[24] S-M I/XI 213. *Labyrinthus medicorum errantium. Das XI. capitel.*

[25] S-M I/IX 238. *Entwuerfe zu den vier Buechern des Opus Paramirum.*

[26] S-M I/I 50. *Elf Traktat. 3. Cura.*

[27] *Ibid.*, p. 145. *10. Causa.*

[28] Pagel, *Das Medizinische Weltbild*, p. 1 and *Paracelsus*, p. 314.

[29] S-M I/VI 235. *Von allen offenen Schaeden. Das drit Buch;* also, S-M I/VI 52. *Drei Buecher der Wundarznei. Vorrede.*

CHAPTER XIV

CURE BY OPPOSITION BETWEEN FLAVORS: THE ALCHEMICAL PURIFICATION OF MEDICINES

If every disease has five different forms, and the organism is the matrix of all the minerals of the universe, the identification of any one disease with a particular material substrate becomes difficult.

The alternative is to regard diseases as spiritual entities—the bodily signs and symptoms being the effects of the spiritual disease and not the disease itself.

Hence the remedy must also be spiritual, since a spiritual entity could not be affected by a material substance.

This further level of abstraction in the Paracelsan cosmology gives rise to a new interpretation of cure by similars: each mineral substance contains a harmful and a beneficial component, the former causing disease and the latter curing it.

Spirituality of Disease

The gradual spiritualization of disease is seen in Paracelsus' progress from the four Aristotelian elements, and the Hippocratic (Group IV) doctrine of an infinity of elements in the body, to his own view that the ultimate components of matter are mercury, sulphur, and salt.

We have already seen that Paracelsus assimilates the four Aristotelian elements to his own duality of earth and stars. And he states that the four elements are not substances at all, but spiritual entities. What is significant is their "nature, course, essence, fruits, qualities."[1] The ultimate level of abstraction and spiritualization of the doctrine is his hypothesis that all of creation is composed of the three elements: mercury, sulphur, and salt:

> The mysteries of the Great and the Little World are distinguished only by the form in which they manifest themselves; for they are only one thing, one being. Heaven and earth have been created out of nothingness, but they are composed of three things – *mercurius, sulphur,* and *sal* . . . . Of these same three things the planets and all the stars consist; and not only the stars but all bodies that grow and are born from them. And just as the Great World is thus built upon the three primordial substances, so man–the Little World– was composed of the same substances. Thus man, too, is nothing but mercury, sulphur, and salt.
>
> (S-M I/VIII 280. *Von den hinfallenden Siechtagen. Der ander paragraphus.*)
>
> . . . basically there are only three kinds of medicine and three kinds of illnesses . . . each *medicus* will remember to give mercury to mercurial diseases, salt to saline diseases, sulphur to sulphuric diseases, to each illness that which is appropriate and fitting.
>
> (S-M I/III 7. *Von den ersten dreien Principiis. Das V. capitel*)

That mercury and sulphur are essential components of all *metals* was ancient alchemical doctrine, receiving its most thorough elaboration in the writings of Geber (8th century, A.D.). Mercury, the primal substance of all metals, reveals itself in their molten state. Sulphur, in turn, was the principle of color: yellow, the color of gold, was the most perfect, while all other colors were degenerate forms of the original yellow.

Paracelsus, however, extends the alchemical theory of metals to matter in general.[2] He therefore adds the third principle–salt–standing for the irreducible ash which remains when organic matter is tried by fire.[a] The mercury, sulphur, and salt are thus spiritualized into principles. Although they at the same time stand for the substances themselves, their

[a]Salt is also called alkali by Paracelsus (S-M I/I 486), and the alkalis of the later Iatrochemical School thus stem from Paracelsus' salt. In Arabic, alkali (*al-qaliy*) originally meant the calcined ashes of certain plants.

major role in Paracelsus' philosophy is to characterize certain observed processes and phenomena:

> Sulphur is that which burns, mercury is that which embodies the virtue, and salt is that which holds the body together.
>
> (S-M I/IX 658. *Von des Bades Pfaeffers Tugenden, Kraeften, und Wirkung. Uslegung der Lateinischen synonyma*)

> Sulphur is the fire, mercury the smoke, and salt the ash [*alcali*].
>
> (S-M I/IX 83. *Die drei (vier) Buecher des Opus Paramirum. Bk. II. Cap. I.*)

Sulphur represents the organization of matter, mercury its activity, and salt its mass.[3]

The rubric, salt, enables Paracelsus to incorporate the Hippocratic (Group IV) doctrine that the elements of the body are infinite.

Ancient Medicine (cap. XIV) had held that "there is in man salt and bitter, sweet and acid, astringent and insipid, and a vast number of other things, possessing *dynameis* of all sorts . . ." In one of his earliest writings Paracelsus paraphrases this passage: "Now there are four tastes in the body as there are in the earth: sourness, sweetness, bitterness, and saltiness."[4] He notes that these tastes are non-material and have nothing to do with the Galenic substances: "cholera starts with bitterness, and everything that is bitter is hot and dry, without, however, being associated with fire. For the fire in question is neither hot nor dry . . . Acidity is melancholy, for whatever is sour is cold and dry. That goes by the name of melancholy and does not concern the earth,[b] inasmuch as earth and melancholy are far apart."[5]

In the same writing the flavors are assimilated to the mineral matrix: "Thus the four temperaments [i.e., sourness, sweetness, bitterness, and saltiness] are in the body as in a garden in which grow amarissa, polypod, vitriol, and salnitre.

[b] In the Galenic tradition both earth and black bile were cold and dry.

In like manner may they all reside in the body, while one alone will come to the fore."[6]

Paracelsus' selection of the word, "taste" (Latin: *gustus*)—an alternative translation of the Greek *chymos*—indicates his desire to get away from the substantial "humors" to a more spiritualized doctrine of the organism's elements, one resembling the "vast number of other things" mentioned in *Ancient Medicine.*

Eight years later, in another writing, he increases the number of flavors to seven and assimilates them to the salty component of the *iliadus*:

> Now, as for the effects of the salts, there are seven different kinds of salts, and each causes its own particular kind of pain. These seven kinds are seven flavors, and the seven flavors make seven different kinds of pain [*wetagen*]. For example, sour and bitter make two kinds of pains, biting and sharp also two kinds, and none of these is identical with the other. For in the same way as a flavor is obnoxious to the tongue, so also is it in open lesions obnoxious to the flesh. For, although there is no sense of taste in these places, they still feel the pains.
>
> (S-M I/VI 241. *Von allen offenen Schaeden. Das Viert Buch*)

Ultimately sulphur is associated with the colors of the body, mercury with its different masses, and salt with its various tastes:

> Note that there are four kinds of sulphur. There is a red one which is red in the body and also threefold: in the flesh, in the blood, in the principal members, heart, liver, kidneys, gallbladder. Then the next is yellow and also threefold: in the fat, in the marrow, and in the grease. Then there is the white one in the brain, in the bones, in the veins. Then there is the green one in the bile.
>
> And what burns there is sulphur. Thus we have red, white, yellow, and green sulphur. It follows that some of the mercury is heavy, as in the flesh, some of it is light, as in the lungs, some of medium weight, as in the bones. For it has the weight.

> Now with the salt: part of it is sweet, as in the flesh; part of it is salty, as in the blood; part of it is bitter, as in the bile; part is sour, as in the thymus, for it has the taste.
>
> Thus the *iliadus* is divided into three parts: into color, weight, and taste. . . .
>
> (S-M I/IX 238. *Entwuerfe zu den vier Buechern des Opus Paramirum*)

> *Anatomia materialis* . . . reveals what blood is, what kind of sulphur, mercury, or salt, and thus also what the heart is—what kind of sulphur, what kind of salt, and what kind of mercury—and thus also with the brain and whatever else there is in the whole body.
>
> (S-M I/IX 67. *Die drei (vier) Buecher des Opus Paramirum. Erster teil. Das erste Buch. Caput sextum)*

When the mercury of the body is colder and less volatile, it causes tremors of the hands and feet and of the ligaments, arteries and joints. When it is sharper and more purified, it generates mania, phrenesy, and syncope—the illnesses which the Galenists associate with melancholy but which are actually due to the spirit of mercury ascending to the head and seeking an outlet there. Sulphur is not volatile but putrefactive and causes such diseases as pleurisy, fevers of the praecordium, stomach, and spleen; also hemicrania and pains of the eyes, teeth, and ears. Salt generates disease when its spirit rises and coagulates in various parts of the body; it is associated with calculi and sand in the veins and cavities of the body, with gout, arthritis, sciatica, fluxes of the stomach and intestines, ulcers, scabies, pruritus, erysipelas, cancers, fistulas, and the like.[7]

> Thus there are also many kinds of holes and *pruritus* according to their contents of the various kinds of salts. Some *dulcia*, that is, holes without pain, compare to the honey salt, sugar salt, liquorice [*suessholz*] salt; some *ardentia*, compare to pepper, ginger, and paradise grain salt, some *eschara*, compare to the arsenical salt and auripigmental salt and others. Some *corrodentia*, compare

to the salt of the alkali, to vitriol, the *plumosum*, etc., some styptic, compare to the *alumina*, etc.

(S-M I/X 551. *Von Oeffnung der Haut, Ein Fragment. Liber I. Caput VI.*)

Thus mercury, sulphur, and salt are an important tool of analysis, enabling the physician, by observing external phenomena, to ascertain what is occurring inside the body. There is a parallel, a correspondence, between mineral processes in the macrocosm and the same processes in the microcosm:

> And the same way as you see that in *saturnus* [lead] there lie the colors red, white, and yellow, while the lead itself is not these colors, nor are they in it. To understand the paradigm look as follows: just as these colors are made manifest through the separation, so in the same way are the salts recognized. And as the red from lead colors red, and the yellowness makes a yellow out of the strength of the separation, the same way *alumen* yields an *alumen* and salt a salt here in the ulcers. And if you may wonder how the *alumen* or salt, etc. may be invisible in that way inside the bodies, just remember how vinegar is contained in wine and yet is never noticed, or copper in vitriol.
>
> (S-M I/VI 130. *Drei Buecher der Wundarznei. Bk. II, Cap. V.*)
>
> Since man has in him such simples, these simples being the ones which cause the falling sickness, then I say that the body contains sulphur of vitriol . . . the sulphur is such a one that, when exalted by its ascendant, causes this falling sickness. The reason is that the minerals lie in man and outside of him too.
>
> (S-M I/I 143-144. *Elf Traktat. 10. Causa*)
>
> Nothing else needs to be known to you in order to understand the matter, *corpus*, etc. of the disease then what the natural things of the earth and the elements indicate to you. If now you know the same, then you know the illness. Herein lies the anatomy, herefrom follows the medicine. For the medicine grows like the illness, and same and same yield each other's theory.

(S-M I/I 320. *Liber de podagricis et suis speciebus. Anatomia*)

The reason is that the (mineral) form of the disease is identical with its (mineral) origin and indicates its origin:

> It behooves the physician, as philosopher and theoretician, well and honestly to recognize the origin of the form [*die form*], and, then what makes the form and what indication springs from the form, as the chief *materiam* to be recognized. . . .
>
> There is no other cause or origin, for as these things grow, so also the *fistulae* form themselves here according to the same cause. For no other cause may be taken but from the salt which gives the form to the one as well as to the other, so that out of this form the *materia primitiva* shall be recognized. It also behooves each physician to recognize the form and note the *materiam peccantem* of the same illness. For how would one recognize man or woman without the form of both. This is a crude example but still gives the name; in the same way, with the illnesses the form indicates the cause to the same extent. That it is which makes the illness and should be recognized by all physicians.
>
> (S-M I/VI 284-285. *Von allen offenen Schaeden. Das VI. Buch. Von den fistulen.* Also, p. 282)

A great variety of salts, sulphurs, and mercuries lies within the body, and each provides insight into one of the manifold kinds of disease process. Although only a symbolic characterization of the disease, they are all the physician needs to treat the disease, since they indicate the mineral form of the disease and thus its origin.

Spirituality of the Remedy

If the disease is spiritual, the remedy must be spiritual also.

In the language of similars this idea is expressed as follows: like cures like because the beneficial element in the substance, when extracted and used as a medicine, expels the harmful element of the (same) substance acting as disease cause.

Here Paracelsus introduces alchemy. He directed the alchemists' attention away from the transmutation of lead into gold and focused it on the discovery of remedies: "Many have said of alchemy that it is for making gold and silver. For me such is not the aim, but only to consider what virtue and power may lie in medicines . . . here the purpose is to make *arcana* and to direct them against all diseases."[8] He urges physicians to learn alchemy and use it in preparing medicines:

> I praise the art of medicine, but how can I praise those who are physicians and not alchemists at the same time? If the art of medicine were found among those who are only alchemists, they would not understand it, and if it were found among those who are only physicians, they would not be able to make use of it, for they do not hold in their hands the key to the mysteries. Thus I can only praise him who knows how to induce nature to be helpful, that is to say, is able to recognize what lies hidden in nature. For never must knowledge and preparation, that is to say, medicine and alchemy, be separated from each other.
>
> (S-M I/X 67. *Das erste Buch der Grossen Wunderznei. Das XIII. capitel.* Also, p. 278. *Das zweite Buch der Grossen Wundarznei. Beschlussred*)

The fundamental alchemical procedure was the "purification" of metals—meaning not only the extraction of metals from their ores but also the separation of the pure metal from its outer "husk." Indeed, the primary meaning of "purification" was extraction of the one pure metal—gold—from all the other metals, regarded as imperfect forms of gold.[9]

In its medical application this meant removing the narcotic *corpus* of the substance and releasing its spirit:

> And the whole *summa* of preparing medicines is that the narcotic is removed in the way described.
>
> (S-M I/VII 281. *Vom Ursprung and Herkommen der Franzosen. Das IV. Buch. Das erste capitel*)

> The medicine shall be prepared so that it will be a food for the hunger and not a narcotic of the same (i.e., by the flatulence and seizures which come from the *corpus* only), since the *corpus* is left behind. My purpose here is only that the medicine shall be separated from the narcotic *corpus*.
>
> (S-M I/VII 264. *Vom Ursprung und Herkommen der Franzosen. Das IV. Buch. Das drit capitel*)

> For in the body nothing should sleep; everything should be awake and joyfully and merrily desire and take that which is its own. . . . As long as the *corpus* is attached to the essence, that is, its flatulence, impurity, and rawness, then these are ingested with the essence, i.e. the *esse essatum* remains bound in the *corpus* and goes unbroken into the effect with the *essentificativum*, which effect is stupefying and stupefies the place of the illness. Thus the medicine is a narcotic.
>
> (S-M I/VII 263. *Vom Ursprung and Herkommen der Franzosen. Das IV. Buch. Das ander capitel*)

This is ordained by God:

> For it is not God's design that the remedies should exist for us ready-made, boiled, and salted, but that we should boil them ourselves, and it pleases Him that we boil them and learn in the process, that we train ourselves in this art, and are not idle on earth but labor in daily toil. For it is we who must pray for our daily bread, and if He grants it to us, it is only through our labor, our skill, and preparation.
>
> (S-M I/X 277. *Das zweite Buch der Grossen Wunderznei. Das XII. capitel*)

Furthermore, the technique of extracting the virtue of the remedy is learned only through experience: Paracelsus defines "*arcanum*" (i.e., the essence of the remedy) as "that which is given by experience."[10]

> Marvellous virtues are inherent in the remedies. One would hardly believe that nature contained such virtues. . . . For only a great artist is able to discover them,

not one who is only versed in books, but only one who has acquired his ability and skill through the experience of his hands. . . . It is an important art, and therefore it cannot be clearly described, but can only be learned by experience.

(S-M I/II 430. *Das siebente Buch in der Arznei, von den Krankheiten die der Vernunft berauben, de morbis amentium. Methodus secunda. Caput I.*)

This actually intensifies the remedy's inherent power. Paracelsus defines "quintessence" as "the result of operations strengthening nature beyond her grade."[11]

The remedy's powers are intensified because it is purified:

Alchemy makes pure that which was impure.

(S-M I/XI 189. *Labyrinthus Medicorum Errantium. Das V. capitel*)

Thus you shall understand of the *quinta essentia* that is small and little, sheltered in a piece of wood, an herb, a stone, or the like. The other is a pure *corpus*. From which we learn separation of the elements. And it is thus also to be understood that the *quinta essentia* is not a fifth entity above the elements, for it is an element. . . .And although it is true that *quinta essentia* heals all diseases, it does not happen by tempering but because of the great property which is in it and the great pureness which is found in it, by which it is more than miraculous to the body, and makes a change and a purification.

(S-M I/III 119. *Neun Buecher Archidoxis. Liber quartus*)

Paracelsus compares strengthening the medicine to growing a tree from a seed:

Therefore, this is the first step in the preparation, the breaking up of the earth.[c]

(S-M I/VII 277. *Vom Ursprung and Herkommen der Franzosen. Das IV. Buch. Das XI. capitel*)

[c]In other words, separating the metal from the ore is like plowing a field.

Thus shall we heighten the *gradus*; in that lies the graduation and the number of degrees—as between a grain that weighs a drachm and the fir tree that grows from it. As many thousands of times this substance is greater than the grain, so many thousands of times more useful it is than the grain. Therefore the strength arises and grows *in arcanis* invisibly, not by virtue of the quantity, but by virtue of the quantity which it would possess if the seed grew to its full extent.

(S-M I/VII 279. *Vom Ursprung and Herkommen der Franzosen. Das IV. Buch. Das XII. capitel*)

That way also the medicine is in your hand. In it you see nothing, but you know that there is something in it similar to a seed which does not look like the ultimate stage of its development. The earth nonetheless brings it there, and if it does not get there, that means it was dead from the beginning. Thus also the medicine in your hand is nothing but a seed. That seed you must cause to grow so that you will bring it to the point of its ultimate development.

(S-M I/VII 265. *Vom Ursprung und Herkommen der Franzosen. Das IV. Buch. Das drit capitel*)

Once extracted from its *corpus*, the medicine is and acts like a spirit:

That *quinta essentia* . . . is a spirit like the spirit of life.

(S-M I/III 118. *Neun Buecher Archidoxis. Liber quartus. De quinta essentia*)

It is not because of the body but because of the strength that the fifth essence is invented, to make out of 20 pounds one ounce and the ounce exceed the 20 pounds. Therefore, the less of body, the higher the virtues in the medicine. If man can make the 20 pounds into one ounce, then the invisible ones can do it still better.

(S-M I/IX 325. *Die Buecher von den unsichtbaren Krankheiten. Ingang des vierten Buchs*)

The medicine itself nobody may see, for it is an invisible thing, but the medicine's body, that one sees. The same way as a soul in man, there also only the body is seen, while the soul is not.

(S-M I/X 91. *Das erste Buch der Grossen Wundarznei. Der ander tractat. Das erst capitel*)

But if you ever were good physicians, as your writings and recipes in no way demonstrate, then you would . . . leave aside the *corpus* and extract the virtue; for on both sides, in the microcosm and in the medicine, the *corpus* has no function, but life in life.

(S-M I/VI 349. *Von Blattern, Laehme, Beulen, Loechern, und Zittrachten der Franzosen und ihres gleichen. Das ander Buch. Das XI. capitel*)

What the eyes see in the plant, or in the stones or the trees, is not the medicine. All they can see is the dross. Inside the dross, however, the medicine lies.

(S-M I/XI 187. *Labyrinthus Medicorum Errantium. Das V. capitel*)

But now it is not the dose swallowed that matters, for what the teeth chew is not the medicine. Nobody sees the medicine. Since nobody sees it, the medicine's body is not needed. But our eyes see it bodily, because without the body we could not use it. If death can sneak up and strangle us and kill us, then the medicine can do it too.

(S-M I/IX 325. *Die Buecher von den unsichtbaren Krankheiten. Ingang des vierten Buchs*)

For the body accepts with pleasure nothing that is not spiritual to it.

(S-M I/III 155. *Neun Buecher Archidoxis. Liber sextus*)

Paracelsus also compares its action to fire:

Now although I speak of the weight of the drug, it is still not to be considered as a dose; for that is not medicine-like. For not in its weight, but outside its weight, the medicine shall be given. For who can weigh the light of the sun? Who can weigh the air, who shall weigh the spirit of the *arcanum*? Nobody. Now the medicine lies in the latter and not in anything heavier. . . . The medicine shall act in the body like fire, and shall that way act as mightily in the illnesses as fire in a pile of split wood. Now know that this is the form of the dose (as you call it). Is it possible to weigh the fire? How much of it would be required to burn a pile of wood or a house? No one can weigh the fire, yet a little spark is heavy enough to burn a forest. But the little spark is without weight. . . . Just as the spark acts in the wood and makes itself big or small, according to the quantity of the wood, so the medicine acts in the same way. It becomes big in the body if the disease is big, and little if the disease is little. Who would undertake to attribute that to the weight? Nobody. For it belongs to the virtues. . . . The virtues cannot be weighed and cannot be placed on the scale against the illness, as if the illness were lying on one side and the medicine on the other.

(S-M I/VII 300. *Vom Ursprung und Herkommen der Franzosen. Das V. Buch. Das XI. capitel*)

The quintessence, when extracted, can even be put into another body: "Some medicines are brought from their *corpus* into another *corpus* and are more effective in a strange *corpus* than in their own."[d]

The remedy's spirituality has a number of consequences.

In the first place, the spirit of the remedy acts against the spirit of the disease, not against the material substance of the body. Hence the Galenist purging and sweating are improper procedures:

The medicine is given to drive out the spirit of the disease, not the matter which you [the Galenists] call peccant. . . . Not the matter but the peccant spirit shall be driven out; then the matter, which you want to drive

[d]S-M I/X 91-92. *Das erste Buch der Grossen Wundarznei. Der ander tractat des ersten Buchs. Das erst capitel.* By the same token, some substances are more effective in their own *corpus* and cannot be extracted. (*Ibid.* Also S-M I/XI 108. *Das Buch von den tartarischen Krankheiten. Das XVIII. capitel*). Paracelsus here has in mind the practice of making alcoholic tinctures of various medicinal substances, and also the fact that some substances do not lend themselves to this kind of processing (one of the distinctions between "foods" and "medicines").

out, and which you regard as something deathlike, will remain healthy and fresh in the body . . .

(S-M I/VII 296. *Vom Ursprung und Herkommen der Franzosen. Das V. Buch. Das VIII. capitel*)

And as little as it would be fitting, if the air had been poisoned by the stars, to take away the air, that little in this case is it fitting to take away the matter. For it is the same with the matter as if you made a smell in a closed room, and the air of that room were dominated by that smell. Now you would not drive away the smell by driving out the air, which is but the *corpus* of the smell, you would do better to drive away the smell from the *corpus* while the *corpus* itself remained in the room. . . . For which reason medicine shall be given so that the body will remain unhurt but the spirit which harms the body will be driven out of it.

(S-M I/VII 296. *Vom Ursprung und Herkommen der Franzosen. Das V. Buch. Das VIII. capitel*)

The disease is what does not have a *corpus*; and what has a *corpus* is not disease.

(S-M I/VIII 161. *Das Buch Paragranum. Der ander tractat. Von der astronomia*)

As the snow goes away from the summer, who grasps its *corpus*? Nobody. But if you mean to count the snow as a malady and say that it is the *corpus* of the malady, then even so that which makes the snow is not a *corpus* but a spirit. The snow is the *corpus*. And the excretions, the faeces which you call humors, those are not the maladies. The malady is that which makes them. Who sees the malady? No one. Who grasps it? No one. How then can the physician look for the maladies in the humors and assign their origins to them, since they are produced by the malady and not the malady by them? The snow doesn't make the winter, but the winter the snow, for when the snow is removed the winter is not made to go away.

(S-M I/VIII 178. *Das Buch Paragranum. Der ander tractat. Von der astronomia*)

Since the remedy's true action is spiritual, the crude laxative, styptic, and other effects employed by the Galenists are not part of the *arcanum* but represent the narcotic effect of the *corpus* which is left behind during alchemical preparation of the medicine.[12]

Furthermore, some substances which have no effect on the body in their crude form, but are apparently quite inert, will develop medicinal effects when properly processed by the alchemist.[13]

The second consequence of the medicine's spirituality is that dose size is unimportant. The spirit of the remedy can as well be in a small part of the substance as in a larger quantity. The full strength of the remedy is in every drop, and Paracelsus talks of doses of a single drop, half a drop, or even less.[14] The physician does not achieve a more powerful effect by increasing the dose but by using a different remedy, one with a more powerful essence.

> The right order of nature demands that anatomy is looked at against anatomy, member against member, but neither stronger and weaker, nor stronger and still stronger; for the maladies are not graded in this way, nor, on the other hand, is medicine.
>
> (S-M I/VIII 155. *Das Buch Paragranum. Der erste tractat. Von der philosophia*)

Since poisons affect the body most powerfully, the best medicines are prepared from poisons. "Consider, a spider is the supreme poison, on the other hand, also, the highest *arcanum* in chronic fevers."[15]

> The medicine . . . is as strong as the illness. A stroke is one of the strongest illnesses, therefore this root also is one which is equal in degree against it. It therefore follows that something severe is always to be directed against something severe, in order that same will find its same.
>
> (S-M I/II 10. *Herbarius. Erklerung der wurzen. Zum schlag*)
>
> Since *pustulae* is the most malignant illness, and none like it is born in the nature and has its origin over the nature,

we shall remember that we also use that medicine which is the very most obnoxious to the nature, so that concordance will be observed; it is according to philosophy that that which is against the nature and a poison to the nature shall be driven away with that which is obnoxious among the elements, and that which the elements themselves hate will be made into a medicine for that which the body hates.

(S-M I/X 501. *Drei chirurgische Buecher. Liber tertius. Caput III.*)

By the same token, even the smell of some medicines is sufficient to cure certain diseases, or at least to prepare the patient for cure, since the essence of the remedy is also found in its smell. "For there are many smells which awaken the epileptic, many which awaken the apoplectic, and not so that they completely cure the illness, but they prepare the way."[16]

Because the remedy is spiritual it acts as a whole, upon the whole body—another aspect of Paracelsus' holism. The medicine must act as a whole, since the essence of every substance has the same wholeness as the substance itself:

> Thus understand me that the entire strength is in one simple and not divided into two, three, four, or five, etc., but in one whole one, and that simple does not need anything but only the alchemy, which is nothing other than what the ore miner, ore smelter, ore man, or miner does. It lies in the extracting and not in the composing. It lies in the recognizion of that which lies in the same, and not in making it from put-together and mended pieces.
>
> (S-M I/VIII 84. *Paragranum. Vorrede und erste zwei Buecher. Entwuerfe und I. Ausarbeitung in Berezhausen. Der erste grund der arznei, welcher ist philosophia.* Also, S-M I/VI 129)
>
> When we want to administer medicaments, we administer the whole earth, that is, all virtues of the sky and earth, of the air and water, which is because when there is an illness in the body, all healthy members must fight against it, not only one but all of them; for one illness is

> the death of all of them. . . . Thus also your medicine will have to be, that it would have in itself the whole firmament of the upper and lower spheres.
>
> (S-M I/IX 94. *Die drei (vier) Buecher des Opus Paramirum. Liber secundus. Caput secundum*)

Being a whole, the medicine makes its way through the body and permeates the whole, giving what is appropriate to every part:

> As little as the sun is divided up, one part to the flowers, one part to the trees, one part to the stones, etc., that little may we divide up the strength of the medicine. That is, we cannot walk the path of medicine if we try to seek out in the body what belongs to this part and what to that. What is healthy to one part is another's happiness, and what is the one's happiness is the other's health.
>
> (S-M I/VII 269. *Vom Ursprung und Herkommen der Franzosen. Das viert Buch. Das sechst capitel*)

Paracelsus formulates the same idea in another way when he states that his medicines are "universal," meaning that they cope with all aspects of the disease in all parts of the body. The Galenic medicines, on the contrary, are "particularistic," since the Galenic physicians try to prescribe a medicine for a particular part of the body, leaving the rest unattended.

> The medicine in the body shall serve all the members. For they have the power of attraction and the desire to avert harm. Now if you pour in a particularistic medicine, you give to one part and let the others stand around empty, without knowing which part of the body needs the medicine the most. Therefore, health consists in giving to all in proportion, as the sun lights the day, and not as the moon lights the night.
>
> (S-M I/VII 270. *Vom Ursprung und Herkommen der Franzosen. Das viert Buch. Das VI. capitel*)
>
> The narcotic is removed in the way described and the particularity is removed—leaving a universal cure.
>
> (S-M I/VII 281. *Vom Ursprung und Herkommen der Franzosen. Das viert Buch. Das XIII. capitel*)

The remedy is universal because it matches the mineral origin of the disease.[17] It does so because it is under the guidance of heaven:

> Once you have effected this separation, then the medicine is in the power of the stars and is led and ruled by them.
>
> (S-M I/VIII 183. *Das Buch Paragranum. Alchimia der dritte grund medicinae*)

The idea of wholeness is seen further in the concept that the medicine restores health rather than driving out the disease: "In restoring the body the medicine restores health; thus the illness departs."[18e] This resembles the alchemical "purification" of metals.[19] And when the body has been cured, it stays cured; the person does not fall sick again soon:

> When the body is restored to health by the medicines described, no further breakdown will follow. This precribing is distinguished from that which allows the disease to return again.
>
> (S-M I/VII 282. *Vom Ursprung und Herkommen der Franzosen. Das viert Buch. Das XIV. capitel*)

And just as the philosopher's stone could transmute any metal into gold, some quintessences can heal all diseases.

Finally, Paracelsus expresses the remedy's wholeness by calling it "food." Just as the nourishment from food is carried from the stomach to all parts of the body, so the medicine makes the body whole by feeding it:

> Medicine shall be prepared so that it will be a food for the hunger and not a putting to sleep of the same.
>
> (S-M I/VII 264. *Vom Ursprung und Herkommen der Franzosen. Das viert Buch. Das drit capitel*)
>
> The nature wants its desire to be gratified and the medicine should fulfill that desire, and not be matched to a fullness. For just as a lust is fed and sated, in the same way illnesses are sated and fed. Therefore it is my

[e]Cf. the comment of Caelius Aurelianus on Herakleides' remark that treatment is designed to save the patient, not to break down the disease (*supra,* p. 256, note.).

> purpose that the medicine should be prepared in such a way that it will be accepted by the illness with such hunger and thirst as food is by the empty stomach.
>
> (S-M I/VII 262. *Vom Ursprung und Herkommen der Franzosen. Das viert Buch. Das erst capitel*)

> For since the nature itself is the physician and desires only an outside help from outside nature by virtue of an alliance, which both natures together have desired, therefore the same outer nature shall be put together with the inner one. Therefore, nature has in her some growing thing [*gewechs*] which shall be brought into another *corpus* and in that *corpus* applied to the body, and that same *corpus* shall be of the potion which the nature accepts as a food. For thus by means of the food the medicine unites itself into one, and thus in such shape that it heals the wound.
>
> (S-M I/X 94. *Das erste Buch der Grossen Wunderznei. Der ander tractat. Das ander capitel*)

These last passages bring out what has been implicit in the whole preceding discussion: the preparation of medicines by "purifying" metals is only an alchemical version of the Hippocratic "coction." The Greeks hypothesized coction as the organism's fundamental restorative process—it makes the morbific matter assimilable by the organism just as cooking food renders *it* palatable. Paracelsus extends the theory of coction to encompass the cooking of metals: "alchemy is an external bowel which prepares its own sphere for the star."[20f] Metals and minerals are made palatable by alchemical cooking.

Thus Paracelsus progresses from the Hippocratic "flavors" (in *Ancient Medicine*) to his own view that diseases are spiritual entities. The alchemical tradition that purification of a substance releases its quintessence supports his view that medicines also act spiritually. The outcome is a formulation of the doctrine of similars holding that (1) any mineral or metal contains a beneficial and a harmful component, (2) the

[f]This point is discussed further below, pp. 475-476.

former may be applied curatively to a disease originating in the latter.

NOTES

[1] S-M I/VIII 164. *Das Buch Paragranum. Das ander tractat, von der astronomia.* Also, S-M I/IX 474. *Von der Bergsucht und anderen Bergkrankheiten. Bk. I, Tract. II, Cap. IV.*

[2] Alan F. Titley, "Paracelsus: A Resume of Some Controversies," *Ambix: The Journal of the Society for the Study of Alchemy and Early Chemistry* (London), I: 3 (March, 1938), 166-183, at page 182.

[3] Pagel, *Paracelsus*, p. 87; Hopkins, *op. cit.*, p. 16.

[4] S-M I/I 211. *Volumen Medicinae Paramirum, Bk. III, Cap. X.* See Pagel, *Paracelsus*, p. 132.

[5] *Ibid.*, p. 212.

[6] *Loc. cit.*

[7] S-M I/IX 234-235. *Entwuerfe und Ausarbeitungen zu den (vier) Buechern des Opus Paramirum. Theophrastus Hohenheim de origine morborum und sanitatis. De sanitate et aegritudine. Tractatus II.*

[8] S-M I/VIII 124. *Aufzeichnungen zum I. und 3. Abschnitt des Paragranum.*

[9] S-M I/XI 187. *Labyrinthus Medicorum Errantium. Cap. V.*

[10] S-M I/IX 658. *Uslegung der Lateinischen synonyma.*

[11] S-M I/IX 658. *Uslegung der Lateinischen synonyma.*

[12] S-M I/VIII 192-194. *Das Buch Paragranum. Alchimia der dritte grund medicinae.*

[13] S-M I/X 94. *Das erste Buch der Grossen Wundarznei. Der ander tractat. Das ander capitel.*

[14] S-M I/IV 55. *De Gradibus et Compositionibus Receptorum et Naturalium Libri VII. Liber sextus. Caput septimum.*

[15] S-M I/VI 129-130. *Drei Buecher der Wundarznei. Das ander Buch. Cap. V.*

[16] S-M I/III 173. *Neun Buecher Archidoxis. Liber septimus. Von specifico odorifero.*

[17] S-M I/VII 328. *Vom Ursprung und Herkommen der Franzosen. Das VII. Buch. Das drit capitel.*

[18] S-M I/IX 205. *Die drei (vier) Buecher des Opus Paramirum. Liber quartus de matrice.*

[19] S-M I/III 119. *Neun Buecher Archidoxis. Liber quartus.*

[20] S-M I/VIII 59. *Paragranum. Vorrede und erste zwei Buecher. Entwuerfe und I. Ausarbeitung in Berezhausen. Vorred.*

CHAPTER XV

ANATOMY OF THE REMEDY
AND
ANATOMY OF THE DISEASE

Paracelsus' statement that cure by similars is based on identity of the disease anatomy and the anatomy of the remedy,[a] reflects his concern with the problem of remedy selection. If the remedy and the disease each have an "anatomy," they both present distinguishing characteristics to the physician's observation. If he knows these characteristics, the physician can identify the disease and select the correct remedy:

> You there bring together the same anatomy of the herbs and the same anatomy of the illness into one order. This simile gives you an understanding of the way in which you shall heal.
>
> (S-M I/I 375. *Weitere Verstreute Bruchstuecke ueber das Podagra*)

The problem is to know what are the characteristics of the disease and the remedy, and how the physician employs them to cure the patient. He does it generally by observing the parallels between microcosm and macrocosm. The disease is part of the microcosm, and the remedy is part of the macrocosm. But the doctrine of similars provides a particular key to the analysis of the microcosm and the macrocosm in directing attention to certain specific and identifiable features of the illness and the remedy which the physician can use for therapeutic purposes.

The primary path to knowledge of the microcosm is through knowledge of the macrocosm:

[a]See above, p. 388.

> No brain can fully encompass the structure of man's body and the extent of his virtues; he can be understood only as an image of the macrocosm, of the Great Creature. Only then does it become manifest what is in him. For what is outside man is also inside; and what is not outside man is not inside. The outer and inner are *one* thing, *one* constellation, *one* influence, *one* concordance, *one* duration . . . *one* fruit.
>
> (S-M I/VIII 180. *Das Buch Paragranum. Der ander tractat, von der astronomia*)
>
> He who studies the sun and the moon and knows with his eyes closed how the sun and the moon look, bears them within himself in the same form as they shine in heaven. Philosophy teaches that they are intangibly imprinted upon man, just as in the firmament, one like a mirrored image of the other. Just as a man can see himself reflected exactly in a mirror, so the physician must have exact knowledge of man and recognize him in the mirror of the four elements, in which the whole microcosm reveals itself.
>
> (S-M I/VIII 71. *Paragranum. Vorrede und erste zwei Buecher. Entwuerfe und I. Ausarbeitung in Berezhausen. Der erste grund der arznei, welcher ist philosophia*)

Hence Paracelsus urges the physician to study the macrocosm and to understand the microcosm from it:

> The condition of urine must be read from the outer world, the pulse must be understood in relation to the firmament, physiognomy to the stars, chiromancy to the minerals, the breath to the east and west winds, fever to earthquakes, etc.—If the physician understands things exactly and sees and recognizes all illnesses in the macrocosm outside man, and if he has a clear idea of man and his whole nature, then and only then is he a physician. Then he may approach the inside of man; then he may examine his urine, take his pulse, and understand

where each thing belongs. This would not be possible without profound knowledge of the outer man, who is nothing other than heaven and earth. It would be bold and presumptuous to approach the study of man without such knowledge and to defend the sandy ground of speculation, which is more unstable than a reed in the wind.

> (S-M I/VIII 76. *Paragranum. Vorrede und erste zwei Buecher. Entwuerfe und I. Ausarbeitung in Berezhausen. Der erste grund der arznei, welcher ist philosophia*)

The physician's supreme task is to observe the outer *naturalia*. For the inner ones want to be governed and treated according to these.

> (S-M I/VI 271. *Von allen offenen Schaeden. Das VI. Buch. Von anderen ofnen scheden in der gemein*)

Those who don't know [the metals] will not know what the diseases are.

> (S-M I/VIII 147. *Das Buch Paragranum. Der erste tractat, von der philosophia*)

And further, we have no knowledge of diseases, only what the heavens indicate.

> (S-M I/VIII 175. *Das Buch Paragranum. Der ander tractat, von der astronomia*)

Impossible it is for us to see and to learn what there is in the body, also no truth on how one thing or another comes about, but just what the great world indicates to us.

> (S-M I/VII 269. *Vom Ursprung und Herkommen der Franzosen. Das viert Buch. Das VI. capitel*)

He who now is a philosopher, he shall enter into the faculty of medicine and convert the external into the internal. The conversion makes the physician, as out of the large world comes the small world. He should so order things that he learn not from the inner man, for there is nothing but seduction and death. He could analyze all the patients there are and still not understand the inner man unless he invokes the outer man.

> (S-M I/VIII 86. *Paragranum. Vorrede und erste zwei Buecher. Entwuerfe und I. Ausarbeitung in Berezhausen. Der erste grund der arznei, welcher ist philosophia*)

The necessary knowledge of the microcosm and macrocosm is given by sense-perception.

> Every mineral there is, opens up its effects, both bad and good, visibly before the eyes; thus they also manifest themselves in the body.
>
> (S-M I/IX 242. *Entwuerfe zu den vier Buechern des Opus Paramirum*)
>
> Inasmuch as the physician is nothing but a guide dog, the same smells the game and smells its footsteps from one to the next until he finds the game itself. Let that be an example to you. As the dog has it in the nose, that you have just as much in the eyes. Learn to recognize the equivalent formations of the anatomy, so that it will not resist you. For only by following this trail will you be able to prescribe the recipes, and you must keep no other method but that which the trail indicates to you.
>
> (S-M I/VIII 365-366. *Von hinfallenden Siechtagen der Mutter. Par. IX.*)

The problem is how the physician obtains this knowledge solely through sense-perception.

Discovery of the Anatomy of the Remedy

By "anatomy of the remedy" Paracelsus means the pattern of spiritual forces within it, not its external form:

> Just as man has his own parts [*glider*], one in one place, another in another, as anatomy indicates, thus the growing things also have their parts: a heart, a liver, a gall-bladder, etc. just as in man. But every such heart is not visible to the eyes, but is a force and a power like that of the heart. . . . Just as every *corpus* has several

> parts but only one body, there you have only one growing thing but numerous forces in it. Just as in the firmament, there are the seven parts as in a man: heart, kidneys, stomach, lungs—not perceptible [*greifliche*] parts but forces and powers without a *corpus* . . . the body is not the *spiritus*, the body is the physician's help.
>
> (S-M I/XI 204-205. *Labyrinthus Medicorum Errantium. Das IX. capitel*)

The physician must comprehend and use this pattern of spiritual forces. Since he cannot observe it directly, he must learn from the macrocosm:

> As little as we can see in a plant what is inside, so little can we see into a man. . . . To know what is hidden in the nature, you must go outside the nature and there find the teacher. Out of this grows experience.
>
> (S-M I/VII 370. *Spital-Buch. (Erster Teil). Dr. Theophrastus allen aerzten seinen gruss*)

One way to obtain knowledge of the remedy is from its signature. The doctrine of signatures held that the medical power of a plant is revealed by its external form; the sidereal body of the plant is congruent with its corporal body.[1]

> Learn to recognize the spouse inside, that is, the form of the medicine, which its equivalent physiognomy indicates to you of its power [*kraft*] and shape.
>
> (S-M I/I 366. *Von den podagrischen Krankheiten und was ihnen anhaengig* (*zwei Buecher*). *Liber secundus Physionomia*)

> There is no illness but has a structure [*austeilung*] and members. If now that is the case, then her enemy also stands in the same image; thus is found something equal, which will be that which drives away the other, as for example: in all measure and shape as the eyes hold their anatomy, thus also *euphragia* holds it. From that it now follows that *euphragia* does not let anything damaging stand to the eyes; for they are on terms of friendship and united in the blood, both sprung from one seed and changed merely in the visible sphere. Therefore the friendly blood strengthens its cousin.

> (S-M I/X 260. *Das ander Buch der Grossen Wundarznei. Das XII. capitel*)
>
> By the art you know the *signatum*, by which everything there is is marked after that out of which it is and to which it belongs, so that therefore every time like and like is found, as then is indicated by the *ars signata*, which a physician shall especially know because of his understanding.
>
> (S-M I/XI 71-72. *Das Buch von den tartarischen Krankheiten. Das XI. capitel*)
>
> In the same way, further arts are also taken from anatomy, that form and form agree, and that the form indicates that for which the locked-up power—which lies hidden under the form—is good.
>
> (S-M I/VIII 304. *Von den hinfallenden Siechtagen. Von corallen*)
>
> Everything that is inside, both in sensitive and insensitive animals, yields a sign of this on the outside, by which figure or sign that which is inside may be sufficiently understood.
>
> (S-M I/X 301. *Das zweite Buch der Grossen Wundarznei. Der ander tractat. Das viert capitel*)

Oswald Croll indicates that the crown of the poppy plant (representing the head) is valuable in diseases of the head; the walnut (resembling the brain) is for brain diseases; haematites (bloodstone), red coral, and burnt calcanthum are all valuable for arresting hemorrhage; the dross of slag from melting iron, "having the signature of the scaly lips of ulcers," is to be used in the same.[2]

Diseases caused by tartar deposits in the body are cured by medicines made from stones:

> To drive out the tartar in its foundations, roots, herbs, seeds, etc. are not enough, but only the corresponding stones. . . . Therefore, then know that the science of signatures proves such things and indicates by the signatures lying in the stones named that they have the power to drive away the tartar. Therefore, one who wants

to be a physician shall know the signature of tartar, and after that the signature of the medicine, so that both signatures will get together in one anatomy, in one cosmography.

(S-M I/XI 108-109. *Das Buch von den tartarischen Krankheiten. Das XVIII. capitel*)

This is the simple way of recognizing the medicinal powers of a substance. The more important question is whether or not Paracelsus proposed other procedures for ascertaining the medicinal powers of metals and minerals.

A clue is given in his comments on physiognomics and chiromancy (palmistry)—the two bodies of learning which systematize his conviction that the internal is revealed by the external:

Through the art of chiromancy and the art of physiognomics . . . it is possible to tell by the shape, form, and color, and nothing more, the qualities and virtues of each herb and root; these are their signs. And for this we need no other test [*probirung*] or long study. For God has carefully differentiated all His creation from the beginning, and has never given to different things the same shape and form.

(S-M I/XIII 376. *Liber de Imaginibus, Caput IX.*)

Physiognomics is the art of discovering what is within and hidden in man . . . . It tells us in what relation his heart stands to God and his neighbor, what eyes are those of a rogue and what eyes are not, which tongue is cunning and which is not, which ears are open to evil and which to good.

(S-M I/XII 343. *Astronomia Magna. Der ander Buch. Das viert capitel. Was signatum coeleste, was coelistis signatum sei*)

Physiognomics, however, is developed by Paracelsus to include what a person reveals of himself *in action*:

If we want to make a statement about a man's nature on the basis of his physiognomy, we must take everything into account; it is in his distress that a man is tested, for then his nature is revealed. For *in extremis*, things reveal their nature and become visible.

(S-M I/XIV 183-184. *Philosophia Magna. Liber artis praesagae*)

By [physiognomics] we know a man's temperament and his attitude toward God and his fellow men. . . . For his conduct toward God, his ways of acting, hearing, and seeing, all these are signs by which his heart can be known. . . . For it is written: by their fruits ye shall know them.

(S-M I/XII 343. *Astronomia Magna. Der ander Buch. Das viert capitel. Was signatum coeleste, was coelistis signatum sei*)

Taking an example from man, no natural virtue is in him without it being marked on him externally, either in his nature or in his proportions, *or in his gestures*, or in his tongue, eyes, ears, etc.

(S-M I/X 300-301. *Das zweite Buch der Grossen Wundarznei. Der ander tractat. Das viert capitel*)

There are four ways by which the nature of man and of all living things can be discovered. . . . First, chiromancy; it concerns the extreme parts of man's limbs, namely the hands and feet . . . . Second, physiognomics, it concerns the face and the whole head. . . . Third, the *substantina,* which refers to the whole shape of the body. . . . And fourth, the customs and usages, that is to say, *manners and gestures in which man appears and shows himself.*

(S-M I/XII 174-177. *Astronomia Magna. Bk. I. Das Buch der Philosophei des himlischen Firmaments. Das XII. capitel. Probatio particularis in scientiam signatam*)

It is difficult to know if this was extended by Paracelsus to include the physician's discovery of the powers of plants and minerals. He states frequently that such powers are revealed by experience based on knowledge of external signs:

Therefore, whoever wants to be experienced in medicine and to understand that which he ought to understand,

> shall learn to recognize the external signs and know what they mean.
>
> (S-M I/X 300-301. *Das zweite Buch der Grossen Wundarznei. Der ander tractat. Das viert capitel*)
>
> Who can believe that in the seed of the *euphragia* be such colors, form, herb, and leaves? Nobody but he who sees what it becomes. *The works make it be believed, for they reveal what is in it.* Thus the physician shall know that the invisible things in it are in knowledge, just as the visible ones. To him, however, who does not know the visible things, the invisible are not credible.
>
> (S-M I/I 57. *Elf Traktat. 3. Von farbsuchten. Andere Redaktion*)
>
> Seek knowledge of the *quinta essentia* through experience. In that you will understand the degrees of its division.
>
> (S-M I/IV 25. *De Gradibus et Compositionibus Receptorum et Naturalium Libri VII. Liber tertius. Caput tertium*)

This is fully consistent with his view that knowledge comes from experience. It is also consistent with the distinction made in Greek medicine between the indicative and the commemorative sign. But what sort of "experience" is he referring to? He objects strenuously to the Galenist practice of haphazardly administering one medicine after the other, until finally the patient gets well:

> How many graveyards must you fill up with this testing [*prob*] before you will learn the man from the inner man? Is this physician-like or murderer-like? A truly wise man could judge whether God intended us to occupy ourselves on earth with this kind of murder or not, for our health. . . . And you say that medicine is so ordered by God, and that the physician should proceed in this way, i.e. through this murdering. In your view it is so, but God did not ordain it in this way—you only imagine it so. God wants us to learn from the outer man, so as not to murder.

(S-M I/VIII 154. *Das Buch Paragranum. Erste tractat.* Also, S-M I/VIII 86-87 and I/X 401)

And, furthermore, he was himself seeking a technique for ascertaining *a priori* what medicine should be prescribed in a given disease.

The healing properties of medicines could be determined *a priori* in two ways—through alchemy and by giving them to healthy persons.

Paracelsus suggests that alchemy is used not only to prepare medicines but also to discover their curative powers. It is "an adequate explanation of the properties of all the four elements . . . and an introduction into the art of their transformation."[3] "I praise the art of alchemy because it reveals the mysteries of medicine."[4]

> The great virtues that lie hidden in nature would never have been revealed if alchemy had not uncovered them and made them visible. Take a tree, for example; a man sees it in winter, but he does not know what it is, he does not know what it conceals within itself, until summer comes and discloses the buds, the flowers, the fruit. . . . Similarly, the virtues in things remain concealed to man, unless the alchemist discloses them, as the summer reveals the nature of the tree.
>
> (S-M I/VIII 191. *Das Buch Paragranum. Alchimia, der dritte grund medicinae*)

Precisely how alchemy was supposed to reveal the therapeutic uses of medicines, however, remains a mystery. In one passage Paracelsus mentions "testing" the remedy:

> And tell me what the corals may do. You know it and babble much and at length about their powers, but when it comes to testing [*probiren*] them, you don't in the least know how to test the powers of the corals, and this is because the process of the *arcanum* is not written in the books. But when the process is over, then its virtues are there.
>
> (S-M I/VIII 189. *Das Buch Paragranum. Alchimia, der dritte grund medicinae*)

The "testing" or "trying" (*probirung*) of substances was a standard alchemical procedure, designed to reveal their inherent properties.[5] Alchemy was also used to isolate the medicinal power in plants and minerals once the power had been recognized by the signature. But could alchemy disclose the existence of a property which could not first be seen from the signature? We do not know.

The second technique available to Paracelsus for determining the therapeutic properties of substances was observation of their effects (especially poisons) when ingested by healthy persons. Such a procedure is described in his work on miners' diseases: he noted the symptoms of different kinds of poisoning and on this basis was able to ascertain the mineral origin of diseases whose symptoms resembled these poisonings.

Others of his writings mention the effect on the body of the external application of plants and minerals.[6] Since he did not distinguish between internal and external lesions—subsuming both under surgery—he might have been expected to investigate the effect of their internal administration.

Thus his next step would have been to administer metals and minerals *in a systematic way* to healthy persons (as had been suggested by Galen).[b] This step was, in fact, taken by Samuel Hahnemann, the founder of homoeopathic medicine, possibly through inspiration from Paracelsus, but we cannot say whether or not Paracelsus did the same.

Discovery of the Anatomy of the Disease

Paracelsus maintains that diseases arise out of the mineral matrix of the body. And since every mineral has a variety of possible forms, each illness has its own specific form which Paracelsus calls the disease "anatomy":

> The illnesses are forged and made in the same way as man is; for that reason, then, each illness is a man, that is, in the property and form of a man, thus also the medicine.

[b] K XVI 86-87. See above, p. 313.

(S-M I/I 363. *Von den podagrischen Krankheiten. Liber secundus. Communis interpretatio morborum*)

Furthermore, the enemy and his conqueror have manifested themselves by anatomy, chiromancy, and physiognomy.

(S-M I/X 260. *Das zweite Buch der Grossen Wundarznei. Eingang des ersten Buchs von den dingen, so dem menschen aus dem glauben zufallen*)

Since [the disease] is now a man and yet invisible, its physiognomy must be taken as it will reveal it and then be matched with the medicine, so that one physiognomy stands on both sides. Thus look for that physiognomy, not of the bodily *corpus*.

(S-M I/I 366. *Von den podagrischen Krankheiten und was ihnen anhaengig. Liber secundus. Physionomia*)

When the physician can observe a certain set of symptoms, how does he know the mineral at the base of this syndrome?

Here Paracelsus proposes three possible solutions. In the first place, the underlying mineral component can sometimes be recognized directly—through the obvious identity between the form of the illness and the properties or form of the mineral. Thus:

Don't you see that *persicus ignis* or *prunus* is a resin? For whatever burns or accepts to be burned is subject to the resin?

(S-M I/VI 118. *Drei Buecher der Wundarznei. Das ander Buch. Vom missbrauch und irrung der alten arzet und scribenten*)

As nature prefigures to us externally the mineral's nature in the rushes, in woods, and other plants, accordingly we shall also know that the salt in the body by its operation gives similar forms; from which it now follows that like heals its like, which is to say, equals form equal kinds of holes. And it has been shown with all types of holes that its like form has been its like medicine. Therefore it behooves the physician to know the anatomy of matching one thing with another.

(S-M I/X 551. *Von Oeffnung der Haut. Ein Fragment. Liber primus. Caput VI.*)

As the *arundines*, etc. take their growing out of the earth, in that way also the saltpeter takes the form in the body out of the kind of salt which also makes *aristolochia rotunda* hollow. For of such effects there are many in the salts, but they do not concern the physician. And in the same way as there are many kinds of tastes in the *arundines*, one sweet, one sour, etc., thus there are also many kinds of flows and waters which grow out of the fistulas. . . . Therefore understand thus about the fistulas; they stand where they want to, in that the differences among them are not to be considered, and they are all equal or similar to their *generata*.

(S-M I/VI 286-287. *Von allen offenen Schaeden. Das VII. Buch. Von den fistulen)*

Now for this *theorica* pay attention to the burning herbs, namely that it is possible to bring by *urtica, flammula*, etc. such a wildfire into the thighs, also by *cantharides*, also by realgar, arsenic, and others. In that way, too, if the *iliadus* lets a mineral go from its chains, then such illnesses originate. Since we have in the body all the minerals. For with anyone whose thighs bite and are mangy with watery acid, this is matched with the powers of *urtica*. What goes to the waterpocks is matched to the powers of *flammula* etc. If now such a thing is possible, that *that flammula which is in the body makes the same operations as the outer one*, who then is going to contradict the theory of minerals out of which the physician derives his strength and recognizes the content of the universe?

(S-M I/VI 276. *Von allen offenen Schaeden. Das VII. Buch. Vom wilden feuer)*

It will be recognized by the physician which burning and blisters are made by the *urtica*, which scales and scratching are caused by the *plumosum*, which indications by *siva rubea*, etc. and similarly, all *salia, aerugines*, and whatever else is corrosive hidden in the external salts.

And just as these same minerals give rise to external *pruritus,* so do their equivalents in the microcosm break out in the same colors, forms, pains, swellings.

(S-M I/VI 280-281. *Von allen offenen Schaeden. Das VII. Buch. Von den umfressenden loechern)*

Astrological concordance provides a second path to knowledge of the disease, and of the remedy also. In medical astrology the parts of the body, diseases, and certain common metals and minerals are associated with the sun, the moon, the planets, and the signs of the zodiac. Thus Aries governs the head and face, Taurus the throat and neck, Gemini the hands, arms, shoulders, collarbone, lungs, and nervous system, Cancer the breast and stomach, Leo the heart, sides, and upper part of the back, Virgo the solar plexus and bowels, etc. Saturn is associated with lead, sulphur, and alum (minerals) and with dropsy, paralysis, leprosy, and hypochondria (diseases). Jupiter is associated with tin, green jasper, emerald, and governs apoplexy, pleurisy, heart disease, jaundice, and gout. Mars rules red copper and iron and causes plague, burning fevers, dysentery, and others.

Knowing the patient's date and time of birth, the physician knows the house of the zodiac in which the sun was located at this moment (the sun sign) as well as the zodiacal sign rising above the eastern horizon (the ascendant). Certain organs of the body, medicines, and diseases are also associated with these two factors.

By reading the movements of the planets, the sun and moon, the signs of the zodiac, etc. the physician can diagnose disease and prescribe remedies.[c]

A third way to discover the disease anatomy is through observation of poisonings. This has already been discussed in connection with the anatomy of the remedy, but the same procedure discloses the anatomy of the disease.

[c] Astrology and the movement against astrology, which was just beginning at this time, are discussed in great detail in Lynn Thorndike's *A History of Magic and Experimental Science* (6 vols., New York, 1923-1958).

However, the curative process itself yields the most information on the disease anatomy. The physician's therapeutic experience leads him to an understanding of disease:

> The physician . . . shall compose the recipe out of his great knowledge, and this leads to the nature, to the anatomy of the members, and *after that to the anatomy of the malady*. . . . Just as a game animal runs ahead of the dog and yet leaves behind such a scent that the dog finds his way, so are the *arcana* game running ahead of all maladies. The physician shall be a hunting dog and find the trail . . .
>
> (S-M I/VIII 365-366. *Von hinfallenden Siechtagen der Mutter. Par. IX.*)
>
> The man and the outer things are matched with one another inasmuch as they accept each other. That is to say, *as soon as the physician comes to understand what things accept one another, then he has the record of the anatomy.*
>
> (S-M I/IX 94. *Die drei (vier) Buecher des Opus Paramirum. Liber secundus. Caput secundum*)
>
> Where now the malady lies there the medicine has its form and its essence and property. That is how the spiritual, essential, medicinal man is recognized—by the place in which the cure lies. For it is *homo cancri, homo lupi, homo guttae, homo pestis, homo febris, homo hydropsis, homo profluvii, homo menstrui, homo vermium*, etc. in all illnesses.
>
> (S-M I/XI 211. *Labyrinthus Medicorum Errantium. Das X. capitel*)
>
> For thus the recipes act, that if one knows the symptoms of the disease, *then they indicate to him the cause* and that cause and the symptoms [the physician] finds by the light of nature.
>
> (S-M I/X 553. *Von Oeffnung der Haut, Ein Fragment. Liber primus. Caput VII.*)

Any systematic exposition of the Paracelsan teachings gives the impression of moving in a circle, since the point of departure lies outside the teachings themselves.

The physician's practice is both the starting-point and the culmination of all doctrinal exposition, since the proof of doctrinal truth is found only in the favorable response of patients to treatment. If the patient recovers, doctrine is assumed to be correct.

Hence the various aspects of the Paracelsan cosmology all arise out of the matrix of practice. They cannot be developed from one another, and they are not necessarily consistent with one another. Since the process of cure is ultimately a mystery, the different ways in which it can be symbolized need not be mutually consistent.

And since all doctrine necessarily refers back to the fact of cure, this fact is the ultimate proof of doctrinal truth. One doctrine cannot be proven correct by another, and the argument ultimately becomes tautological, seeking authority only in fact, not in other doctrine. The anatomy of the medicine is given by practice, as is the anatomy of the disease. The cause of the disease is identical with its cure. "There the ground lies where the remedy lies; in the latter lies the recognition, understanding, and knowledge, and that which leads to them."[7]

Doctrinal Corollaries

This method of defining disease and remedy has important consequences for two of the problems which exercised the Rationalist and Empirical schools of antiquity: the number of symptoms to be taken into account in treating disease and the number of possible diseases.

Since each disease is determined by the mineral which generates it, the number of possible diseases is a function of the number of species and sub-species of minerals. "The species of earths are species of illnesses; thus, not seventy kinds of fevers, but so many kinds of [minerals] against the fevers, that many kinds of fevers. The *genera* [of minerals] give the *genera* of division and in the same are also the divisions of the illnesses."[8] "The nature of the elements is such that any illness made by the nature of the body has its equivalent in the nature of the element. . . . For which reason the *genera* of diseases may be recognized out of the *genera* of the elements."[9]

> There are as many species of jaundice as there are medicines for jaundice; hence, there must be as many different anatomies, i.e., different species, of this illness, which, except for the differences in the medicines, you would not be able to find.
>
> (S-M I/I 375. *Weitere verstreute Bruchstuecke ueber das Podagra. I.*)

> No physician can describe the least illness so that it should straitly follow his letter. For which reason not for nothing shall the philosophy of minerals be known, out of which all [disease] generations are understood.
>
> (S-M I/VI 371. *Von Blattern, Laehme, Beulen, Loechern, und Zittrachten der Franzosen und ihres gleichen. Das viert Buch. Das ander capitel*)

The number of possible diseases, while not infinite, is nonetheless very great, and Paracelsus is thus closer to Empiricism than Rationalism in this respect: "You will have trouble learning one mineral, and just think how hard it will be to learn the more than 1000 of them."[10]

From this the physician knows how many symptoms he must take into account in his diagnosis and treatment: the only symptoms with a right, as it were, to recognition are those which form part of the symptom-complex of one of the mineralic diseases:

> You see how the salts yield all forms; furthermore, that all of them are corrosive but that some corrode with pain and others without pain. But this fact shall not be used to justify another method of cure or another theory, but the physician should proceed according to the ulceration and regard neither form nor species.
>
> (S-M I/VI 284. *Von allen offenen Schaeden. Das VII. Buch. Von den fistulen*)

Hence the "unimportant" symptoms may be disregarded by the physician. This is the more true in that excessive preoccupation with symptoms may lead the physician to a "symptomatic" treatment, whereas the correct treatment is causal:

> The nature and force of a disease must be discovered by their cause and not by their symptoms . . . for we must not merely extinguish the smoke of the fire but the fire itself. If we want the earth to produce better grass, we must plow it and not merely tear out the bad grass. Similarly the physician . . . should direct his thought to the origin of the disease and not only to that which his eyes see. For in this he would see but the symptoms and not the origin. Similarly, smoke is only the symptom of the fire, not the fire itself.
>
> (S-M I/X 274. *Das zweite Buch der Grossen Wundarznei. Das XVIII. capitel)*
>
> These, however, since they don't make the illnesses, but the illnesses make them, I don't let them stand as signs.
>
> (S-M I/I 50. *Elf Traktat. 3. Von farbsuchten. Signa*)
>
> The *materia peccans* is nothing but a seed. Just as the simples mentioned above grow out of a little seed, so the same thing happens here. But what grows from the seed is not considered a disease; but the root, which keeps the seed's strength, that is the object of the cure.
>
> (S-M I/VI 287-288. *Von allen offenen Schaeden. Das VII. Buch. Von den fistulen*)
>
> The symptoms are to be taken only in that respect that by them the *corpus*, i.e. the substance, is recognized. He who incorrectly introduces the signs and causes will err in his whole practice.
>
> (S-M I/IX 69. *Die drei (vier) Buecher des Opus Paramirum. Erster teil. Das erste Buch. Caput sextum*)

Thus Paracelsus deviates in a very interesting fashion from the Empirical doctrine of antiquity. To the extent that he emphasizes the disease cause—even a formal cause—he must neglect the symptoms. There is an inherent conflict in medical thought between stress on the symptoms and stress on the disease cause.

Since the cause is given by the disease cure, Paracelsus proposes a new approach to naming diseases—after the cure rather than after the cause:

> Now if you will say, this [disease] is Jovic, that is Saturnic, then I cannot act against you. If you say, that is *acorina aegritudo* and this disease is *anthera,* then I will say that you are learned doctors, and will be telling the truth. For thus it goes out of philosophy. If you also say, that disease is *pulagii*, that is *melissae*, then I see that you have sense in those maladies. But if you say, that is *cholera,* that is *phlegma,* then I know that you don't have sense but are born out of speculation and fantasy, which never has given birth to anything with truth in it. Therefore, this is not medicinelike, but speculative and fantastic, since any fool can think up such a ground. Now in dysentery you say "This is *sanguis.*" It is not true. If you say, "It is *vitium stomachi,*" again it is not true. It is only imagining with you, for only the imagination needs the choleric, the phlegmatic, the melancholic, and the sanguinic. But if you would say, "This is *morbus hermodactyli,*" "This is *morbus coloquinthidis,*" "This is *morbus helleborinus,*" then I would have to commend you and say good things of you; for you would be on the right ground and would partake of truth. Thus the name should be based on and rooted in the right ground and not in fantasy. For *colica* is named *sibethina, iliaca* is named *moschata.* Why that? Because it is learned from the philosophy of the macrocosm, which to the philosophy of the microcosm gives, teaches, and shows every name, kind, property, and sign.
>
> (S-M I/VIII 142. *Das Buch Paragranum. Der erste tractat. Von der philosophia*)
>
> I am concerned only with finding out the origin of a disease and its treatment and with relating the name to this.
>
> (S-M I/XI 135. *Sieben Defensiones. Second Defense*)
>
> The names are properly given when based on therapy, such as *caducus viridellus morbus* (since this species of

epilepsy is cured by *viridellus*). But if it is not done that way, with these distinctions, then it is an error, since the distinctions remain nonetheless.

> (S-M I/XI 70. *Die drei (vier) Buecher des Opus Paramirum. Erster teil. Das erste Buch. Caput sextum*)

> The physician shall divide all illness according to the names of his medicines . . . and say thus: He shall not say, "This is *icteritia*." That is unmasterly, for any peasant's hand knows that much. But thus he shall speak: that is *morbus leseoli*, and for this reason—you thereby comprehend *cura,* property, name, quality, disposition, and art and science in one name. For *leseolus* cures *icteritia* and nothing else.
>
> (S-M I/III 8. *Von den ersten dreien Principiis. Das sechste capitel*)

He even urged that a fracture or a broken bone be called *morbus consolidativus* instead of the Galenic "solution of continuity."[11]

Finally, it may be noted that Paracelsus fails to solve the problem of the uniqueness and specificity of the individual constitution. Sometimes he maintains that the individual is unique:

> The same way as you dye a piece of cloth yellow and dye a piece of wood yellow, that is, one color, that is one illness but two bodies. Since now there are two bodies and yet one color, one *signum*, the medicine must be conformed to the body and not to the color, in the same way as a piece of wood is mastered by a planer, a piece of iron by a hammer. Attention needs to be had in these things, so know that the body shall lie under the physician's eyes. If he does not take it for itself, he will not drive out the illness. Although he may come with the medicine that takes away the color, still the body is there.
>
> (S-M I/IX 203. *Die drei (vier) Buecher des Opus Paramirum. Liber quartus de matrice*)

But more often the disease takes precedence over the uniqueness of the individual constitution:

> Each man is capable of *lepra, apoplexia,* and all illnesses, but the [mineral] anatomy gives to each one his particular illness . . . as many classes of earths, that many classes of men. And just as each kind of earth has its own *procreationes,* so each man carries his own *morbum.*
>
> (S-M I/VI 336-337. *Von Blattern, Laehme, Beulen, Loechern, und Zittrachten der Franzosen und ihres gleichen. Das ander Buch. Das viert capitel.* Also S-M I/VIII 86, S-M I/I 180, and S-M I/I 206)

> Thus also know, if vomiting, tightness around the chest, and many other such symptoms in limbs and the like occur, don't let yourself be bewildered or led to assume other causes of the illness; for thus is that man's nature, his to vomiting, his to tightness, his to fullness, his to paralysis, to pressing, his to flowing, his to constipation, etc. And although manifold different symptoms occur, to the one in this way, to the other in another way, yet this is not the fault of the illness. For the wood has one kind of fire, the oil another, the resin a third, and yet all are just the element fire.
>
> (S-M I/I 60. *Elf Traktat. 3. Von farbsuchten. Andere Redaktion. Signa*)

And in the *Volumen Medicinae Paramirum* he expressly denies that individuality is conferred by the horoscope.[12]

Paracelsus' difficulty here stemmed from the same source as his ambiguity with respect to the number of symptoms to be taken into consideration by the physician. A defined (as opposed to an unknowable) disease cause is incompatible with the specificity of the individual case. To the extent that Paracelsus veered toward definable causes he had to belittle the significance of the symptoms and of the individual constitution.

NOTES

[1] S-M I/XI 210. *Labyrinthus Medicorum Errantium. Das X. capitel.*

[2] O. Croll, *Bazilica Chymica and Praxis Chymiatricae* (London: John Starkey, 1670). Royal Chymistry, pp. 76-77. Of Signatures of Plants, Representing Human Members, pp. 1, 11, 17.

[3] S-M I/VIII 55-56. *Das Buch Paragranum. Vorred.*

[4] S-M I/X 66-67. *Das erste Buch der Grossen Wundarznei. Das XIII. capitel.*

[5] S-M I/XIV 415. *Coelum philosophorum sive liber vexationum (fixationum).*

[6] S-M I/VI 276, 280-282. *Von Allen offnen Schaeden. Das sibend Buch: Vom Wilden Feuer, Heilung, Von den umbfressenden loechern.*

[7] S-M I/VIII 83-84. *Paragranum. Vorrede und erste zwei Buecher. Entwuerfe und I. Ausarbeitung in Berezhausen. Der erste grund der arznei, welcher ist philosophia.*

[8] S-M I/I 321. *Liber de podagricis et suis speciebus. Liber primus. Anatomia.*

[9] S-M I/III 5. *Von den ersten dreien Principiis. Das dritte capitel.*

[10] S-M I/VIII 147. *Das Buch Paragranum. Der erste tractat. Von der philosophia.*

[11] S-M I/III 455. *Tabellarisch gruppierte Uebersichten allgemeiner Krankheitstypen.* Also, S-M I/VI 59.

[12] S-M I/I 177-182. *Volumen Medicinae Paramirum. Bk. I. Cap. 2-5.*

CHAPTER XVI

CURE BY THE HEALING POWER OF NATURE

Finally Paracelsus presents cure by similars as the body's natural healing power seizing the remedy and wielding it against the disease. The remedy is effective against the disease because it is like the disease:

> Therefore, then the nature takes a weapon against the illness which looks like the illness and is like the illness, and uses the mastery like a warrior who wields his weapon depending on how his enemy meets him. The nature is like this, and I recommend that the physician understand her skill if he wants to make good on his allegations.
>
> (S-M I/II 325. *Von den natuerlichen Wassern, Buch III-V. Das IV. Buch. Der vierte tractat*)
>
> And the physician should let that be his example how two enemies set themselves against each other, who are both cold, who are both hot, who are both in armor, who both enter the fight with the same weapon. As now there victory is sought, thus you should also know that in man the two fighters demand natural help from one mother, that is, from one strength. With such strength also the *arcana* do act.
>
> (S-M I/VIII 106. *Paragranum. Vorrede und erste zwei Buecher. Entwuerfe und I. Ausarbeitung in Berezhausen. Der ander grund der arznei, welcher ist astronomia*)

This is merely a detailed statement of his general thesis that the major role in healing is played by the body's own forces:

Then our own nature is itself our physician, which is to say, it has in itself what it needs.[a]

(S-M I/IX 92. *Die drei (vier) Buecher des Opus Paramirum. Liber secundus. Caput secundum*)

Where the nature itself does not want to be a medicine, there all illnesses are mortal.[b]

(S-M I/XI 91. *Das Buch von den tartarischen Krankheiten. Das XIV. capitel*)

That also the physician should know, that the body by itself drives away more illness than the physician and his medicine.

(S-M I/IX 359. *Vorlaeufige Ausarbeitung zum vorstehenden Entwurfe der fuenf Buecher von den unsichtbaren Krankheiten. Caput de morbis somnii*)

When there is an illness in the body, all healthy members fight against it, not only one, but all of them; for one illness is the death of all of them. That the nature notices, and therefore it strikes out against the illness with all the might of which it is capable.

(S-M I/IX 95. *Die drei (vier) Buecher des Opus Paramirum. Liber secundus. Caput secundum*)

This natural healing power is found crystallized in *mumia* (mummy)–desiccated human flesh, originally prepared from the bodies of travelers who had died of thirst in the desert.[1]

Mumia is a liquor which is spread through the whole body and which causes parts to heal . . . the wounds are to be filled with the inner *mumia*.

(S-M I/VI 62, 71. *Drei Buecher der Wundarznei. Das erste Buch, Cap. II, VI.* Also, S-M I/III 249, 251. *De Vita Longa. Liber primus, Cap. I, II, III.* S-M I/IX 310. *Die Buecher von den unsichtbaren Krankheiten. Ingang des vierten Buchs*)

The *mumia* is the sweet mercury of the organism, which is identical with elemental mercury:

[a]Cf. *Nutriment*, cap. XV (Jones, I, 347).

[b]Cf. Celsus, *De Medicina*, III, 1: 4.

> *Mumia* is sweet mercury, as sweet mercury heals all wounds.
>
> (S-M I/VI 62. *Drei Buecher der Wundarznei. Das erste Buch. Cap. I.*)
>
> This balsam which is used to heal ulcers lies in the outer elements and is the balsam which prevents them from rotting . . . the outer balsam of the elements is the *liquor mercurialis* in which all healing lies.
>
> (S-M I/VI 135. *Drei Buecher der Wundarznei. Das ander Buch. Cap. VII*)

Paracelsus' confidence in the body's natural healing capacity owed something to his observation that wounds heal more rapidly when kept clean and otherwise left alone. In his *Chirurgia Magna*, published in 1535, he opposed the cauterization and filthy dressings of the Galenists—a reform in the treatment of wounds for which Ambroise Pare (1509-1590), writing ten years later, is usually given credit.[c]

Reliance on the natural healing power leads to interpretation of symptoms as signs of the body's struggle against disease. Hence they tell the physician precisely what the organism's healing power is doing to overcome the disease:

> Whichever signs occur, after which the patient must die, are the complaint of the nature; they ask for help the same way as a captain surrounded by enemies who cries for help by the sign *cito, cito, cito*, not meaning that the enemy has conquered him but only that he fears it; when it has conquered him, he no longer gives a sign for help; only before, nothing afterwards.
>
> (S-M I/VII 321. *Vom Ursprung und Herkommen der Franzosen. Das VI. Buch. Das XI. capitel*)

Hence the symptoms are not to be repressed but encouraged and stimulated by the physician:

> Here Hippocrates gives good instructions on how to drive out what is not fitting and suitable to the nature. For some want to drive out all that is obnoxious to the nature

[c]Pare's *La Methode de traicter les playes faictes par hacquebutes et aultres bastons a feu* appeared in 1545.

by the stool, some by the urine, some by sweat, etc. All that, however, shall no longer be, such thoughts shall be abandoned as not medicinelike. Know that the physician should first of all know where the nature wants to get out; for it is the first physician, the man is the second. Where now the nature starts, there the physician shall also help, so that it may go out in that place. That is to say, the nature is a better *medicus* than man, knows best where to go out is most useful. If it wants to get out by the sweat, and if you find the signs in *virtute expulsiva*, then help that it may go out by the sweat.

(S-M I/IV 523. *Deutsche Kommentare zu den Aphorismen des Hippokrates. Aphorismus XXI. Quae ducere oportet etc.*)

Consider well what you do, for if you heal up the flux, then you murder; if you direct it wrongly, if you heal up the self-healing lesions, then you murder.

(S-M I/X 556. *Von Oeffnung der Haut, Ein Fragment. Liber primus. Caput VIII.*)

These ideas fit naturally into the theory of mineral causes and cure through similars. Since the disease results from activation of one of the minerals in the body's matrix, the symptoms and visible lesions represent the effort made by the organism's archeus to drive the offending mineral out of the body. Cure must come from the similar medicine—the one which intensifies the symptoms and thereby furthers the organism's effort to expel the disease. Repressing the symptoms by administering a "contrary" medicine merely perpetuates the existing mineral disturbance. Paracelsus calls this "blocking" (*oppilatio*)—the body's natural outlets are stopped up, preventing the egress of the morbific substance or vapor. Fevers and plague fall into this category.[2] Certain manias are caused by the spirit of mercury rising to the head and seeking an outlet there.[3] Cancer is caused by *oppilatio* of the natural outlets for discharge of the realgar of hemorrhoidal or menstrual blood; thereupon the nature seeks another outlet, and this causes cancer. Cure must be sought in medicines which unblock these outlets.[4]

> But whatever is seeking passages of elimination is due to the diversification of the nature in the method of elimination. Thus, in expelling poison, the alchemist expels each poison by the passage proper for it: white sulphur through the nose, arsenic through the ear, the excrements through the anus, and likewise all other poisons, each according to how its passage has been arranged for. If one of these poisons is obstructed by inability of the nature, by conditions peculiar to it, or the like, then it also becomes a hearth of disease if you are afflicted.
>
> (S-M I/I 196. *Volumen Medicinae Paramirum. Bk. II. Cap. IX.* Also, *Cap. XII.*)

Even stones cleanse themselves inwardly in the same way: the moss on a stone is its "excrement" (*stercor*) which comes from the inside.[5]

In his work on miners' diseases, Paracelsus prescribes sweating as a general therapeutic method.[6]

The process of cure is not only from inside out, but also from upwards down:

> Where there are such lesions, there are good healthy eyes, and light heads. But before that and before they break open, there is a bad face, heavy heads, tightness of chest, stinging pain in the side, bad digestion in the stomach. All of which, however, goes away by the breaking open, not that the fluxes are setting down from above, but that the vitriols rise upwards to the higher parts and cause the illness described, which rising ceases to happen after the breaking open. For which reason the breaking open is the health of the same, and shall not be healed except after all the vitriol in the thigh is resolved away and melted.
>
> (S-M I/X 311. *Das zweite Buch der Grossen Wundarznei. Der ander tractat. Das IX. capitel*)

Hence medicines should be suitable to the power of the heart:

> Every cure should proceed from the power of the heart; for only thereby can all diseases be expelled. Therefore, and take good note of this, it is particularly absurd to act

in opposition to the heart. The heart wants to dispel the diseases, then why do you drive them toward the heart? . . . After all, the curative power must come from the heart, and the disease must be driven into the remotest corner. . . . Every medicine should act outward from the heart, and not in the direction of the heart. It starts from the heart and is made to work by the heart's own power.

(S-M I/VII 241-243. *Vom Ursprung und Herkommen der Franzosen. Das dritte Buch. Das IV. capitel*)

In the veneric *luxus* you shall act so that the medicine be appropriate to the heart and promote the natural expulsion.

(S-M I/VII 244. *Vom Ursprung und Herkommen der Franzosen. Das dritte Buch. Das V. capitel*)

The doctrine of the healing power of nature is psychologically related to the doctrine of long life. God, who created human beings, wanted them to live a long time and for that reason endowed them with a natural healing power:

> God alone preserves the body in life; He wants us to have a long life and therefore provides us with many kinds of help and support.
>
> (S-M I/IX 329. *Die Buecher von den unsichtbaren Krankheiten. Das V. Buch. Eingang*)
>
> . . . thus many dropsies are healed, many consumptions, and many other illnesses, without the patient knowing why, as he recovers from it out of natural inborn medicine. For God protects man in all ways from death, for the refreshment of his life. For in long lives of men God has pleasure.
>
> (S-M I/XI 198. *Labyrinthus Medicorum Errantium. Das VII. capitel*)

NOTES

[1] Multhauf, *op. cit.*, p. 105.

[2] S-M I/XIV 639. *De pestilitate. Von der cur und heilung der natuerlichen und ubernatuerlichen pestis, und das in 16 partikel geteilet. Caput primum.*

[3] S-M I/IX 234-235. *Entwuerfe und Ausarbeitungen zu den (vier) Buechern des Opus Paramirum. Theophrastus Hohenheim de origine morborum und sanitatis. De sanitate et aegritudine. Tractatus II.*

[4] S-M I/VI 264-266. *Von allen offenen Schaeden. Das VI. Buch. Vom Krebs, ursprung und heilung.*

[5] S-M I/IV 446. *De modo pharmacandi: erstes Buch. Tractatus II.*

[6] S-M I/IX 487-488. *Von der Bergsucht und anderen Bergkrankheiten. Bk. I. Tractat IV. Cap. 6.*

CHAPTER XVII

PARACELSUS THE PHYSICIAN

Having set forth the gist of Paracelsus' medical teachings in the form of comments upon his various formulations of the doctrine of similars, we may summarize the discussion, indicating the practical import of some of these ideas and their relevance to scientific method.

Paracelsus' Doctrine of Perception: The Importance of the Visible

Paracelsus sought a medicine of experience founded on visible knowledge. He wanted to bypass the speculative Galenic pathology by establishing a direct relationship between the (visible) symptoms and the (visible) formal cause. His writings are full of references to the visible, and many have been mentioned above.[a]

He stressed the visible for the same reason as the Empirical School: the visible is trustworthy because agreed upon by all and is thus a reliable guide to practice:

[a]If more are needed, the following passages and their contexts may be examined. "Thus the nature teaches the physician to recognize that lesion by her things which she exhibits, and to heal by those which heal these" (S-M I/X 544. *Von Oeffnung der Haut, Ein Fragment. Liber primus. Caput III.*). "Since [the disease] is now a man and yet invisible, its physiognomy must be taken as it will reveal it and then matched with the medicine" (S-M I/I 366. *Von den podagrischen Krankheiten und was ihnen anhaengig. Bk. II.*). "The physician shall derive his knowledge from things external and not from man. If he finds an illness in a man, he will not and may not recognize what it is and how from its location, but he must get his knowledge from outside" (S-M I/VIII 83. *Paragranum, Vorrede und erste zwei Buecher. Der erste grund der arznei*). "The nature possesses the knowledge and makes the meaning of all things visible; it is the nature that teaches the physician" (S-M I/VIII 70. *Paragranum. Vorrede und erste zwei Buecher. Der erste grund der arznei*). Also, S-M I/VI 179; S-M I/VIII 70, 144-145, 152, 179; S-M I/IX 44, 253; S-M I/X 260; S-M I/XI 205).

> This is my vow . . . not to guess, but to know.
> (S-M I/VI 181. *Entwuerfe, Notizen und Ausarbeitungen zur Bertheonea. Jus jurandum*)

Our understanding of Paracelsus differs from the customary view of this great thinker. It has been traditional to classify him as a magician, an astrologer, or, at best, a neo-Platonic philosopher, and scholars have lost sight of the important fact that he was above all a practicing physician. While he used the language of astrology and magic and borrowed concepts from contemporary philosophical discourse, his aim in so doing was to find the most suitable vehicle for expressing his medical and therapeutic insights. The essential problem for Paracelsus, as for any physician, was how to make intelligible the hidden and apparently unknowable processes occurring within the organism. The key to his thought is to be found only in an analysis of the therapeutic problems which he was trying to solve, and these were identical with the problems confronting the ancients.

Hence the matrix of his thought is supplied by the series of interlinked therapeutic problems which had exercised the Empirical and Rationalist Schools. In this conflict Paracelsus stood squarely on the side of the Empirics, agreeing with their assumption that the inner workings of the organism are not knowable *a priori*. His whole philosophy of the microcosm and macrocosm aims to find correspondences in the great world for the processes occurring in the body. He reinterprets the Rationalist *logos*—which to this school meant the physician's capacity to perceive the inner workings of the organism directly—as the "light of nature," meaning the abiiity to *learn from experience.*

The idea that medicine should be based on the visible is fully consonant with his religious views. Paracelsus notes in several places that nothing is so concealed that it may not be made visible,[1] a clear reference to the New Testament, for example, *Matthew* X:26 "Nothing is so secret that it cannot be made apparent." He states further:

> I must not speak and tell of the unseeable, but of the visible. For the doctor should bear in mind that we have

God visibly and perceptibly before our eyes . . . . Hence far more does medicine stand visibly before us and they should receive it visibly and not in a dream, perceptibly and not in the shadows.

(S-M I/IX 44. *Die drei (vier) Buecher des Opus Paramirum. Das I. Buch. Cap. I.*)

God, through the Holy Spirit, has given us sufficient mortal light to illuminate and complete our work and task, our talents and doctrine.

(S-M I/XII 13. *Astronomia Magna. Vorrede in die ganz philosophiam sagacem;* also, S-M I/I 300. *Ein Buechlein (Philosophia) de generatione hominis*).

By this he means that the Holy Spirit has granted man the light of nature which enables him to learn from experience.

His reliance on the visible gives rise to his major criticism of Galenic medicine. Their logic and dialectic "detract from the light of nature."[2] He is particularly incensed by their claim to possess *a priori* knowledge of physiological processes:

Who is there that could see a pestilence through the skin? . . . The Bacchants speculate through a wall and see the hidden which is not to be seen.

(S-M I/VIII 179-180. *Das Buch Paragranum. Der ander tractat.* "Bacchants" are Galenists. Also, pp. 164, 173.)

You must acknowledge that our eyes do not pass through the skin; hence we should not indulge in too much speculation, but base ourselves powerfully on the four elements.

(S-M I/VI 286. *Von allen offenen Schaeden. Das VII. Buch. Von den fistulen*)

Everything invisible should be removed from medicine. What the eyes of fire [i.e., alchemy] do not possess is the source of error. Out of this the unfounded medicine has been formed. It is hard to believe that the body contains four humors and expells them; this is only imaginary [*es stet im glauben*]. But medicine should not be imaginary

> but should be based on the eyes. Nothing is in the imagination but the diseases of the soul. All medicine of the body is visible, without any imagination.
>
> (S-M I/IX 44. *Die drei (vier) Buecher des Opus Paramirum. Das erste Buch. Caput primum*)

And, indeed, their assumed ability to comprehend the hidden workings of the organism is an extension of the ancient Rationalist view that physiological knowledge is given by the manipulation of logical categories.

Part of his attack on this aspect of Galenism was his assimilation of medicine to surgery—that part of healing which deals with the visible.[3]

Furthermore, reliance on the visible is fully in accord with Paracelsus' social attitudes. He scoffed at the superior airs of the school physicians who thought they understood the invisible: "You speak in such a strange language that no honest man can follow you. Thus medicine is separated from all professions and from all learned men. Hence I want to teach philosophy in German so that it will be accessible to all. By the same token, everything needed for the body can be discovered outside and tested [*probirt*] outside, passed through the fire and purified. When you have experienced everything outside, then you can go into the body."[4] In this passage, which typifies his thinking, he draws a parallel between speaking German so that even the uneducated will understand, and basing medicine on the visible—for the same reason. Since medicine is needed by all, it should be accessible to all. It should not be formulated as occult knowledge in the exclusive possession of a social minority whose interests are not necessarily in harmony with those of the patient, or of society as a whole.

Thus denial of the physician's capacity to perceive directly the workings of the organism is more than a detail in Paracelsus' medical doctrine. With him, as with the Greek physicians, this problem is fundamental, and its solution determines the whole structure of his medical philosophy.

This leads to our only criticism of Walter Pagel's works on Paracelsus. Pagel interprets the "light of nature" as the capacity of man's "astral body" to look directly into the objects of nature or, in other words, to commune directly with the "astral bodies" of other animate and inanimate things.[b] This leads him, in effect, to place theory before practice: he has endeavored to work Paracelsus' theory into a coherent structure and to base his medical practice upon this. "Paracelsus' persistent plea for homoeopathic and isopathic measures, and his doctrine of signatures so closely connected with this plea, *is the outcome of his quest* for knowledge through union of the object with something alike in the observer, and for the 'magnetic' forces and 'sympathy' in nature at large as expressions of the fundamental unity of all its objects and phenomena."[5] "The invention of remedies *hence follows from* a study of the correspondences between man and the world outside."[6] We maintain the contrary—Paracelsus' theory is derived from his practice and not his practice from his theory. Pagel's attempt to present the theory as the basis of the practice leads to a doctrine of perception which, in our view, Paracelsus never espoused. He did not think that he could perceive beneath the skin and directly into the interior of animals, plants, and minerals.

[b]See Pagel, *Paracelsus,* pp. 50, 52 (n. 39), 120; *Medizinische Weltbild,* pp. 55, 125. Pagel writes (in a communication to the author, February 23, 1966), "I take this to mean that something is received from the object and incorporated in the observer, i.e., a union (more or less close) with the object. In my opinion this exceeds mere empirical observation as well as what you can get by book-learning or from reading astrological tables of correspondences." He supports this view with references to *Philosophia Sagax,* Book III: *"nun der imaginiert, zwingt die kreuter"* [He who imagines, forces the plants] (S-M I/XIII 484), and *Philosophia Magna, Book III, Tractatus III, Caput I: "so ist mein geist im himel zu erfaren die kreuter, so ist mein geist in kreutern. Nun sind geist im himel, geist in kreutern, also im luft, also im wasser, dieselbigen geist und mein geist, die komen zusammen"* [As my soul is in heaven experiencing the herbs, so my soul is in the herbs. Now there is a soul in heaven and in the herbs, thus in the air and the water; this same soul and my soul come together.] (S-M I/XIV 58). But in the *Labyrinthus Medicorum Errantium* Paracelsus equates "Imagination" with the light of nature: *"was got fuer ein scienz geben hat den vitriolatis, durch welche scientiam kranke gesunt werden, das also scientia vitriolata, durch die der vitriolum operirt, in euch selbst sei wie in vitriolo imaginative imprimirt. das ist impressio luminis naturae und sind die radii, so sie in dich imprimirn"* [What God gave to the *vitriolata* as a science through which the sick are made well, i.e., the *scientia vitriolata* through which the *vitriolum* operates, is impressed imaginatively in you yourselves just as in the *vitriolum.* This is the impression of the *lumen naturae,* and the same rays make the impression on you.] (S-M I/XI 194).

Pagel's view is epitomized in his discussion of the following passage from the *Labyrinthus medicorum errantium:*

> . . . when you learn [*ablernen*] from the scammony the knowledge [*scientia*] which it possesses, it will be in you just as in the scammony.
>
> (S-M I/XI 191. *Labyrinthus medicorum errantium. Das VI. capitel.*)

He states that *ablernen* here means *ablauschen,* i.e., to overhear, adding that this yields a deeper knowledge of the thing than what is obtained through mere eyesight and that only the physician who is "called" can achieve it.[7]

Thus, to the word, *ablernen*—which means only "to learn" in any number of a variety of ways—Pagel attributes the sense of direct perception. The passage and its discussion exemplify the contrast between his interpretation of Paracelsus and our own view that the whole intent of Paracelsus' philosophy was to elaborate a method through which the physician could *ablernen* the mysterious ways of disease and health *without* being able to "overhear" them or perceive them directly. Even though Paracelsus occasionally makes statements such as: "[the physician] is the one who knows the invisible, which has no name and no matter but yet has its effect," he does not mean by this that the physician has a sixth sense which is denied to others. He only means that, *by employing the light of nature,* the physician can come to understand the invisible as well as the visible.[8] And when he claims that the *scientia* which is in nature is revealed by "*magica* in the three methods" he has in mind the application of philosophy, astrology, and alchemy—all of which yield knowledge through the light of nature.[9]

Thus Paracelsus relied entirely on sensory observation as a source of medical knowledge and did not allow the senses to penetrate below the surface of objects or of living beings.

We stress this conflict in interpretations of Paracelsus—as exemplified by Pagel's attempt to extend the meaning of *ablernen*—not for trivial reasons but because it represents the very point upon which the Empirical and Rationalist traditions were unalterably opposed, upon which no compromise could be allowed. We feel that the same is true for Paracelsus. Either he did or he did not allow the physician to perceive directly into the organism, and into other natural objects. We maintain that he did not, and from this flow the remaining doctrines of his therapeutic *weltanschauung*.

Underlying all of this is his conviction that medicine is visible because it should be, and must be, accessible to all—not merely to those who are "called" or have studied in the schools. And this, in turn, is the outcome of that love of his fellow man which is the cornerstone of his whole philosophy.

Paracelsus as a Scientist

To Paracelsus *scientia* means the unchanging laws of nature. And, like Hippocrates and the Empirics, he held that the physician will be successful only insofar as he obeys these laws: "For the nature is the master, but the physician is the servant. And the nature is such a master that she does not soon let herself be commanded by any servant."[10c]

The laws of nature are the "*practica globuli* or *sphaerae*," and they can be ascertained by man through the use of his senses and the light of nature. Even the stars have their own reason (*vernunft*), and man can comprehend their *scientia* by observing their movements. Hence astrology is for him the purest science—being based exclusively on observation and the light of nature.[11]

The physician cures disease through his knowledge of the *scientia* of plants and minerals. In other words, he takes the place of the archeus inside the body, which acts through *its* knowledge of the *scientia*. The correct remedy cures the disease because *it* knows the *scientia*. The remedy, the archeus, and the physician can all cure disease only insofar as they follow the laws of *scientia*.[12]

The question to be resolved now is how man comprehends the *scientia* of the universe. In general, this is possible because he is made of the same matter as the universe: "Thus

[c]Thus he anticipates Bacon's dictum: "Nature is commanded by obeying her."

the body of man accepts the body of the world, as the son accepts the blood from the father, for it is one blood and one body, separate only in soul, but not separated in the *scientia*. It therefore follows that sky and earth, air and water, are one man in the *scientia*, and man is one world with sky and earth, with air and water also in the *scientia.*"[13] Man does not obtain this information directly, however, as has been explained already. He must follow a rigorous routine and discipline: "Just as a teamster cannot go across shrubbery and mountains, thus also you cannot with the medicines. Therefore it is a *scientia* which goes out of the art of the light of nature, not out of speculation, within which no *scientia* has ever been.[14]

The physician comprehends *scientia* through the practice of medicine, that is, through his experience. But all experience is not equally valid. Paracelsus makes a very interesting distinction between "true" and "false" experience. The false experience he calls "*experimentum*" and maintains that it must be supplemented by *scientia* before it can become true experience—*experientia.*

Thus, in discussing *Aphorisms* I: 1, he states the following about the passage, "experiment is fallacious" (*experimentum fallax*):

> Hippocrates means that experience [*erfarnheit*] can be deceitful . . . . He means that it contains something but doesn't contain something, it is not to be trusted. And the same with experiments [*experimenten*].
>
> But *experientia* is the art and the help of the patient, and it must not be false. It must be valid and certain. For it is from God. The physician is from God—thus both were so created. If medicine now were deceitful, that would be neither honorable nor praiseworthy but would be the abrogation of medicine and would make it a nullity.
>
> It is far from being this. Like a woman who lives honorably in matrimony and thus has her husband—so should medicine be wedded to the physician. Hence it is not deceitful.

What preserves a marriage? Only knowledge of the heart, that is the beginning and the end. This the physician and the medicine should also be. One comes to the other, so there is nothing deceitful. But where such an understanding is absent, then all is false on both sides.

But things weren't this way in the times of Hippocrates. Then coloquinth was taken for all horses. It helped one and ruined another. Hence it was called by him deceitful, meaning that the knowledge of the two natures was lacking.

Thus in the beginning medicine had no theory [*theorica*] but only experience [*erfarnheit*]: this is a laxative, this other constipates. What worked and how they worked was hidden. Thus what harmed one helped the other.

Now we have theory, however, and things are not this way any more. Science [*scientia*] is there and no longer fallacious experiment [*experimentum*]. This is the effect of the medical theory which consists of four pillars: philosophy, astrology [*astronomia*], alchemy, and physic.

(S-M I/IV 496-497. *Deutsche Kommentare zu den Aphorismen des Hippokrates, Aphorismus I. Experimentum Fallax*)

Thus *scientia* transforms *experimentum* or *erfarnheit* into *experientia.* Paracelsus' discussion, in the *Labyrinthus medicorum errantium,* of the relations between *scientia, experimentum,* and *experientia* is even more revealing. He notes that medicine is nothing but a "certain great experience" *(experienz, erfarnheit).* But this is not the same as *experientia.* Nor are experiments (*experimenta*) the same as *experientia.* Through *scientia* the experiments are transformed into *experientia.* Where there is no *scientia,* there is just experiment. Without *scientia* it is just *experimentum ad sortem,* haphazard experimentation. *Scientia* is needed if experience is to be certain and reliable. "For *scientia* is the mother of experience, and without *scientia* nothing is there."

A pear tree bears fruit out of the *scientia* which God gave it. Scammony purges through the *scientia* given it by God.

This *scientia* includes not only the fact that it purges ("*alein das sie scheissen macht das weistu iezt, hast von ir nichts mer als von einem wort, das du nicht weisst was ist*"), but also the *what* and *how* ("*was er purgiren sol und wie*"). When you know as much as the scammony, then you will have experience with *scientia* and not just experiment alone. Unless you know as much as the scammony knows, you have only *experimentum* without *scientia.*

This is like being a German and hearing French spoken. You hear the words and recognize them but don't know what they mean.

The eyes give experiment, but experience arises from the understanding ("*sie sehen experientiam nicht, welche also verstanden sol werden*").

If God has given the *scientia* to all the growing things, how much more willingly does He give it to the physician, so that he will make his patients well, to honor him. "They will fall from him just as a pear tree lets the ripe pears fall to the ground."[15][d]

Science is the mother of experience, and Paracelsus deprecates the value of mere haphazard experimentation. The experience of the Galenists is a deceitful experience (*vermeinte erfarnheit*), since they do not know *scientia.*[16] Their doctrine is not a true science but only "*particular experimenten* which any peasant can do."[17] True experience must be born of philosophy.[18]

This seems to contradict his earlier position that experience is the test of all things and the source of all knowledge. But the contradiction is only apparent. His use of the categories, *scientia* and *experientia,* and his insistence that reliable experience (*experientia*) must incorporate *scientia,*

[d]Oswald Croll, who wrote a compendium of his doctrines in the early seventeenth century (translated into English as *Philosophy Reformed and Improved in Four Profound Tractates* (London, 1657), states that Paracelsus opposed "those that follow the rule of their experience" and "inveigh[ed] against empirics who have no skill at all" while the true physician has the "true knowledge and experience of Nature's light," the "theory and the practice" (pp. 128, 140, 141). This work is an excellent exposition of Paracelsus' medical doctrines.

are equivalent to asserting that scientific method must rest upon a hypothesis. Experimentation without a hypothesis yields no knowledge at all, for the experimenter cannot interpret the results of experiment without a hypothesis. If we take a passage such as "*scientia* is contained in the object in which God has provided it; *experientia* is knowledge of cases in which *scientia* has been put to the test,"[19] and replace the second "*scientia*" by "hypothesis," it becomes clear that those who have called Paracelsus a pioneer of scientific method are correct.[e]

The "hypothesis" here is Paracelsus' whole doctrine of the microcosm and the macrocosm, the *anatomia mineralis,* the mineral origin of diseases, and cure through similars.

A method based on hypothesis does, in fact, proceed by testing the hypothesis against experience. But the hypothesis itself must be formulated *a priori,* that is, deductively. Nonetheless, it is not simply invented out of thin air, but must itself be based on analysis of the situation and on other prior experience.[20]

One further comment may be made on the scientific element in Paracelsus' thought. The purpose of scientific method is to discover new knowledge, and the Empirical School emphasized this aspect of their method. Paracelsus draws attention to this aspect of his own philosophy, contrasting it with the procedures of the Galenists: "Speculation is just wishful thinking. The basis which I lay down is not speculation but discovery [*inventio*], not speculation but the properties of nature."[21] Paracelsus characterizes his own therapeutic procedure as the *inventrix magicae artis.*[22]

[e]Pagel denies that Paracelsus' therapeutic method is as close to scientific method as I have maintained. He writes that although Paracelsus is "inspired by a deep distrust of the power of human reasoning and is thus related to those trends of scepticism and empiricism which were soon to contribute to the foundation of modern science," and that this "yielded unexpected fruit, first in a negative critical sense by exposing the weakness and unreality of the ruling elemental and humoral doctrine and secondly in the adoption of experimentalism and empiricism," so that "in consequence, important proto-scientific ideas and findings already emerge in the works of Paracelsus," "their importance and range have been grossly overestimated," and Paracelsus "is not a scientist in the modern sense." (*Paracelsus,* pp. 51-53).

Duty and Responsibility of the Physician

Paracelsus is rancorous against the Galenists because they debase the vocation of physician—who is God's surrogate on earth and the channel of His mercy to mankind. "God has created medicine and the physician even though He Himself is the physician and operates through the physician and works nothing Himself without the physician."[23]

This suggests an important limitation on the physician's powers. He can do nothing against God's will; in particular, he cannot heal unless God so wills. "A physician should remember and be aware that he should not presume to know the hour when health is reinstituted, or the hour when his medicine is taking effect. For that lies in God's hand. But if the predestined course of events does not agree with what you physicians are about to do, you will not make the patient well with any medicine."[24]

The physician is limited in a second way: he must act in agreement with the natural healing effort of the organism (*die natur*): "The physician comes from the nature, from the nature he is born. Only he who receives his experience from the nature is a physician and not he who writes, speaks, and acts with his head and with ratiocinations aimed against the nature and her ways."[25] "You cannot contend against the nature and force it against its will. For which reason anyone will consider that a physician is merely the nature's servant and not its master."[26] "The art of healing comes from the nature, not from the physician. Therefore the physician must grow out of the nature with perfect understanding."[27]

In accepting these constraints on the physician's power Paracelsus might appear to be seeking an excuse for failure, but this would be incorrect, for (somewhat inconsistently) he does not admit any disease to be beyond the power of God or the nature to cure. In fact, he places a heavy burden of responsibility upon the physician. "Every disease has its own remedy . . . if you would love your neighbor, you must not say, 'You cannot be helped.' You must admit that *you* cannot do it and that *you* do not understand his illness. Only such truthfulness can free you from the curse that is decreed against those who are false. Therefore take good care . . . to continue your studies until you discover the art which is the foundation of good works."[28] "All diseases can be cured, without exception. Only because we do not know how to deal with them properly, because we are unable to understand life and death in their essence, can we not defend ourselves against them."[29] "No disease is so great that God has not created a remedy against it."[30]

The Galenists are the ones who maintain that their art is perfect but that God sometimes prevents the cure: "so then the hand of God is stretched like a veil over their imposture and ignorance, and they justify themselves but accuse God." When their medicines fail, they say: "By God, [the remedy] is written down right here. I have done just the right thing. It must be a plague sent by God."[31]

The physician has two possible approaches to healing, which Paracelsus calls "defensive" and "curative" medicine. The best example of the former was Paracelsus' procedure with wounds: shielding them from injury or contamination and allowing them to heal undisturbed.[f] But this technique is also applicable to internal illnesses:

> For thus it is also in the body with its maladies. If it is just defended, then it heals all its maladies by itself, for it knows how it should heal these, while the physician may not know it, for which reason he is merely the one who shields the nature . . . . If we defend the nature, then she must herself use her *scientia;* for without *scientia* she does not recover. But if we use the *scientia* beyond the defending, then we are the healers . . . therefore there are two kinds of physicians, those who commit the *scientia* to the nature, and use *defensoria* only . . . then there are the *curatores,* i.e. those who themselves use the *scientia* of the nature.
>
> (S-M I/IX 93. *Die drei (vier) Buecher des Opus Paramirum. Liber secundus. Caput secundum.* Also, I/VII 238.)

[f]Thus Paracelsus' "defensive medicine" has nothing in common with the 20th-century procedure of the same name—designed to shield the physician from injury and not the patient.

He castigates the Galenists for pretending to take the place of the body's own healing power:

> The false [physician] proceeds as follows: he begins slowly and gradually to doctor [the patient], spends much time on syrups, on laxatives, on purgatives, and oatmeal mushes, on barley, on pumpkins, on melons, on julep, and other such rubbish, is slow, and frequently administers enemas, does not know himself what he is doing, and thus drags along with time and gentle words until he comes to the term. Then he ascribes the spontaneous end to art.
>
> (S-M I/XI 129. *Sieben Defensiones.* First Defense)

Curative medicine, the second procedure, is more complicated than the Galenists allow. It means helping the nature to do what it would do of its own accord, but more slowly and imperfectly, if left alone:

> Any physician should watch how the nature wants to get out, and there drive out and help. He who knows how to do it industriously and intelligently, he then consummately knows the third part of medicine . . . I do not mention the fact that he cannot direct the nature differently at first, but only by greater perspiring and the like.
>
> (S-M I/IV 525. *Deutsche Kommentare zu den Aphorismen des Hippokrates. Aphorismus XXI.*)
>
> That is the right medicine which drives an illness out as it desires to be driven out.
>
> (S-M I/VII 110. *Von der Franzoesischen Krankheit 3 Buecher. Das ander Buch. Das viert capitel*)

The true physician promotes the development of the disease, the ripening of the mineral which has escaped from the matrix and needs to be expelled from the organism. He must take care not to deflect the disease from its natural course:

> No untimely thing may be healed before its time; and if a healing should occur, it is a suppression. In all these things the nature must be moved ahead toward its own voluntary consummation.

> (S-M I/VII 222. *Vom Ursprung und Herkommen der Franzosen. Das ander Buch. Das X. capitel*)

> When a crisis arises in an illness, the physician shall observe attentively to see if the break in the disease is announced by the crisis or entirely consummated, so that the crisis be not worse that the *status,* and have held itself equal. Then the physician shall not start to do anything, but stand still with all his medicines and not do anything new, but let the nature alone do the work.
>
> (S-M I/IV 523. *Deutsche Kommentare zu den Aphorismen des Hippokrates. Aphorismus XX.*)

The true physician does not promote just any secretion or excretion of the body which seems to him suitable (i.e., after the fashion of the Galenists). If the liquids (minerals) are not already being expelled by the body, the physician should not endeavor to promote them. "For where outlets are made without a prior indication or desire on the part of the nature, diseases become fatal or chronic and lasting."[32] Since the nature always acts for the best, Paracelsus advises the physician not to select the patient's diet for him but to allow him to eat what he wants: he will instinctively select the right food.[33]

This is all eminently Hippocratic, and it is interesting to note how Paracelsus has reinterpreted the Hippocratic theory of coction. He notes that the universal archeus or alchemist is responsible for the maturation of plants and minerals in the macrocosm. "What makes the pears ripe? What makes the grapes? Only the natural alchemy. What makes grass into milk? What makes wine out of dry earth? The natural digestion . . . . Thus what nature has in her she cooks, and when it is cooked, then is nature whole."[34] In the same way the body can, by alchemical processes which it knows, mature a substance and make it spiritual, that is, medicinal:

> If you drink a medicament, then the belly, which is your alchemist, is compelled to prepare this for you. But if the belly can reduce the medicament to such a condition that it is received by the stars, then that medicament is

> directed. If not, it remains in the belly and passes off with the excrement.
>
> (S-M I/VIII 185. *Das Buch Paragranum. Alchimia der dritte grund medicinae*)

The physician can further this process through his alchemical knowledge which transforms the substance *outside the body* prior to its administration. "In this respect alchemy is an *external bowel* which prepares its own sphere for the star."[35] Thus alchemy is fused with the Hippocratic theory of coction.

In prescribing the remedy which is to help the natural healing powers of the organism, the physician is guided by external signs. Specifically, he relies on the concordance between the anatomy of the remedy and the anatomy of the disease. By his knowledge of these external indications he knows which medicine is suitable for which illness, *but he does not know how the remedy cures the illness.*

> Therefore let the mercury work according to its nature; it knows how to lead the man according to his idiosyncrasy and nature, which the physician cannot understand completely. Therefore, it is an error for the physician to say "that patient must recover with perspiration or vomiting." He thus disregards the manifold kinds of men and does not realize that the medicine shall not be told what to do.
>
> (S-M I/I 16. *Elf Traktat. I. (Andere Redaktion) Cura:* also, S-M I/II 431.)

> We shall act according to it; it does not act according to us.
>
> (S-M I/IV 482. *Bruchstueckweise Ausarbeitungen zum I-3 Buch des Modus Pharmacandi. Liber secundus. Tractatus tertius*)

> Just as all art, strength, and might lie in the fencing master, the same lie in the illness. And as the fencing master wields his weapon according to the need, so the illness does with the medicine in the body . . . . Since now the physician is not more than that, his pharmacy

also is not more than a smithy in which they are forged. What now follows from that? Nothing, except to give the nature that which it desires in the fencing game.

(S-M I/VII 239. *Vom Ursprung und Herkommen der Franzosen. Das dritte Buch. Das ander capitel.* Also, S-M I/VIII 106. *Paragranum. Vorrede und erste zwei Buecher. Entwuerfe und I. Ausarbeitung in Berezhausen. Der ander grund der arznei*)

The *medicine* possesses the *scientia* and *not* the *physician.* Thus Paracelsus overturns the traditional Aristotelian argument that the physician produces health just as a carpenter makes a house—from the preexisting idea in his head:[g]

> The medicine is to be likened to a carpenter . . . the same thinks of a house as it should be, and thus he makes it. But not the physician: he may not imagine how the illness develops, for he does not make it. The nature makes it. If now the physician wants to know the same too, then he must first ask the nature and understand this out of her; as much as she teaches him, that much he knows. A carpenter cuts down the tree and works it according to his need and pleasure, but not the physician. The medicine cannot be fashioned as he wants it, it stays as it is, and thus he must use it.
>
> (S-M I/X 544. *Von Oeffnung der Haut. Ein Fragment. Liber primus. Caput III*)

The medicine acts in the appropriate way because it knows the *scientia.* The physician can determine which remedy knows the *scientia* by observation of externals, but he cannot direct the medicine himself. "Hence it follows that he does not have *scientia curandi* but *scientia administrandi* only. Thus he is compelled by the administering to seek in the medicine the *scientia* which lies in it."[36]

The correct remedy is the *specific* for each disease. The specific strikes at the disease and at nothing else in the body. "But this tapping shall be done only by the mercurial

[g]*Parts of Animals* 639b 16-640a 8. Discussed above at page 148.

essence. For the other drives out not only the dropsy, but with it much more which should rather be avoided. For this disease the mercury shall be fitting, as wood for the fire."[37]

The specific remedy is suitable because it has the same anatomy as the disease.

> If the same is taken, then the nature of the macrocosm, the same image, stands in man. Thus the medicine gets to the place where it belongs.
>
> (S-M I/XI 210. *Labyrinthus medicorum errantium. Das X. capitel*)

The Galenists are wrong in thinking that remedies are effective through their hot or cold qualities. "In the specifics there are many rare virtues which do not take their origin from the fact that they are hot or cold, but have a nature and an essence outside of all of these."[38] "Where the concordance does not exist and is not found, then all compounded remedies are futile and in vain."[39] "For which reason I justly reject the ineffectual recipes composed by ineffectual physicians who claim to make the nature whole by their composing and do not consider that she herself is the compounder. These physicians do not know the pharmacy of the nature and despise it, claiming to bring about better medicines by their jars than the nature in her *arcana.*"[40] "You are all so simple-minded that you think that nothing more is needed but pounding and *cribrentur et misceantur, fiat pulvis cum zuccaro.*"[41]

The Galenists falsely claim to be able to add to the prescription an ingredient which will direct the medicine to a certain part of the body. "I have often seen that they talk of *dirigentibus* and *directoriis,* that is, of the additive which shall lead the medicine to its place, which yet has no ground to it. For they say that *salvia, lavendula, maiorana* are *ducentia* to the head, which shall lead the medicine there as a guide leads another man who does not know the way. But this is not medicinelike. For not in this way does the medicine go, but it leads itself by the strength of its image."[42]

This assumed ability to know and direct that action of the medicine in the body is all part of the proud, pagan attitude of the school physicians who think they know more than the nature and can guide the natural processes in the organism. "In no way be too sure of yourselves in your art, although you are expert at it, for that is a pagan attitude."[43]

> All this I want to have indicated to you to make you realize that the medicine must follow the illness and not the Polyphemus-like rams-heads of the academies who shortsightedly want to be fencing-masters themselves and to direct the medicine according to their heads . . . . The physician must discard his wisdom, insofar as he undertakes to govern the same according to his own head; he must aim to know what the nature desires, and not what he himself desires. For the physician himself often desires something cold when the nature is hot. But since he is not the physician but the nature is the physician, then he has no business giving this medicine. He must ask the nature whether what is in his head is pleasing to it or not. When he has learned that, then it falls to the ground that hot is driven away by the cold, or cold by heat . . . . Therefore the nature shall be given its weapon, that is, the specific.
>
> (S-M I/VII 239. *Vom Ursprung und Herkommen der Franzosen. Das dritte Buch. Das ander capitel*)

The Galenists use emetics and cathartics. But "purging is the physician's weapon and not that of the illness, and therefore it does not help."[44] "The humors are from the disease, and not the disease from them."[45] The purgative effect of the medicine is not even part of the *arcanum* but belongs to the narcotic part of the medicine which should be cast aside. "If it were the right weapon of medicine, then the illness itself would strike, and you would not comprehend how the stroke was done."[46]

Not only are the Galenic remedies useless in disease, they actually harm the patient, since they attempt to cure the disease in an unnatural way:

> And note in yourselves that this power must have an outlet or it will break open the vault [of the body]. Thus, when the pustules are formed in the body in a certain way, if they are suppressed and choked off, they will break through into the center of the body from which they have come and will cause death.
>
> (S-M I/VI 365. *Von Blattern, Laehme, Beulen, Loechern und Zittrachten der Franzosen und ihres gleichen. Das ander Buch. Das IX. capitel*)

> Then now also know that if it should happen that warts or similar growths arise from another cause, that this is not harmful but useful. But these are often suppressed by alleged physicians, using caustics and cutting, and afterwards there arise the complaints and lesions described which would not have happened if these alleged physicians had not employed their unfounded arts.
>
> (S-M I/X 318. *Das zweite Buch der Grossen Wundarznei. Der ander tractat. Das XII. capitel*)

These physicians do not understand the doctrine of similars and erroneously think that the symptoms of disease are harmful signs, to be suppressed. "For the nature seeks outlets and seeks ways and bridges to preserve the man. And that which she does for the good of man, that you say is for death."[47] Or else they use narcotic medicines which only deaden the symptoms, and that temporarily.[48] Hence they ruin their patients' lives and health and leave the wreckage for Paracelsus to try and cure.

> Why do you throw it in my face if I cannot cure impossible things, when you cannot cure the possible? But rather you ruin it so that I must build it up against you.
>
> (S-M I/XI 157. *Sieben Defensiones*. Seventh Defense)

The only true cure is through similars. Although an apparently cold medicine may cure an apparently hot disease, this is not because of the coldness "but because of the other nature which we distinguish from the first," that is, the similarity between the anatomy of remedy and disease.[49]

When the Galenists do effect a cure, it is only because they have hit upon the correct remedy accidentally. "And thus you often use ten or fifteen remedies or more, one after the other, and none accomplishes anything, until perhaps in the end one comes who hits it by accident. Without realizing it, he gives the similar medicine and thus heals, *which also would have happened if you had inquired in this manner from the beginning.*"[50] If it is not a similar, then "the seed of health is not in it, then all your prescribing is in vain; just as when it rains or dews on a piece of wood or on a rock."[51] Everything other than cure by similars is "the ineffectual theory—false and abhorrent to nature—of the four humors, of cholera, phlegms, etc . . . a speculative undertaking which derives from no experience, reason, or truth, and is against philosophy, against the nature, against the microcosm, and against the illness itself—a vain *durchribne leckerei.*"[52][h]

[h] "Rubbed-through licking."

NOTES

[1] S-M I/XI 192. *Labyrinthus medicorum errantium. Das VI. capitel;* S-M I/XII 92. *Astronomia Magna. Bk. I. Cap. IV. Was signatum und was der signator sei.*

[2] S-M I/VIII 321. *Von hinfallenden Siechtagen der Mutter. Par. I.*

[3] S-M I/VI 179. *Entwuerfe, Notizen, und Ausarbeitungen zur Bertheonea. Argumentum III.*

[4] S-M I/VIII 144-145. *Das Buch Paragranum. Der erste tractat.*

[5] Pagel, *Paracelsus,* p. 52 (stress added).

[6] *Ibid.,* p. 43 (stress added).

[7] *Ibid.,* pp. 51-52, 60-61.

[8] S-M I/VIII 177. *Das Buch Paragranum. Der ander tractat;* also, S-M I/XI 204. *Labyrinthus medicorum errantium. Cap. IX.*

[9] S-M I/XI 192. *Labyrinthus medicorum errantium. Das VI. capitel.*

[10] S-M I/IV 525. *Deutsche Kommentare zu den Aphorismen des Hippokrates. Aphorismus XXI.*

[11] S-M I/XII 26-27. *Astronomia Magna. Bk. I. Das Buch der Philosophei des himlischen Firmaments. Das I. capitel.* (Cf. Pagel, *Paracelsus,* p. 57); S-M I/IX 578. *De peste libri tres cum additionibus. Imaginatio impressionis.*

[12] S-M I/IX 93. *Die drei (vier) Buecher des Opus Paramirum. Liber secundus. Caput secundum.* S-M I/VII 265. *Vom Ursprung und Herkommen der Franzosen. Bk. IV. Cap. III;* S-M I/VIII 140. *Das Buch Paragranum. Der erste tractat.* S-M I/XI 194-195. *Labyrinthus medicorum errantium. Das VI. capitel.*

[13] S-M I/IX 94. *Die drei (vier) Buecher des Opus Paramirum. Liber secundus. Caput secundum.*

[14] S-M I/I 37. *Elf Tractat. 2. Vom schweinen oder schwintsucht (Andere Redaktion).*

[15] S-M I/XI 190-195. *Labyrinthus medicorum errantium. Das sechst capitel.*

[16] S-M I/VII 372. *Spital-Buch. Erster Teil. Dr. Theophrastus allen aerzten seinen gruss.* Their spiritual father, Pliny, was a mere "experimenter." S-M I/VIII 171. *Das Buch Paragranum. Der ander tractat. Von der astronomia.*

[17] S-M I/I 366. *Von den podagrischen Krankheiten und was ihnen anhaengig (zwei Buecher). Liber secundus. Physionomia.*

[18] S-M I/IV 36. *De Gradibus et Compositionibus Receptorum et naturalium Libri VII. Caput tertium.*

[19] S-M I/XI 192. *Labyrinthus medicorum errantium. Sechst capitel.* Pagel, *Paracelsus,* p. 60.

[20] F.S.C. Northrop, *The Logic of the Sciences and the Humanities* (New York, 1959), contains a discussion of the various stages of scientific method.

[21] S-M I/VIII 142. *Das Buch Paragranum. Der erste tractat. Von der philosophia.*

[22] S-M I/XI 212. *Labyrinthus medicorum errantium. Das X. capitel.*

[23] S-M I/I 231. *Volumen Medicinae Paramirum. Bk. V, Cap. VIII.*

[24] *Ibid.,* p. 227. *Bk. V, Cap. III.*

[25] S-M I/VI 52. *Drei Buecher der Wundarznei. Vorrede.*

[26] S-M I/VII 150. *Von der franzoesischen Krankheit 3 Buecher. Das drit Buch. Das X. capitel.*

[27] S-M I/VIII 70. *Paragranum. Vorrede und erste zwei Buecher. Entwuerfe und I. Ausarbeitung in Berezhausen. Der erste grund der arznei.*

[28] S-M I/XI 129-130. *Sieben Defensiones.* First Defense.

[29] S-M I/II 430. *Das siebente Buch in der Arznei, von den Krankheiten die der Vernunft Berauben, de morbis amentium. Methodus secunda. Caput I.*

[30] S-M I/VIII 269. *Von den hinfallenden Siechtagen. Der I. paragraphus.*

[31] S-M I/VIII 171. *Das Buch Paragranum. Der ander tractat.* Also, p. 195.

[32] S-M I/IV 525. *Deutsche Kommentare zu den Aphorismen des Hippokrates, Aphorismus XX.*

[33] S-M I/I 20. *Elf Traktat. I (Andere Redaktion). Cura;* S-M I/XI 104. *Das Buch von den tartarischen Krankheiten. Das XVII. capitel.*

[34] S-M I/VIII 59. *Paragranum. Vorrede und erste zwei Buecher. Entwuerfe und I. Ausarbeitung in Berezhausen. Vorred.* Also, S-M I/VII 265. *Vom Ursprung und Herkommen der Franzosen. Das viert Buch. Das drit capitel.*

[35] *Loc. cit.*

[36] S-M I/XI 194-195. *Labyrinthus medicorum errantium. Das sechst capitel.*

[37] S-M I/I 8. *Elf Traktat. I. Cura.*

[38] S-M I/III 169. *Neun Buecher Archidoxis. Liber septimus.*

[39] S-M I/I 324. *Liber de podagricis et suis speciebus. Liber primus. Chiromantia.*

[40] S-M I/VI 138-139. *Drei Buecher der Wundarznei. Der ander Buch. Cap. VII.*

[41] S-M I/VIII 189. *Das Buch Paragranum. Alchimia der dritte grund medicinae.*

[42] S-M I/XI 210. *Labyrinthus medicorum errantium. Das X. capitel.*

[43] S-M I/I 232. *Volumen Medicinae Paramirum. Bk. V, Particle I.*

[44] S-M I/VII 240. *Vom Ursprung und Herkommen der Franzosen. Das dritte Buch. Das ander capitel.*

[45] S-M I/XI 202. *Labyrinthus medicorum errantium, Cap. VIII.*

[46] S-M I/VII 241. *Vom Ursprung und Herkommen der Franzosen. Das dritte Buch. Das drit capitel.*

[47] S-M I/I 19-20. *Elf Traktat. I. (Andere Redaktion). Cura.*

[48] S-M I/IX 200. *Die drei (vier) Buecher des Opus Paramirum. Liber quartus de matrice;* S-M I/XI 296. *Consilium von dem Bruch an Franz Boner, Salzburg.*

[49] S-M I/IX 236. *Entwuerfe zu den vier Buechern des Opus Paramirum. Tractatus II.*

[50] S-M I/X 401. *Das zweite Buch der Grossen Wundarznei. Der drit tractat. Der drit teil. Das erst capitel.*

[51] S-M I/VII 396. *Spital-Buch (erster teil). Der ander tractat.*

[52] S-M I/VI 276. *Von allen offenen Schaeden. Das VII. Buch. Vom wilden feuer.*

CHAPTER XVIII

CONCLUSION: THE EMPIRICAL AND RATIONALIST TRADITIONS IN GREEK AND RENAISSANCE MEDICINE

The preceding pages have described the conflict between the Empirical and Rationalist therapeutic philosophies which first emerged in the oldest works of the Hippocratic Corpus, from the fifth and early fourth centuries B.C.

Aristotle strengthened the intellectual foundations of Rationalist medicine, while the Sceptics did the same for Empiricism.

Until at least the second century A.D. the two schools led a separate existence. At this time Rationalism received its ultimate formulation by Galen.

The Empirical School disappeared from recorded history in the third century, and thereafter medical thought was dominated by Galen and the Arabs.[a]

In the sixteenth century Paracelsus mounted the first effective challenge to Galenic medicine, accepting the governing tenet of Empiricism—the primacy of experience—and recasting it in terms of the doctrine of similars and Christian love for humankind.

* * * * * * * * *

The corollary of reliance on experience is a vitalist interpretation of the organism. In the Group I and IV Hippocratic

[a]An intriguing problem, yet to be investigated, is the possible doctrinal connection between the Empirical School and the School of Salerno—which first became prominent in the ninth century. Certainly the Salernitan writings, and those of the school of Montpellier established in the twelfth century by professors from Salerno, reveal significant parallels with the teachings of the Empirics. Montpellier remained a focus of vitalist therapeutics up through the nineteenth century.

works the *physis* is the principal agent of cure, while the physician is secondary. The Empirical School also relied on the *physis*, as did Paracelsus—calling it *die natur*, the archeus, or the alchemist.

The key to an understanding of these therapeutic doctrines is thus found in their attitude toward the *physis*.

The Empirics simply postulated its existence and upon it based their whole curative method.

The Rationalists, on the contrary, denigrated the *physis*, denying its spontaneity and reducing its myriad operations to a finite number of patterns which could be analyzed and explained in logical terms. They were uncomfortable with the theory of coction, since it was not subject to formal logical analysis. They could not even accept Aristotle's proposed reduction of coction to a conflict between the "active" qualities (hot and cold) and the "passive" ones (wet and dry). Opposing hot to cold, and wet to dry, seemed to make better logical sense, and this formula was ultimately adopted.

By the second century A.D. the *physis* had largely disappeared from Rationalist thought. Galen observes that they interpreted it in a number of different ways and that many philosophers denied its existence altogether.

This trend in Rationalism was carried to its ultimate by the Methodists who replaced the *physis* by the invisible movement of atoms.

Galen, who was first trained as an Empiric, was shocked by the Methodist position and also by the confusion within Rationalism over the significance of the *physis*. He aimed to restore it to its rightful place in medical thought, and this meant finding a place for it within the pathological theory of *Nature of Man*. Thus he inserted a new stage in the chain of causal relationships accepted by the Rationalists: henceforth coction was effected by a clash among opposed qualities and humors—as expressed through the *dynameis* of the organs.

This synthesis of the Empirical and Rationalist positions, however, was achieved at the price of logical consistency.

The touchstone of the true vitalist doctrine, i.e., of genuine reliance on the *physis*, is the attitude toward the symptoms. Acceptance of the *physis* means interpreting symptoms as signs of the organism's effort to rid itself of disease. Hence they are beneficial, and the physician must follow them in his treatment—administering the similar remedy to promote the natural process of elimination.

In the Group I Hippocratic works such symptoms as hemorrhage, hemorrhoids, skin eruptions, diarrhoea, swellings, pains in the joints, and fevers are all viewed as beneficial. But in the Group III works such symptoms are taken to be morbific, and the physician is to neutralize them by the contrary remedy.

Cure through contraries is fundamental to Rationalism, as cure through similars is fundamental to Empiricism.

Galen's achievement was to provide a new interpretation of coction. The Empirical view was that coction resulted from treatment by similars (the *secunda*), and evacuation followed of itself. Rationalists after Galen, however, produced coction by *contraries* and then called for a new group of medicines to bring about the desired evacuation. They paid lip-service to the Hippocratic coction while interpreting symptoms as morbific phenomena to be removed by contraries.

Even though Rationalists for another 1700 years continued to use emetics, purgatives, and sudorifics in the treatment of disease, this was only an inferior imitation of the natural mode of cure. The Empirics subordinated their whole treatment to the natural impulse of the body, using the same remedy to bring about coction-evacuation and applying it only at the precise moment when the body was prepared to do the same. The Rationalists divided treatment into two stages and, furthermore, codified their practices into a rigid system relying on a cut-and-dried doctrine of critical days.

Thus they were not Hippocratics, despite their theoretical advocacy of the *physis*. The heart of the Hippocratic doctrine was prognosis of the disease, precise discrimination among similar cases, and meticulous individualization of treatment. Galen substituted diagnosis for prognosis, subsumed cases under a limited number of headings on the basis of the humoral proximate cause, standardized treatment by a preformulated doctrine of critical days, and treated with contraries instead of similars.

Paracelsus reintroduced the idea that symptoms are beneficial—being the signs of the struggle of the vital force against disease.

* * * * * * * * *

The conflict between a vitalist and a non-vitalist therapeutics had important corollaries. Empirical acceptance of the *physis* led to the view that the number of diseases is infinite, since the *physis* is spontaneous and self-determined and can adopt an infinite number of different defenses against morbific influences. The number of significant symptoms also becomes infinite, since each defensive action by the *physis* is unique, different from all others, and to be appreciated by the physician in its uniqueness.

Hence the Empirics stressed the *propria* over the *communia* as guides to treatment.

The Rationalist position stemmed from their instinctive desire to limit the natural variety of the phenomena. If the body possesses only four humors and the number of diseases is limited to the combinations of these four humors, the number of useful symptoms must be limited to those arising from the four humors.

Since the humors are identical in every patient, the morbific symptoms common to large groups of patients are most useful to the physician, and the Rationalists stressed the *communia* over the *propria*.

Just as the Rationalists reduced the natural variety of the symptoms to those referable to the four humors, so they reduced the natural variety of the remedies to the same least common denominator: the hot, the cold, the wet, and the dry. The medicine was selected for its contrary effect on the patient's *communia*.

Paracelsus held that the world contains an infinite number of plant and mineral remedies, each with its specific effect on the body. This conviction was the basis of his doctrine of the infinity of diseases in the world. In contrast to the Rationalist desire to limit this variety, he assimilated the number of diseases to the number of possible remedies: "Who knows the number of illnesses but he who knows the number of growing things and of the natural *arcana*?"[1]

But this complicated the problem of whether or not diseases vary throughout history and from one country to another. Paracelsus ultimately maintained that they do vary, some disappearing and others appearing,[2] for this reason advocating German remedies for German diseases,[3] but this was not compatible with the mineral origin of disease, since minerals are eternal and not subject to historical or geographical variation.[b]

Paracelsus was also unclear with respect to the uniqueness of the individual constitution: his instinctive drive toward specificity conflicted with the mineral origin of disease.

Along the same lines is his ambiguity about the number of useful symptoms. He favored a large number but was once more restrained by the theory of minerals and concluded that only those identifiable with a given mineral-determined disease are useful.

Thus the theory of minerals—the idea that diseases are classified according to the curative medicine—permitted an ordered expansion of the number of possible diseases and a methodologically precise limitation on the number of symptoms which the physician must consider:

> Although the enemies are many, and cannot well be numbered by the physician, still this is not necessary. For he who would piece out such things would introduce too much erring into the practice of medicine. For in practice the diseases are cured by the *arcana* . . . He who wants to consider every jaundice separately knows not what the *arcanum* is; for the *arcanum* heals all of those species. If the *particularis medicus* [i.e. the Galenist] should seek for each species its particular diet and recipe, that seeking

[b]This contradiction is noted by Pagel, *Das medizinische Weltbild,* pp. 9ff.

would become too long-lasting for the patient. . . . .Now it is done according to the *arcanum,* and the uncertainty concerning the many species of the same illness has been taken away.

(S-M I/IX 481-482. *Von der Bergsucht und anderen Bergkrankheiten. Das erste Buch. Der dritte tractat. Das viert capitel*)

No illness occurs without a poison, for poison is the beginning of each illness. . . . That you shall recognize; thus you find that to the arsenic are to be attributed more than 50 illnesses and still another 50, of which none is the same as the other, and yet all are from the arsenic. Many more still come from salt, and still more from mercury, still more from realgar and sulphur. . . . You in vain learn of each particular illness its particular origin, since one thing makes so many illnesses. That is what you should seek after, and then you will find the cause.

(S-M I/I 186. *Volumen Medicinae Paramirum. Bk. I. Cap. IX.*)

The theory of minerals yields a unique solution to another of the problems perplexing the Empirics and Rationalists—whether the organism is ultimately knowable or unknowable. Paracelsus abolished the Galenic proximate (material) cause by assimilating it to the mineral "form."

This formal cause is knowable because it becomes externalized in the symptoms during the course of the disease. The mineral form is knowable because it is *visible.*

Hence diagnosis is not needed and, like the Empirics, Paracelsus calls for prognosis: "He is a physician who indicates future operations. The present operation is shown by the eyes. But that which is evident to the eyes, that shall be prognosticated in advance—that a proper physician can do, but never a one has been examined in this."[4]

Paracelsus rooted the exciting (procatarctic) cause in more solid doctrinal ground with his general theory of microcosm and macrocosm. Here, again, his position is identical with that of the Empirics.

This school saw disease and health as a continuum

representing the ongoing interaction between organism and environment. The *physis* functions in both states, differing only in the pattern and strength of its movements. Since the body's vital reactions are influenced by every change in environmental conditions, the Empirics regarded such information as essential to correct therapeutic method, and they included the exciting causes as essential components of the symptom-syndrome.

Just as the thrust of Empirical doctrine led to exaltation of the exciting cause, the thrust of Rationalism led to its neglect.

These physicians subordinated the exciting cause to the proximate cause because the latter could be hypostatized into an independently existing entity, while the former could not be so objectified.

Thus the Rationalists demarcated health from disease. Health was the condition in which no disease could be found in the organism; disease was the state in which the physician could diagnose the presence of a disease entity.

For the Empirics disease was not an entity but a dynamic process. Health was also a process. Both reflected the interaction between the organism and its environment.

The processes of disease and health were encompassed in Paracelsus' doctrine of the macrocosm and microcosm. The macrocosm causes the diseases of the microcosm through the five *entia*. Since microcosm and macrocosm are in continuous interaction, sickness and health are aspects of the same process. "There where diseases arise, there also one can find the roots of health. For health must grow from the same root as disease, and whither health goes, thither also disease must go."[5] "Just as the sun and moon are separated from each other, although formerly were one thing, so health and disease were one thing, and later they were separated from each other, as the sun was from the moon. And just as these wane and wax in the sphere of heaven, and now one or the other appears, so also are all the stars woven into the body—this you should know—and similarly distributed, and the same is true of the forms in which health and disease are manifested. For all of them must be present in the body in order that the 'inner firmament' may be whole and that the number of the parts may be full."[6]

The Empirics held that remedies were discovered only by trial and error. Paracelsus' correspondences between microcosm and macrocosm, and especially his doctrine of signatures, seem an effort to circumvent this Empirical position and find a direct route to the remedy. The doctrine of signatures and the microcosm-macrocosm correspondences seem to provide the physician with *a priori* knowledge of the remedies. However, these are only *guides to the physician's practice.* Hence, the true value of the remedy is only revealed by its use, whatever its signature may indicate: "The signature points to the place, and the place indicates the need, and the need is satisfied through discovery [*durch inventricem*]."[7 c]

Paracelsus' signatures are closer to the commemorative signs of the Empirics than to the indicative signs of the Rationalists.

And in the controversy over the relative importance of *logos* and experience Paracelsus also takes the side of the Empirics. He assimilates *logos* to experience when he defines the "light of nature" as the capacity to learn from experience and condemns traditional logic as valueless for medicine.

Thus Paracelsus agrees with *Ancient Medicine* that knowledge of the *physis* arises from medical practice—rather than, as the Rationalists put it, that medical practice is the application of *a priori* knowledge of the *physis*:

> It is the physician who reveals to us the diverse miraculous works of God. . . . What is in the sea that he should not bring to the light of day? Nothing. He should make it manifest, and not only what is in the sea, but also what is in the earth, in the air, in the firmament . . . but if they are not brought to light, it is a sign that the intelligence capable of discovering them is still lacking.

[c]Therapeutics is the *inventrix* or *inventrix magicae artis* (S-M I/XI 212. *Labyrinthus medicorum errantium. Das X. capitel*).

(S-M I/IX 70. *Die drei (vier) Buecher des Opus Paramirum. Erster Teil. Das erste Buch. Caput sextum*).

He even carries the argument further. Medical practice *based on the doctrine of similars* yields knowledge of nature. "Thus all things are against us which are for us. Therefore we have medicine—to get to know them."[8]

* * * * * * * * *

Paracelsus' attitude toward his predecessors shows sympathy for the Empirical tradition. He includes them among the "specificists" (*specifici*) who "treat all diseases specifically as to form as well as essence."[9][d]

He probably took some of his ideas from Celsus and the Empirical fragments preserved in Galen, although this cannot be proved or disproved. In any case, it is unimportant, since the Empirical and Rationalist ideologies are perennial and can arise spontaneously at any time.

His name, however, suggests homage to the author of *De Medicina*. Being greater than Celsus would be pointless unless Celsus himself were great (otherwise Paracelsus would have taken the name, "Paragalen").

Paracelsus followed the Empirical School in his attitude toward the ancients. He condemned the teachings of Galen. He called Aristotle a "sharp fantasist who has left some considerable work on generation" but was "kept in the dark by the unpropitious constellation prevalent at his time and so much fettered by animal nature that nothing remained but the impression of a sharp seed that fell among thorns." He was "subtle in a perverse way" and in him the "kernel of nature remained a dust and a withered flower."[10] "It

[d]He observes that the Galenists "cynically" call them "empiricists," thus alluding to the perennial Rationalist view that the ancient Empirics were uneducated and in a class with lay and folk practitioners (*loc. cit.*). See also S-M I/V 64. *Nachschrift aus der Vorlesung ueber tartarische Krankheiten. 2 Buecher. Liber secundus, Tractatus I. Caput sextum.*

would take a long time to show how far the Aristotelian, Stoic, and Platonic philosophy is from mine."[11]

That the Galenists who were his contemporaries reacted to his theories in the same way the Rationalists of antiquity reacted to the Empirics may be seen from Erastus' criticism of him.

There can be no doubt, however, of his admiration for Hippocrates. He does not include him among the Pagan "*naturales*,"[12] and his writings contain many favorable references to the Father of Medicine:

> God suffered the spirit of medicine to emerge in its fundamentals through Apollo, through Machaon, Podalirius, and Hippocrates. . . . No one has been able to advance as far in the work as Machaon and Hippocrates did. And in medicine what is not proved with works has lost its disputation.
>
> (S-M I/XI 125. *Sieben Defensiones.* Preface. Also, S-M I/IV 523.)

He wrote a book of comments on the Hippocratic *Aphorisms*—his only commentary on any of the writings of his predecessors. And he even seems to identify himself with Hippocrates in the following passage:

> The laudable province of Carinthia . . . represents Maecenas, and gives *asylum Hippocraticorum* in our times, protecting and sheltering. For this may God give recompense, peace, and unity.
>
> (S-M I/XI 160. *Sieben Defensiones.* Conclusion. This was written at a time when he had sought refuge in Carinthia—one of his childhood homes.)

Oswald Croll gives further details on Paracelsus' attitude toward Hippocrates: he approved of those elements in the Hippocratic Corpus which we have characterized above as Empirical and disapproved of those which we have characterized as Rationalist. Hippocrates "wrote many things which most Galenists reject at this day."[13] Croll notes further that Paracelsus and Hippocrates both combined the theory of medicine (physic—"the knowledge of all diseases") with the practice (surgery—"the curing of the same"), and the latter, "like the carpenter's work, cannot be done without hands." They are interdependent, and every physician should be a surgeon, and vice-versa. "That there may be a sound bridegroom for a sound bride."[14]

> Paracelsus therefore, doth not find fault with Hippocrates for saying that hunger is to be cured with meat, thirst with drink, fullness with evacuation, inanition with refection, labor with rest, idleness with labor; and generally that contraries cure contraries. But he is point blank against Galen who applied that contrariety of Hippocrates chiefly to those bare and naked qualities which Hippocrates utterly disclaimed, for he by an unhappy mistake referred the first and principal ideas of cures to refrigerations, calefactions, humectations, exsiccations, with their companions.[15][e]

And finally, Croll places the whole development of Empirical medicine by Paracelsus in its proper perspective, urging the good physician to "learn of Paracelsus and other chymists to prepare and make up their medicines, but to observe the method of Hippocrates in curing diseases, as it agreeth with their own judications and inventions; for by this means these two schools of Old and New physic may be reconciled without contradiction."[16]

* * * * * * * * *

Throughout this volume we have contended that the elements of a scientific approach to therapeutics are found in the Empirical system, that these physicians were the first practitioners of a scientific medicine.

To understand why this is so we may expand upon our earlier discussion[f] and note that scientific method includes the following steps: (1) the investigator must accurately

[e]See *Aphorisms* II: 22 (Jones, IV, 113).

[f]See above, Introduction.

record the data of observation; (2) preliminary analysis of these data permits the formulation of a hypothesis for further investigation; (3) the hypothesis is tested for accuracy and reliability by experimental trials; (4) the body of knowledge thus disclosed, which is assumed to reflect the laws of nature, must be coherent and consistent, but it is also only hypothetical, subject to modification at any time through further observation and experiment.

In the light of this definition of scientific method the Empirics are seen to have been scientific, while the Rationalists were not.

Clearly the Empirics were better observers than the Rationalists: Sprengel writes that Galen's "predilection for theory seems to have prevented him from becoming a good observer."[17] His writings are full of boasting about his cleverness in diagnosis and treatment but contain not a single careful description of a sick person.

The Empirical talent for observation was rooted in their love for the patient. Einstein observed that the man who would seek "those highly universal laws" which govern the processes of reality must possess a quality of "intuition based upon something like an intellectual love [*Einfuehlung*] of the objects of experience."[18] The object of medical experience is the patient, and precise observation of the patient is the absolute prerequisite of a scientific therapeutics. Thus it was not frivolity or personal hostility, but genuine insight into the requirements of scientific method, which led the Empirics to describe the Rationalists as "dull of heart and blind of eye." The Empirical Hippocratic work, *Precepts*, observes: "Where there is love of man, there is also love of the *tekhnę*" (cap. VI: Jones, I, 319). And Paracelsus was making the same point when he held that medicine is rooted not only in experience but also in Christian love: application of disciplined observation to the patient's needs makes the physician the agent of God's mercy on earth.

Their preliminary observation led the Empirics to hypothesize that the organism contains a reactive force which effects cure through an infinite variety of coction processes.

Their therapeutics, designed to promote coction of the crude humor and its ultimate evacuation, was an effort to delineate these various processes. The *physis* served as a hypothesis, with the same role and function as any scientific hypothesis —that of revealing new knowledge. Each time the physician administered a medicine to a sick patient he was testing the validity of this hypothesis, and each recorded cure supplied knowledge of one further way in which the *physis* could be aided to overcome disease.

Thus their initial hypothesis of the existence of a vital force was developed into a body of *a posteriori* knowledge of the ways taken by this force to protect and heal the organism.

Proof that the *physis* of the Empirics was only an operating hypothesis is seen in their tentative formulation of it. The author of *Ancient Medicine* refuses to describe the humors or even to specify their number. He employs the term merely as an operational definition of perceived physiological and pathological processes. And, as we have noted, the Empirics themselves "refused to investigate the *physis*." Although they postulated the existence of this force, they had no *a priori* knowledge of how it would operate in any individual case of disease. Careful observation and treatment of sick persons enabled them to develop a body of knowledge of the various procedures adopted by this force in coping with different morbific stimuli. Thus the initial hypothesis could be modified by the results of experience.

It could be argued that the Rationalists also had a hypothesis: the four-humor doctrine. Disease was supposed to arise from the isolation of one of the humors from the *krasis*, and cure resulted from expulsion of this humor or restoration of the *krasis* through administration of the "contrary" medicine.

But the static four humors could not serve as a hypothesis for investigation in the same way as the *physis* of the Empirics: the latter accepted the variety of nature, admitting that the manifestations of disease are infinite since the *physis* is spontaneous and autonomous, but the four humors of the Rationalists served only to restrict the field of observation. The signs and symptoms of disease were cut and spliced to fit these preexisting categories. Diseases were distinguished from one another, and "important" symptoms from "unimportant," on logical grounds alone, in isolation from the therapeutic process. Where the Empirics relied on the *propria*, the Rationalists eliminated them from consideration (because they could not be logically connected with any proximate cause).

No practical experience could lead the Rationalists to alter their operating hypothesis of the four humors. Hence an essential element of scientific method was absent. The Rationalists saw these humors as concrete entities, ascribed to them certain powers and qualities, and even based therapeutic practice on these definitions. While the Empirical knowledge was *a posteriori*, Rationalist doctrine was *a priori* and not subject to modification by practical experience.

The difference between the two doctrines can be discussed in terms of the relations between theory and practice. Empirical therapeutics was a *method* based upon a hypothesis. The theory of the organism was developed out of the method, out of practice. Both the author of *Ancient Medicine* and Paracelsus hold that knowledge must originate in practice, specifically, in the practice of medicine. The idea that therapeutics is primary, and itself yields knowledge of the organism, is one of the great Empirical contributions to medical philosophy.

Since the theory is generated by practice, the problem of the bridge between theory and practice does not exist in Empiricism. The contrast here with Rationalism is fundamental: since this theory was developed in abstraction from the therapeutic process, it needed an additional postulate for its application, and these physicians relied instinctively on the concept of "contrariety." It seemed normal and natural to assume that "cure" was equivalent to opposing or neutralizing the disease "cause."

In Empirical therapeutics the place of the *a priori* doctrine of contraries was taken by their *a posteriori* records of cures. The discovery of remedies was the purely "empirical" element in their medical doctrine, and they maintained that no *a priori* knowledge could or did exist in this domain.

The question of the scientific basis of Empiricism and Rationalism can be approached in yet another way. Scientific method deals with the raw material of observed phenomena. Its aim is to establish laws and relations among them, and to this end the phenomena must be transformed into "facts," into data which will permit the elaboration of a body of laws. But "facts" do not exist in themselves. The variety of the universe presents the observer with certain phenomena which appear as self-evident "facts" depending upon his operating assumptions. The "facts" change their shape and configuration in function of the hypothesis adopted for investigating them. The Empirical postulate of a vital force which could operate autonomously and spontaneously led them to view as significant a broader range of phenomena than did the Rationalists—for whom the variety of nature was necessarily confined within the narrow categories of the four humors. Instead of fighting the infinity of symptoms and diseases, the Empirics accepted this fact and made it a keystone of their system. By relying on *propria* over *communia* they incorporated into their method precisely the characteristics which distinguish the individual patient from all others like him.

Here again the Empirics were scientific. Although scientific method introduces order and regularity into the observed phenomena, this must not be at the expense of the phenomena. It must not infringe upon or violate the natural relations among the phenomena. The true scientist must have profound respect for the data of experience.

While, in theory, the possible combinations of four humors are unlimited—since different proportions of each humor can be assumed in each combination[g]—Rationalist doctrine was still a *psychological* obstacle to the physician's willingness to accept a large variety of symptoms and

[g]Galen suggests the possibility of fifteen different "moist" constitutions, each requiring a different "dry" remedy (K X 209).

diseases. Furthermore, *it did not propose any method* for elucidating these pathological subtleties.

All elements of the Empirical ideology are present in Paracelsus' doctrine, but he altered this ideology in two ways. In the first place, the requirement of precise observation (which for the Empirics needed no further justification) was rooted by Paracelsus in Christian love. Only by loving the patient can the physician observe him properly.

This religious underpinning only reinforced the Empirical precept and did not alter it. His second change, however—acceptance of the doctrine of similars as a general governing principle—led to a fundamental reconstruction of the whole theory of medicine and therapeutics.

Three stages are thus to be discerned in the development of Empirical therapeutics. In the Hippocratic Corpus the theory of coction is central. The teachings of the Empirical School were based on an analysis of medical experience. With Paracelsus the whole ideology is generated by the doctrine of similars.

Each element reappears in each stage of the development of Empiricism. Only its relative doctrinal weight changes from one era to another.

Even though Paracelsus gave a different structure to the Empirical therapeutic precepts, his system was scientific for the same reasons that the Empirical system itself was scientific.

In the first place, Paracelsus denied the relevance of logic to the investigation of nature: the laws of nature have their own logic, their own internal consistency. He describes this ordered structure of nature as the "*practica globuli* or *spherae*"—a definition which reveals the significance of practice, i.e., experience. This *practica* he calls *scientia*. Man can come to understand *scientia* through his light of nature, *provided he follows the proper method.*

As with the Empirics, this method consists of practicing medicine in the light of the correct hypothesis. It is medical experience illuminated by the hypothesis of a relationship between the microcosm and the macrocosm which, in turn, relies on pervasive application of the doctrine of similars. When the physician treats his patients on the basis of this hypothesis, he acquires genuine experience (*experientia*). If he treats his patients haphazardly, i.e., without the guidance of this hypothesis, he does not acquire experience—since this sort of experience is not true experience, but merely a series of experiments (*experimenta*).

For Paracelsus, as for the Empirics and for the author of *Ancient Medicine*, the practice of medicine is a method of investigating nature—and here "nature" can be taken in its restrictive sense of the *physis* of man or in the broader sense of the whole universe. The Empirics maintained that the records of their cases gave them knowledge of the workings of the *physis*. Paracelsus calls therapeutics the *inventrix magicae artis*.

Thus the history of the Rationalist and Empirical traditions is the history of the conflict between Aristotelianism and Scepticism as applied to medicine. The Rationalists adopted the Aristotelian analysis of physical reality, and their practice was based upon this analysis. The Empirics, on the other hand, accepted the Sceptical critique of the Aristotelian metaphysic and thus denied the possibility of a reliable physiology and pathology. Instead they established therapeutics as an independent and self-sufficient *method* based on the postulate of the *physis*. Their medical knowledge grew through the accumulated experience of generations of Empirical physicians who also based their practice on the postulated existence of the *physis*.

Paracelsus accepted their critique of the Aristotelian-Galenic metaphysic and of the humoral pathology which it engendered. His own operating hypothesis incorporated the theory of microcosm-macrocosm, the doctrine of similars, and the archeus or alchemist within the organism.

* * * * * * * * *

We stated in the Introduction that medical history represents the interaction between the Empirical and Rationalist systems of thought. This polarity is perennial, recurring in each new age clothed in the medical vocabulary of that age.

All physicians do not adhere strictly to one or the other system. The Empirical end of the spectrum will always contain individuals who veer toward Rationalism, while the Rationalist end will contain some who are moving toward Empiricism.

The private systems of such physicians, however, are internally inconsistent, since only the pure forms of Empiricism and Rationalism are coherent and logically complete.

The Empirical system is scientific (according to the modern understanding of scientific method), while the Rationalist system is unscientific.

The question may be asked why medical practice should contain two opposed systems of thought rather than one. And why is Methodism generated by Rationalism—treatment on the basis of "communities" being even further removed from scientific method than treatment based on the four humors?

These questions touch on the problem of the social determinants of medical thought—which has been adumbrated in the preceding pages but not discussed in depth. The materials for such an analysis are too sparse in the period covered by this volume, and a more comprehensive analysis is found in Volumes Two and Three of this work. At this point we can only give some suggestions.

The perpetuation of either system, and its waxing and waning, are determined by the recruitment to the medical profession of persons of the Empirical or Rationalist psychological type. Representatives of both types are found in every population, and different sets of social, economic, legal, and other conditions will encourage one type or the other to undertake the practice of medicine.

Thus the appeal of the two systems is ultimately psychological—one reason (*inter alia*) why therapeutic experience rarely seems to convince the adherents of either system to abandon it and embrace the opposing one.

However, the recruitment of one or the other type to the medical profession is affected by the other conditions mentioned. And here the differing *functions* of Empirical and Rationalist medicine—as reflected in the different *structures* of these ideologies—enter into play.

Empiricism is a set of rules for medical practice. It is a *method of treating* the sick organism and thus of investigating it. Its function is purely curative, and this ideology is oriented toward the patient—his need to be cured as skilfully, rapidly, and carefully as possible.

Rationalism is a *theory* of the organism. Its function is to *explain* the workings of the organism in sickness and health, and it is oriented toward the needs of the physician.

The author of *Ancient Medicine* was the first to note this contrast in the structures of Empiricism and Rationalism when he attacked those who "abandon the old *method* to rest the art on a postulate" (cap. XV). "Certain physicians and philosophers assert that nobody can know medicine who is ignorant what a man is; he who would treat patients properly must, they say, learn this. But the question they raise is one for philosophy." (cap. XX). This Empiric objects to the attitude emerging in *Nature of Man* (or some similar writing) that practice must be based on an *a priori* theory of the organism: "My view is that all that philosophers or physicians have said or written on the *physis* no more pertains to medicine than to painting . . . clear knowledge of the *physies* can be acquired from medicine and from no other source . . ." (cap. XX). The theory is generated only by medical practice.

The existence of these two ideologies reflects the dichotomy in medicine between the interests of the physician and of the patient.

While the patient's need is to be cured, the physician has other needs—economic, social, and psychological.

He has to earn a living from the practice of medicine. Thus he will prefer a therapeutic doctrine which enables him to earn the best living possible with the minimum amount of work.

He needs a doctrine which elevates him above the patient, that is, one which allows him to deal with the patient from a position of superiority.

Finally, he needs one which binds him to his fellow-practitioners. Given the economic competition among physicians, such support will be forthcoming only if there is common allegiance to a body of knowledge which counteracts these divisive economic forces.

The tie with other members of the profession is needed because of the hostility, real and potential, of the patient. Sometimes sick persons fare poorly under the physician's ministrations. Strong emotions are aroused. The physician may be blamed, rightly or wrongly, for an untoward outcome. He must often look to his colleagues for moral and psychological reassurance, and professional unity is important to him. The greatest source of such group cohesion is adherence to the same body of doctrine, the same ideology.[h]

It is a major thesis of this history that the development of *therapeutic theory itself* has been profoundly affected by the felt need for professional cohesion, as this need generates pressures which are manifested primarily in the area of medical thought.

If proven, this thesis casts doubt upon the easy assumption that an inherently scientific procedure in medicine has an intrinsic advantage over an unscientific one merely because it can produce better therapeutic results. There is no evidence at all that the doctrine which produces the best therapeutic results is the one best suited to ensuring professional unity.

In fact, the best therapeutic results are produced by the Empirical system of practice. That is why this system is oriented toward the needs of the patient. And the doctrine which best meets the need for professional unity is Rationalism. That is why this system is oriented toward the needs of the physician.

[h]When their medicines fail, the Galenists say: "By God, the remedy is written down right here. I have done just the right thing. It must be a plague sent by God." (See above, p. 473).

Medical thought is a part of the knowledge upon which society draws to meet its various needs. It is thus affected by the influences which help shape this body of knowledge. Some of these influences arise from the intrinsic needs of medical practice, i.e., the correct understanding and the cure of the sick person. Others, however, arise from the medical profession's need for cohesion. Medicine is practiced by individuals, but when society contains a large number of such individuals, new forces are generated. The awareness of a common interest in protecting the profession from external assault engenders pressures for group cohesion which make themselves felt in the area of *therapeutic theory*.

Precisely to the extent that it satisfied the needs of the patient Empiricism failed to provide the physician with the desired support and assurance, and we have already noted Deichgraeber's opinion that the Empirical School did not constitute a sociological unity. In the first place, it was (and is) a more difficult system of practice, requiring the expenditure of time and intellectual effort and demanding a degree of emotional involvement with the patient. Since it relied on sensory observation alone—the careful recording of fleeting patterns of symptoms—Empirical knowledge was not qualitatively different from the knowledge applied in many other spheres of activity. It was identical with the knowledge of the cook, the cobbler, the shipbuilder, the architect. Good results in medicine were (and are still) produced by a careful eye, a willingness to work hard, and the skill developed by years of experience. But possession of such knowledge could not be invoked to justify a position of psychological superiority *vis-a-vis* the patient, since any patient with the same ability to observe, the same willingness to make the requisite effort, and the same years of experience could in theory produce the same results. And, indeed, any layman could compete with the physician in observing the patient's symptoms. Finally, being a set of rules for practice and not a theory of the organism, adherence to the Empirical method served more to divide physicians than to unify them.

The reason for this will become clear from the contrast with Rationalism.

While an inherently unscientific procedure and thus poorly adapted to the needs of the patient, this doctrine met all the requirements of the physician. In the first place, it was an easier system of practice, relying on the obvious symptoms (the *communia*) rather than on the more subtle ones (the *propria*) and thus avoiding the need for the time-consuming individualization of treatment demanded by Empiricism.

It elevated the physician above the patient psychologically. Not only did it draw on a body of arcane knowledge which was qualitatively different from any ordinary knowledge possessed by the patient and exclusively the province of the physician, but it strengthened the physician's self-esteem in another way besides—by casting doubt upon the patient's self-healing capacity. Healing by contraries is a form of self-assertion: the physician cures by *opposing* and conquering something within the patient rather than by aiding and cooperating with the patient's own intrinsic healing power.

Finally, Rationalism was an admirable instrument of professional cohesion, and here the contrast with Empiricism is very great. By its concreteness, its hypostatization or objectification of physiological processes, its postulate that these processes stand in a logical relationship to one another, Rationalism held up to the physician a clear and logical doctrinal structure. And in its application to the individual patient this system of thought *could be interpreted in a different way by every physician.* For no results of practice could prove the physician wrong. The essential elements of the doctrine were invisible (the proximate causes), and their relationship to the particular patient was never anything more than a matter of speculation. The hypothesis could never be disproved through experiment.

In contrast, for the Empiric the only proof of the correctness of his procedures was the therapeutic outcome. This system did not supply the physician with an objectified body of knowledge to which all could pay lip-service and each apply differently. It only called for zealous adherence to certain rules of practice. If this was done, the results would be favorable, if not—unfavorable or disastrous. The whole metaphysical structure which provided the Rationalists with professional cohesion was absent from Empiricism.

Hence this doctrine—because it so successfully bound physician to patient—could not bind physicians to one another. And Rationalism promoted professional cohesion precisely to the extent that it isolated the physician from the patient and the medical profession from society.

Thus Empiricism, albeit a scientific approach to therapeutics and one which, we must assume, yielded better therapeutic results than Rationalism, was a weaker social force. Evidence for this will be adduced in later volumes of this history which show that these practitioners have probably been always in a numerical minority. Of interest also is the fact that Rationalism survived the barbarian onslaughts on Rome and emerged as the orthodox medicine of the Middle Ages and Renaissance.[i]

The loss to posterity of the volumes of Empirical observations (apart from the invaluable treatise by Celsus), and the preservation of the therapeutically worthless Galenic writings, are evidence of the true priorities of the medical profession. The Empirical works were of genuine therapeutic value, and physicians today might have succeeded in culling from them items of interest, while the Galenic works were monuments to error. Yet the former were allowed to disappear while the latter survived.

So great is the contribution of logic to professional cohesion! Galen's thought (despite its internal inconsistencies) appears clear and coherent, and his tremendous output prevented critics for many centuries from penetrating to its unstable foundations.

Professional cohesion is engendered by doctrinal coherence. Hence the desire for logical consistency is a hallmark of Rationalism. These physicians stressed theory over practice because a convincing logical theory seemed more important

[i]In this connection Francis Bacon's explanation why the works of Aristotle and Plato survived, while those of the Ionians perished, seems apt: "at a later period, when human learning had, as it were, been wrecked in the inundations of barbarians into the Roman Empire, then the systems of Aristotle and Plato were preserved in the waves of ages, like planks of a lighter and less solid nature" (*Novum Organum*, Book I, Aphorism LXXVII).

to them than success in practice. This led them to substitute the four humors for the *physis*. It led to the assumption that proximate causes were *a priori* knowable. And it led to the doctrine of contraries.

* * * * * * * * *

In conclusion, Windelband's contrast between idiographic and nomothetic forms of knowledge is seen to require modification. Both the Empirics and the Rationalists aimed to establish nomothetic disciplines. Both aimed to develop rules of medical practice. The Empirics, however, did so on the basis of a more comprehensive description of the elemental data. Their doctrine was both idiographic *and* nomothetic. Any scientific interpretation of reality must be the same, formulating general laws based on a thorough appreciation of the individual case.

The Empirical tradition thus offered an initial fusion of idiographic and nomothetic knowledge. While the disease descriptions were complete, however, the nomothetic element was still incomplete. The step from diagnosis to therapy, in particular, was still only "empirical"—founded on the trial-and-error knowledge preserved in historical records. And while Paracelsus promised a more direct route from diagnosis to treatment, he did not spell out the precise way in which a given illness could be identified with a given mineral.

A better fusion of idiographic and nomothetic knowledge was effected by Samuel Hahnemann, the representative of Empiricism in the nineteenth century, whose homoeopathic system is discussed in Volume Two of this series.

Volume Three discusses in detail the socio-economic factors which affect medical practice, showing how they interact with the Empirical and Rationalist ideologies.

NOTES

[1] S-M I/VIII 111. *Paragranum. Vorrede und erste zwei Buecher. Entwuerfe und I. Ausarbeitung in Berezhausen. Der ander grund der arznei.*

[2] S-M I/XI 135-136. *Sieben Defensiones.* Second Defense; S-M I/VII 235. *Vom Ursprung und Herkommen der Franzosen. Das ander Buch. Das XXI. capitel.*

[3] S-M I/XI 142. *Sieben Defensiones.* Fourth Defense; S-M I/IX 474-475. *Von der Bergsucht und anderen Bergkrankheiten. Bk. I. Tract. II. Cap. 5.*

[4] S-M I/I 60. *Elf Traktat. 3. (Andere Redaktion). Signa.*

[5] S-M I/IX 227. *Die drei (vier) Buecher des Opus Paramirum. Liber quartus de matrice.*

[6] S-M I/VII 289. *Vom Ursprung und Herkommen der Franzosen. Das V. Buch. Das IV. capitel.*

[7] S-M I/XI 212. *Labyrinthus medicorum errantium. Das X. capitel.*

[8] S-M I/I 68. *Elf Traktat. 4. Processus.*

[9] S-M I/I 167. *Volumen Medicinae Paramirum, Bk. I of Prologues, Prologue Three.*

[10] S-M I/I 243-244. *Ein Buchlein (philosophia) de generatione hominis. Die erste vorrede.*

[11] S-M I/VIII 72. *Paragranum. Vorrede und erste zwei Buecher. Entwuerfe und I. Ausarbeitung in Berezhausen. Der erste grund der arznei.* Also, pp. 69, 81, 148.

[12] S-M I/I 170. *Volumen Medicinae Paramirum. Bk. II of Prologues. Prologue I.*

[13] Oswald Croll, *Philosophy Reformed and Improved in Four Profound Tractates* (London, 1657), p. 147.

[14] *Ibid.*, p. 151.

[15] *Ibid.*, p. 115.

[16] *Ibid.*, p. 155.

[17] *Histoire de la Medicine,* Vol. II, p. 120.

[18] Quoted in Karl Popper, *The Logic of Scientific Discovery,* p. 32.

BIBLIOGRAPHY

(a) Greek Medicine

Ackerknecht, Erwin H. "A Plea for a 'Behaviorist' Approach in Writing the History of Medicine." *Journal of the History of Medicine and Allied Sciences,* XXII (1967), 211-214.

Alexanderson, Bengt. *Die Hippokratische Schrift Prognostikon.* Stockholm: Almquist and Wiksell, 1963.

Allbutt, Clifford. *Greek Medicine in Rome.* London: Macmillan Co., Ltd., 1921.

Amerio, Adriana. "Considerazioni su Acrone Agrigentino." *Medicina nei Secoli* III (1966), Supp. al #4, 33-37.

Aristotle. *Works.* Edited by W. D. Ross. 10 vols., Oxford University Press.

__________. *Parts of Animals.* Translated by A. L. Peck. Loeb Classical Library.

__________. *Generation of Animals.* Translated by A. L. Peck. Loeb Classical Library.

Athenaeus. *Deipnosophistae.* Translated by C. B. Gulick. 7 vols., Loeb Classical Library.

Berlin, Isaiah. *The Hedgehog and the Fox.* New York: Mentor Books, 1957.

Bevan, Edwyn. *Stoics and Sceptics.* Oxford: Clarendon Press, 1913.

Boas, George. *Rationalism in Greek Philosophy.* Baltimore: Johns Hopkins Press, 1961.

__________. *Some Assumptions of Aristotle.* Transactions of the American Philosophical Society, New Series, LXIX, Part 6, 1959.

Bratescu, G. "L'Hippocratisme et sa Revision dans l'Antiquite," *Studii Clasice* V (1963), 43-67 (in Rumanian).

Brock, A. J. *Greek Medicine.* London: Dent, 1929.

Bourgey, L. *Observation et Experience chez les Medecins de la Collection Hippocratique.* Paris: Vrin, 1953.

Caelius Aurelianus. *On Acute Diseases and on Chronic Diseases.* Translated by I. E. Drabkin. Chicago: University of Chicago Press, 1950.

Castiglioni, Arturo. "Neo-Hippocratic Tendency of Contemporary Medical Thought," *Medical Life* (1934), XLI, No. 3, 115-146.

__________. *A History of Medicine.* New York: Alfred A. Knopf, 1941.

Celsus. *De Medicina.* Translated by W. G. Spencer. 3 vols.; Loeb Classical Library.

Cohen, Morris R., and Nagel, Ernest. *An Introduction to Logic and Scientific Method.* New York: Harcourt, Brace & World, Inc., 1934.

Comte, Auguste. *Cours de Philosophie Positive.* 3rd ed.; Paris, 1869.

Cornford, F. M. *Plato's Cosmology.* London: Routledge and Kegan Paul, 1956.

Coulter, Harris L. *Divided Legacy: A History of the Schism in Medical Thought. Volume II. Progress and Regress: J. B. Van Helmont to Claude Bernard. Volume III. Science and Ethics in American Medicine: 1800-1914.* Washington, D.C.: Wehawken Book Co., 1973, 1975.

Deichgraeber, Karl. *Die Epidemien und das Corpus Hippocraticum.* Berlin: Verlag der Akademie der Wissenschaften, 1933.

———. *Die Griechische Empirikerschule.* Berlin: Weidmann, 1930. Reprinted with additions Berlin/Zurich: Weidmannsche Verlagsbuchhandlung, 1965.

———. *Der Listensinnende Trug des Gottes.* Goettingen: Vandenhoeck und Ruprecht, 1952.

———. " 'Profasis.' Eine terminologische Studie," *Quellen und Studien zur Geschichte der Naturwissenschaften und der Medizin*, III (1933), 1-17.

Diels, Hermann. "Anonymi Londinensis ex Aristotelis Iatricis Menoniis et aliis medicis eclogae," *Supplementum Aristotelicum*, III, No. 1 (1893).

Dierbach, J. H. *Die Arzneimittel des Hippokrates.* Heidelberg: Neue Akademische Buchhandlung von Karl Gross, 1824.

Diogenes Laertius. *Lives of the Philosophers.* Translated by R. D. Hicks. 2 vols.; Loeb Classical Library.

Dobson, J. F. "Erasistratus," *Proc. Royal Soc. of Medicine*, XX (1927), 825-832.

———. "Herophilos of Alexandria." *Proc. Royal Soc. of Medicine, Sect. Hist. Med.*, XVIII (1925), 19-32.

Dow, Sterling. "Two Families of Athenian Physicians," *Bulletin of the History of Medicine*, XII (1942), 18-26.

Duering, Ingemar. "Aristotle's Method in Biology" in *Aristote et les Problemes de Methode.* Publications Universitaires de Louvain, Louvain et Paris (1961), pp. 213-221.

Edelstein, Ludwig. "The Genuine Works of Hippocrates," *Bulletin of the History of Medicine*, VII (1939), 236-248.

———. "Die Geschichte der Sektion in der Antike," *Quellen und Studien zur Geschichte der Naturwissenschaften und der Medizin*, III, No. 2 (1932), 50-106.

———. "Hippokrates," *Pauly-Wissowa, Real-Encyclopedie der Classischen Altertumswissenschaft, Supplementband VI*, (1935), cols. 1290-1345.

———. *Peri Aeron und die Sammlung der Hippokratischen Schriften.* Berlin: Weidmann, 1931.

———. "The Professional Ethics of the Greek Physician," *Bulletin of the History of Medicine,* XXX (1956), 391-419.

Englert, Ludwig. "Untersuchungen zu Galens Schrift Thrasybulos," *Studien zur Geschichte der Medizin* (Leipzig: Barth, 1929), Heft 18.

Faber, Knud. "Nosography in Internal Medicine," *Annals of Medical History*, IV (1922), 1-63.

Farrington, Benjamin. *Head and Hand in Ancient Greece.* London: Watts, 1947.

Favier, Albert. *Menodote de Nicomedie: Precurseur de la Methode Experimentale Moderne.* Paris: Rousset, 1906.

Forster, E. S. "The Pseudo-Aristotelian Problems, Their Nature and Composition," *Classical Quarterly*, XXII (1928).

Fuchs, Robert. "Anecdota Medicorum Graeca," *Rheinisches Museum*, XLIX (1894).

Galen. *Medicorum Graecorum Opera Quae Exstant: Claudii Galeni Opera Omnia.* Edited by Carolus Gottlob Kuehn. 20 vols.; Leipzig, 1821-1833.

———. *In Hippocratis De Officina Medici Commentariorum* (C.M.G. *Supplementum Orientale* I), Translated from the Arabic by Malcolm Lyons. Berlin, 1963.

———. *De Causis Procatarcticis: Libellus a Nicolao Regino in Sermonem Latinum translatus* (C.M.G. Supplementum II). Berlin, 1937.

———. *Scripta Minora.* Edited by I. Marquardt. 3 vols.; Leipzig: Teubner, 1893.

————. *De Subfiguratione Empirica* (in Deichgraeber, *Die Griechische Empirikerschule*, pp. 42-90).

————. *Galen on Medical Experience.* Translated from Arabic by Richard Walzer. Oxford University Press, 1947.

————. *Galen's Hygiene.* Translated by R. M. Green. Springfield, Illinois: Charles C. Thomas, 1951.

————. *Galen's Art of Physick.* Translated by N. Culpepper. London: Peter Cole, 1652.

————. *Oeuvres Anatomiques, Physiologiques et Medicales de Galien.* Translated by Charles Daremberg. 2 vols.; Paris: Bailliere, 1854-1856.

————. *De Methodo Medendi. Galen's Method of Physick Or His Great Masterpiece: Whereto is Annexed a Succinct and Plain Commentary ... by its Translator, P. English.* Edinburgh, 1656.

————. *Les Six Principaux Livres de la Methode Therapeutique de C. Galien.* Lyon, MDCV.

————. *On the Natural Faculties.* Translated by A. J. Brock. Loeb Classical Library.

Harris, C. R. S. *The Heart and the Vascular System in Ancient Greek Medicine: From Alcmaeon to Galen.* Oxford, at the Clarendon Press, 1973.

Heinimann, Felix. "Diokles von Karystos und der Prophylaktische Brief an Koenig Antigonos," *Mus. Helv.*, XII (1955), 158-172.

Herodotus. *The Persian Wars.* New York: Modern Library, 1942.

Hicks, R. D. *Stoic and Epicurean.* New York: Russell and Russell, Inc., 1962.

Hippocrates. *Oeuvres Completes d'Hippocrate.* Translated by E. Littre. 10 vols.; Paris: Bailliere, 1839-1861.

————. *Hippocrates.* Translated by W. H. S. Jones. 4 vols.; Loeb Classical Library.

————. *The Medical Works of Hippocrates.* Translated by J. Chadwick and W. N. Mann. Springfield, Illinois: Charles C. Thomas, 1950.

Hohenstein, Hans. *Der Arzt Mnesitheos aus Athen.* Unpublished Berlin dissertation, Jena, 1935.

Ilberg, J. "Die Aerzteschule von Cnidos," *Ber. Ueber die Verhandlungen d. Saechs. Akad. d. Wiss. zu Leipzig: Phil.-Hist. kl.* 76 Bd. (1924), 3 Hft., 14 ff.

Iskander, A. Z. "Galen and Rhazes on Examining Physicians," *Bulletin of the History of Medicine* (1962), XXXVI, 362-365.

Jaeger, Werner. *Aristotle: Fundamentals of the History of His Development.* 2nd ed.; Oxford University Press, 1962.

————. "Diocles of Carystos: A New Pupil of Aristotle," *Philosophical Review*, XLIX (1940), 393-407.

————. *Diokles von Karystos.* Berlin: Gruyter, 1938.

————. *Paideia: The Ideals of Greek Culture.* Vol. III, Oxford University Press, 1939.

————. "Das Pneuma im Lykeion," *Hermes*, XLVIII (1913), 29-74.

————. "Vergessene Fragmente des Peripatetikers Diokles von Karystos." *Abhandlungen der Preussischen Akademie der Wissenschaften: Philosophisch-Historische Klasse*, No. 4., 1938.

James, William. *Pragmatism.* Cleveland and New York: Meridian Books, 1965.

Joly, Robert. *Recherches sur le Traite Pseudo-Hippocratique Du Regime.* Paris: Societe d'Edition "Les Belles Lettres," 1960.

Jones, W. H. S. "Hippocrates and the Corpus Hippocraticum," *Proc. Brit. Acad.* XXXI, (1945).

————. *The Medical Writings of Anonymus Londinensis.* Cambridge University Press, 1947.

————. "Philosophy and Medicine in Ancient Greece," *Bulletin of the History of Medicine*, Supplement No. 8, Baltimore, 1946.

Kalthoff, Paul. *Das Gesundheitswesen bei Aristoteles.* Berlin/Bonn: F. Duemmler, 1934.

Kapp, Ernst. *Greek Foundations of Traditional Logic.* New York: Columbia University Press, 1942.

King, L. S. *The Growth of Medical Thought.* Chicago: University of Chicago Press, 1963.

Kirk, G. S. *Heraclitus: The Cosmic Fragments.* Cambridge University Press, 1962.

Kirk, G. S., and Raven, J. E. *The Presocratic Philosophers.* Cambridge: The University Press, 1962.

Klibansky, Raymond *et al. Saturn and Melancholy.* London: Nelson, 1934.

Kovner, Saveliy. *Istoriia Meditsiny* [*History of Medicine*]. Kiev: University Press, 1888 (in Russian).

Kucharski, P. "La 'Methode d'Hippocrate' dans le Phedre," *Revue des Etudes Grecques*, LII (1939), 301-357.

Kudlien, F. "Herophilos und der Beginn der Medizinischen Skepsis," *Gesnerus*, XXI (1964), 1-13.

Kuehn, Josef-Hans. *System und Methodenprobleme im Corpus Hippocraticum.* Wiesbaden: Franz Steiner Verlag GMBH, 1956.

LeBlond, J. M. *Logique et Methode chez Aristote.* Paris: Vrin, 1939.

Lesky, Albin. *A History of Greek Literature.* New York: Thomas Y. Crowell, 1966.

Lonie, I. M. "Erasistratos, the Erasistrateans, and Aristotle," *Bulletin of the History of Medicine*, XXXVIII, No. 5 (September-October, 1964), 426-443.

————. "The Cnidian Treatises of the Corpus Hippocraticum," *Classical Quarterly*. N.S. XV, No. 1 (1965), 1-30.

————. "The Hippocratic Treatise Peri diaites okseon," *Sudhoffs Archiv*, Bd. 49, H. I (March, 1965), 50-79.

Margenau, Henry. *The Nature of Physical Reality.* New York: McGraw-Hill Book Co., 1950.

Marx, Friedrich. *A. Cornelii Celsi Quae Supersunt.* Corpus Medicorum Latinorum, Volume I. Leipzig, 1915.

Marx, K. F. H. *De Herophili celeberrimi medici, vita, scriptis, atque in medicina meritis.* Goettingen: Dieterien, 1840.

Mates, Benson. *Stoic Logic.* University of California Publications in Philosophy, No. 26. Berkeley: University of California Press, 1953.

Meyerhoff, Max, "Autobiographische Bruchstuecke Galens aus Arabischen Quellen," *Sudhoffs Archiv* XXII (1929), 72-86.

Michelakis, Emmanuel. *Aristotle's Theory of Practical Principles*, Athens: Cleisiounis Press, 1961.

Miller, H. W. "*Dynamis* and *Physis* in: *On Ancient Medicine,*" *Transactions of the American Philological Association,* LXXXIII (1952), 184-197.

————. "The Concept of *Dynamis* in *De Victu,*" *Transactions of the American Philological Association,* LXXXX (1959), 147-164.

Northrop, F. S. C. *The Logic of the Sciences and the Humanities.* New York: Meridian Books, 1959.

Neuburger, Max. *History of Medicine.* London: Frowde, 1910.

____________. "The Doctrine of the Healing Power of Nature Throughout the Course of Time," *Journal of the American Institute of Homoeopathy*, XXV (1932), 861ff. 1011ff., 1167ff., 1320ff.

Oribasius. *Oeuvres d'Oribase*. Translated by Daremberg and Bussemaker. 6 vols.; Paris: L'Imprimerie Imperiale, 1851-1876.

Petersen, Julius. *Hauptmomente in der geschichtlichen Entwicklung der medizinischen Therapie*. Kopenhagen: Host, 1877.

Paul of Aegina. *The Medical Works of Paulus Aegineta*. Translated by Francis Adams. London: Welsh, Treuttel, Wuertz, 1834.

Plamboeck, Gert. *Dynamis im Corpus Hippocraticum*. Academie der Wissenschaften und der Literatur (Mainz), Abhandlungen der Geistes- und Sozialwissenschaftlichen Klasse, 1964, No. 2, 63-109.

Plato. *The Dialogues of Plato*. Two Volumes. Translated by B. Jowett. New York: Random House, 1937.

Pliny. *Natural History*. Ten Volumes. Translated by W. H. S. Jones. Loeb Classical Library.

Pohlenz, Max. *Hippokrates und die Begruendung der wissenschaftlichen Medizin*. Berlin: Gruyter, 1938.

Popper, Karl. *The Logic of Scientific Discovery*. New York: Harper and Row, 1959.

Randall, J. H. *Aristotle*. New York: Columbia University Press, 1960.

Robin, Leon. *La Pensee Grecque et les Origines de l'Espirit Scientifique*. Paris: Editions Albin Michel, 1963.

Ross, Sir David. *Aristotle*. London: Methuen, 1966.

Rufus of Ephesus. *Oeuvres de Rufus d'Ephase*. Translated by Charles Daremberg. Paris: L'Imprimerie Nationale, 1874.

Russell, Bertrand. *A History of Western Philosophy*. New York: Simon and Schuster, 1945.

Sarton, George. *A History of Science: Ancient Science Through the Golden Age of Greece*. Cambridge: Harvard University Press, 1952.

____________. *Galen of Pergamon*. Lawrence: University of Kansas Press, 1954.

Saunders, J. B. de C. M. *The Transition from Ancient Egyptian to Greek Medicine*. Lawrence: University of Kansas Press, 1963.

____________ and Steuer, Robert O. *Ancient Egyptian and Cnidian Medicine: The Relationship of their Aetiological Concepts of Disease*. Berkeley: University of California Press, 1959.

Schelenz, Hermann. *Geschichte der Pharmazie*. Berlin: J. Springer, 1904.

Schoener, Erich. "Das Viererschema in der antiken Humoralpathologie," *Arch. Gesch. Med.*, Suppl. 4 (1964).

Schubring, K. "Zu Aufbau und Lehre der hippokratischen Schrift De Locis in Homine," *Berl. Med.*, XIV (1964), 739-744.

Senn, G. "Ueber Herkunft und Stil der Beschreibungen von Experimenten im Corpus Hippocraticum," *Sudhoffs Archiv XXI* (1929), pp. 217-288.

Sextus Empiricus. Translated by R. G. Bury. 4 vols.; Loeb Classical Library.

Siegel, Rudolph. *Galen's System of Physiology and Medicine*. Basel and New York: Karger, 1968.

Sigerist, Henry E. "Notes and Comments on Hippocrates," *Bulletin of the History of Medicine: The Johns Hopkins University*, II, No. I (1934), 190-214.

Soranus of Ephesus. *Soranus' Gynecology*. Translated by Owsei Temkin. Baltimore: Johns Hopkins University Press, 1956.

Sprengel, Kurt. *Histoire de la Medicine*. Vols. I and II. Paris: Deterville, 1815.

Steckerl, Fritz. *The Fragments of Praxagoras of Cos and His School.* Leyden: Brill, 1958.

Stephen of Athens. *Stephani Atheniensis Philosophi: Explanationes in Galeni primum librum therapeuticum ad Glauconem, Augustino Gadaldino Mutinensi interprete.* Lugduni, MDLV.

Steuer, Robert O. "Whdw: Aetiological Principle of Pyaemia in Ancient Egyptian Medicine," Supplement No. 10 to *Bulletin of the History of Medicine.* Baltimore: Johns Hopkins University Press, 1948.

Stevenson, Ian. "Why Medicine is Not a Science," *Harpers* (April, 1949), 36-39.

Temkin, Owsei. "A Galenic Model for Quantitative Physiological Reasoning," *Bulletin of the History of Medicine*, XXXV (1961), 470-475.

__________. *Galenism: Rise and Decline of a Medical Philosophy.* Ithaca and London: Cornell University Press, 1973.

__________. "Galen's Pneumatology," *Gesnerus,* VIII (1950), 180-189.

__________. "Greek Medicine as Science and Craft," *Isis,* XLIV (1953), 137.

__________. "The Scientific Approach to Disease: Specific Entity and Individual Sickness," in *Scientific Change.* Edited by A. C. Crombie. London: Heinemann, 1963.

Tertullian, *De Anima.* Edited by J. H. Waszink. Amsterdam: J. M. Meulenhoff, 1947.

Theophrastus. *Enquiry Into Plants.* Translated by Sir Arthur Hort. 2 vols.; Loeb Classical Library.

Thorndike, Lynn. *A History of Magic and Experimental Science.* 6 vols. New York: Macmillan Co., 1923-1958.

Tolstoy, L. *War and Peace.*

Wellmann, Max. *A. Cornelius Celsus: Eine Quellenuntersuchung.* Berlin: Weidmann, 1901.

__________. *Die Fragmente der Sykelischen Aerzte.* Berlin: Weidmann, 1901.

__________. *Die Pneumatische Schule.* Berlin: Weidmann, 1895.

Whewell, W. *The Philosophy of the Inductive Sciences: On the Philosophy of Discovery.* London: J. W. Parker and Son, 1860.

Windelband, Wilhelm. *A History of Philosophy.* Vol. I.; New York: Harper and Row, 1958.

__________. *A History of Ancient Philosophy.* New York: Dover, 1956.

__________. *Geschichte und Naturwissenschaft: Rede zum Antritt des Rektorats der Kaiser-Wilhelms-Universitaet Strassburg.* gehalten am 1. Mai, 1894, Strassburg, 1904.

Zeller, Eduard. *Outlines of the History of Greek Philosophy.* 13th ed. rev. by Dr. Wilhelm Nestle. London: Routledge and Kegan Paul, 1963.

__________. *Stoics, Epicureans and Sceptics.* New York: Russell and Russell, 1962.

(b) Paracelsus

Avicenna (Abnali Ibn Sina). *Kanon Vrachebnoi Nauki* [The Canon of Medical Science]. Four Volumes. Tashkent: Izdatel'stvo Akademii Nauk Uzbekskoi S.S.R., 1954 (in Russian).

Bacon, Francis. *Advancement of Learning. Novum Organum.*

Croll, Oswald. *Bazilica Chymica & Praxis Chymiatricae, or Royal and Practical Chymistry in Three Treatises...* All faithfully Englished by a Lover of Chymistry. London: Printed for John Starkey, 1670.

____________. *Philosophy Reformed and Improved in Four Profound Tractates.* Translated by H. Pinnell. London, 1657.

Hopkins, Arthur John. *Alchemy, Child of Greek Philosophy.* New York: Columbia University Press, 1934.

Jung, C. G. *Paracelsica: Zwei Vorlesungen ueber den Arzt und Philosophen Theophrastus.* Zurich and Leipzig: Rascher Verlag, 1942.

____________. *Paracelsus.* St. Gallen: Tschudy, 1952.

Koyre, Alexandre. "Paracelse," *Revue d'Histoire et de Philosophie Religieuses.* (Strasbourg), III: 1-2 (1933), 46-75, 145-163.

Multhauf, Robert. "Medical Chemistry and 'the Paracelsans,' " *Bulletin of the History of Medicine,* XXVIII (1954), pp. 101-126.

Oosterhuis, R. A. B. *Paracelsus en Hahnemann: Een Renaissance der Geneeskunst.* Leiden: Sijthoff, 1937.

Pachter, Henry. *Paracelsus: Magic into Science.* New York: Henry Schuman, 1951.

Pagel, Walter. *Das Medizinische Weltbild des Paracelsus. Seine Zusammenhaenge mit Neuplatonismus und Gnosis.* Wiesbaden: Steiner, 1962.

____________. "Paracelsus and the Neoplatonic and Gnostic Tradition," *Ambix,* VIII, No. 3 (October, 1960), 125-166.

____________. *Paracelsus: An Introduction to Philosophical Medicine in the Era of the Renaissance.* New York and Basel: Karger, 1958.

____________, and Rattansi, Pyarali. "Vesalius and Paracelsus," *Medical History,* VIII, No. 4 (October, 1964), 309-328.

Paracelsus. *Four Treatises of Theophrastus von Hohenheim, Called Paracelsus.* Translated from the original German, with introductory essays by C. Lilian Temkin, George Rosen, Gregory Zilboorg, and Henry E. Sigerist; edited, with a preface, by Henry Sigerist. Baltimore: The Johns Hopkins University Press, 1941. (Publications of the Institute of the History of Medicine, The Johns Hopkins University, 2nd ser.: Texts and Documents, Vol. I.).

____________. *Hermetic and Alchemical Writings of Paracelsus the Great.* 2 vols. Trans. Arthur Edward Waite. London: Elliott, 1894.

____________. *Paracelsus.* Ed. Franz Spunda. Vienna and Leipzig: K. Koenig, 1925.

____________. *Paracelsus: Leben und Lebensweisheit im Selbstzeugnissen.* Ed. Karl Bittel. Leipzig: Reclam, 1945.

____________. *Paracelsus: Selected Writings.* Edited with an Introduction, Jolande Jacobi. Trans. Norbert Guterman. 2nd ed. New York: Pantheon Books, Bollingen Series XXVIII, 1958.

____________. *Theophrastus Paracelsus' Werke.* Translated Into Modern German by Will-Erich Peuckert. Vols. I and II (Medizinische Schriften). Basel and Stuttgart: Schwabe, 1965.

____________. *Theophrastus von Hohenheim, gennant Paracelsus: Saemtliche Werke. I. Abteilung. Medizinische, naturwissenschaftliche, und philosophische Schriften.* Ed. Karl Sudhoff, Vols. IV-IX. Munich: O. W. Barth, 1922-1925; I-V, X-XIV. Munich, Berlin: R. Oldenbourg, 1928-1933.

———. *Theophrastus von Hohenheim, gennant Paracelsus: Saemtliche Werke. II. Abteilung. Die theologischen und religionsphilosophischen Schriften.* Eds. Karl Sudhoff and Wilhelm Matthiessen. I. Munich: O. W. Barth, 1923.

———. *Volumen Medicinae Paramirum of Theophrastus von Hohenheim, called Paracelsus.* Translated from the Original German with a Preface by Kurt F. Leidecker. Supplements to the Bulletin of the History of Medicine: Supplement No. 11. Baltimore: The Johns Hopkins Press, 1949.

Sudhoff, Karl. *Versuch einer Kritik der Echtheit der Paracelsischen Schriften.* Vol. II. Berlin: G. Reimer, 1899.

Sprengel, Kurt. *Histoire de la Medicine.* Vols. II and III. Paris: Deterville, 1815.

Temkin, Owsei. "The Elusiveness of Paracelsus," *Bulletin of the History of Medicine*, XXVI, No. 3 (May-June, 1952), 201-217.

Titley, Alan F. "Paracelsus, A Resume of Some Controversies," *Ambix*, I, No. 3 (March, 1938), 166-183.

Thorndike, Lynn. *A History of Magic and Experimental Science.* Vol. V: *The Sixteenth Century.* Vol. VI: *The Sixteenth Century.* New York: Columbia University Press, 1941.

Van Helmont, Jean-Baptiste. *Oriatrike, or Physick Refined.* Trans. J. Chandler. London, 1662.

INDEX

LIST OF PASSAGES QUOTED FROM THE HIPPOCRATIC CORPUS AND THE WRITINGS OF ARISTOTLE, GALEN, CELSUS, CAELIUS AURELIANUS, SEXTUS EMPIRICUS, AND PARACELSUS

(Bracketed number indicates page on which passage appears)

(a) Hippocratic Corpus

(b) Aristotle

(c) Galen

(d) Celsus

(e) Caelius Aurelianus

(f) Sextus Empiricus

(g) Paracelsus

* * * * *

Grateful acknowledgment is hereby made to the publishers of the following translations of Paracelsan works for permission to use the passages cited:

ACKNOWLEDGEMENT

I would like to thank the following persons who have read parts of this volume and given me valuable advice and suggestions: George Boas, Richard J. Durling, Rainer Koehne, Paul O. Kristeller, Geoffrey Lloyd, and Walter Pagel.

My thanks go also to Dr. John Blake and Mrs. Dorothy Hanks of the History of Medicine Division, National Library of Medicine, for their unfailing kindness and assistance.

Published by:

WEHAWKEN BOOK COMPANY
5104 Wehawken Road
Washington, D.C. 20016